AF411488

SAPHENOUS VEIN BYPASS GRAFT DISEASE

FUNDAMENTAL AND CLINICAL CARDIOLOGY

Editor-in-Chief

Samuel Z. Goldhaber, M.D.

*Harvard Medical School
and Brigham and Women's Hospital
Boston, Massachusetts*

Associate Editor, Europe

Henri Bounameaux, M.D.

*University Hospital of Geneva
Geneva, Switzerland*

1. *Drug Treatment of Hyperlipidemia*, edited by Basil M. Rifkind
2. *Cardiotonic Drugs: A Clinical Review, Second Edition, Revised and Expanded*, edited by Carl V. Leier
3. *Complications of Coronary Angioplasty*, edited by Alexander J. R. Black, H. Vernon Anderson, and Stephen G. Ellis
4. *Unstable Angina*, edited by John D. Rutherford
5. *Beta-Blockers and Cardiac Arrhythmias*, edited by Prakash C. Deedwania
6. *Exercise and the Heart in Health and Disease*, edited by Roy J. Shephard and Henry S. Miller, Jr.
7. *Cardiopulmonary Physiology in Critical Care*, edited by Steven M. Scharf
8. *Atherosclerotic Cardiovascular Disease, Hemostasis, and Endothelial Function*, edited by Robert Boyer Francis, Jr.
9. *Coronary Heart Disease Prevention*, edited by Frank G. Yanowitz
10. *Thrombolysis and Adjunctive Therapy for Acute Myocardial Infarction*, edited by Eric R. Bates
11. *Stunned Myocardium: Properties, Mechanisms, and Clinical Manifestations*, edited by Robert A. Kloner and Karin Przyklenk
12. *Prevention of Venous Thromboembolism*, edited by Samuel Z. Goldhaber
13. *Silent Myocardial Ischemia and Infarction: Third Edition*, Peter F. Cohn
14. *Congestive Cardiac Failure: Pathophysiology and Treatment*, edited by David B. Barnett, Hubert Pouleur, and Gary S. Francis
15. *Heart Failure: Basic Science and Clinical Aspects*, edited by Judith K. Gwathmey, G. Maurice Briggs, and Paul D. Allen

ADDITIONAL VOLUMES IN PREPARATION

SAPHENOUS VEIN BYPASS GRAFT DISEASE

Edited by

Eric R. Bates
University of Michigan Medical Center
Ann Arbor, Michigan

David R. Holmes, Jr.
Mayo Clinic
Rochester, Minnesota

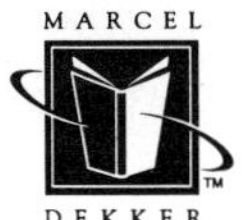

MARCEL DEKKER, INC.   NEW YORK · BASEL · HONG KONG

Library of Congress Cataloging-in-Publication Data

Saphenous vein bypass graft disease/edited by Eric R. Bates, David R. Holmes,
  Jr.
        p. cm.—(Fundamental and clinical cardiology; v. 33)
     Includes index.
     ISBN 0-8247-9902-X (alk. paper)
     1. Coronary artery bypass. 2. Saphenous vein—Transplantation.
I. Bates, Eric R. II. Holmes, David R. III. Series. [DNLM: 1. Coronary
Disease—surgery. 2. Saphenous Vein—transplantation. 3. Coronary Artery
Bypass—adverse effects. 4. Postoperative Complications—prevention &
control. W1 FU538TD v. 33 1998/WG 300 S2405 1998]
RD598.35.C67S27   1998
617.4'12—dc21
DNLM/DLC
for Library of Congress

                                                      98-5321
                                                        CIP

The publisher offers discounts on this book when ordered in bulk quantities. For
more information, write to Special Sales/Professional Marketing at the address
below.

This book is printed on acid-free paper.

MARCEL DEKKER, INC.
270 Madison Avenue, New York, New York 10016
http://www.dekker.com

Current printing (last digit):
10 9 8 7 6 5 4 3 2 1

PRINTED IN THE UNITED STATES OF AMERICA

Series Introduction

Coronary artery bypass grafting has revolutionized the management of coronary heart disease. Although this surgery has reduced mortality and improved the quality of life for millions, it is a procedure that has been vexed by diminishing long-term results. As the saphenous vein grafts age, they become stenotic. For the most part, gradually—but occasionally suddenly—these grafts occlude and cause either unstable angina pectoris or myocardial infarction.

Diagnostic and therapeutic strategies to manage saphenous vein bypass graft disease are scattered in multiple articles published in cardiology and cardiac surgery journals. However, until now, no comprehensive textbook has tackled this problem in a unified manner. I am pleased and honored to include *Saphenous Vein Bypass Graft Disease* in our Fundamental and Clinical Cardiology series published by Marcel Dekker, Inc. As a practicing general cardiologist, I have found this textbook to be most useful in helping me deal with practical, daily clinical problems that arise in my patients who have undergone bypass surgery.

Drs. Bates and Holmes are internationally recognized clinical cardiologists who have provided us with an invaluable contribution. Their book achieves the objectives of our Cardiology series with its excellent text, comprehensive references, and beautiful illustrations.

Samuel Z. Goldhaber, M.D.

Preface

Saphenous vein bypass graft surgery for the treatment of coronary artery disease has been performed for over two decades. The operation is the most commonly performed major surgical procedure in the United States. Over 300,000 operations are performed each year, and over 2 million patients who have undergone this surgery are still alive. Unfortunately, surgery is only a palliative procedure because of either progression of native coronary artery disease or development of saphenous vein bypass graft disease. Importantly, 10% of vein grafts are occluded within 1 month and 20% are occluded within 1 year. The subsequent attrition rate is 2% per year for 5 years and 5% per year for the next 5 years. Only 25% of vein grafts are angiographically normal 10 years after surgery and 50% are occluded.

Controversy exists as to whether improvements in surgical and pharmacological treatment have altered the natural history of saphenous vein bypass graft disease, and it is still not clear whether saphenous bypass graft atherosclerosis differs from coronary atherosclerosis. Graft atherosclerosis usually involves larger plaques which are frequently ulcerated and often have superimposed thrombus. The risk of recurrent ischemia after bypass graft surgery is at least 5% per year. Angioplasty can be performed with high success rates in grafts less than 3 years old, but complications increase with the age of the graft and only 40% of patients are alive and event-free 2 years later. Repeat surgery can be performed in selected patients, but morbidity and mortality are increased, patency rates are decreased, and fewer patients gain symptomatic relief as great as that with the initial operation. Directional, rotational, or extraction atherectomy are alternatives to angioplasty, but have not yet been shown to be superior to angioplasty. Endoluminal stenting is increasingly being performed, but it has not been studied in large randomized studies.

This book represents a unique undertaking in that the treatment of saphenous vein bypass graft disease has not previously been thoroughly reviewed and analyzed. This book will focus attention on an important disease process that affects hundreds of thousands of patients and will serve as an important reference for clinicians and investigators.

Eric R. Bates
David R. Holmes, Jr.

Contents

Contributors

Eric R. Bates, M.D.   Division of Cardiology, Department of Internal Medicine, University of Michigan Medical Center, Ann Arbor, Michigan

Edmund R. Becker, Ph.D.   Department of Health Policy and Management, Rollins School of Public Health, Emory University, Atlanta, Georgia

John A. Bittl, M.D.*   Department of Intervention Cardiology, Brigham and Women's Hospital, and Department of Medicine, Harvard Medical School, Boston, Massachusetts

Martial G. Bourassa, M.D.   Research Center, Montreal Heart Institute, Montreal, Quebec, Canada

Bernard Raymond Chaitman, M.D.   Division of Cardiology, St. Louis University Health Sciences Center, St. Louis, Missouri

Edward T. A. Fry, M.D.   Nasser, Smith and Pinkerton Cardiology, Inc.; The Indiana Heart Institute; and St. Vincent Hospital, Indianapolis, Indiana

Kirk N. Garratt, M.D.   Division of Cardiovascular Diseases and Internal Medicine, Mayo Clinic, Rochester, Minnesota

John McB. Hodgson, M.D.[†]   University Hospitals of Cleveland, Cleveland, Ohio

David R. Holmes, Jr., M.D.   Department of Cardiology, Mayo Clinic, Rochester, Minnesota

Robert J. Lederman, M.D.   Division of Cardiology, Department of Internal Medicine, University of Michigan Medical Center, Ann Arbor, Michigan

---

Current affiliations:
*Ocala Heart Institute, Ocala, Florida
[†]MetroHealth Medical Center, Cleveland, Ohio

Floyd D. Loop, M.D.   Department of Thoracic and Cardiovascular Surgery, The Cleveland Clinic Foundation, Cleveland, Ohio

Bruce W. Lytle, M.D.   Department of Thoracic and Cardiovascular Surgery, The Cleveland Clinic Foundation, Cleveland, Ohio

Patrick D. Mauldin, Ph.D.*   Department of Health Policy and Management, Rollins School of Public Health, Emory University, Atlanta, Georgia

Charles Maynard, Ph.D.   Department of Medicine, University of Washington School of Medicine, Seattle, Washington

William L. Mecca, M.D.[†]   University Hospitals of Cleveland, Cleveland, Ohio

Derek D. Muehrcke, M.D.   Department of Thoracic and Cardiovascular Surgery, The Cleveland Clinic Foundation, Cleveland, Ohio

David W. M. Muller, M.D., F.R.A.C.P., F.A.C.C.   Department of Cardiology, St. Vincent's Hospital, Darlinghurst, New South Wales, Australia

Charles M. Orr, M.D.   Nasser, Smith and Pinkerton Cardiology, Inc.; The Indiana Heart Institute; and St. Vincent Hospital, Indianapolis, Indiana

Cass A. Pinkerton, M.D.   Nasser, Smith and Pinkerton Cardiology, Inc.; The Indiana Heart Institute; and, St. Vincent Hospital, Indianapolis, Indiana

M. Salim Ratnani, M.D.   Department of Thoracic and Cardiovascular Surgery, The Cleveland Clinic Foundation, Cleveland, Ohio

Mark J. Ricciardi, M.D.   Division of Cardiology, Department of Internal Medicine, University of Michigan Medical Center, Ann Arbor, Michigan

William C. Roberts, M.D.   Baylor Cardiovascular Institute, Baylor University Medical Center, Dallas, Texas

Jorge Saucedo, M.D.   Division of Cardiology, Department of Internal Medicine, University of Michigan Medical Center, Ann Arbor, Michigan

Bruce F. Waller, M.D.   Departments of Pathology and Medicine, Indiana University Medical School, and Cardiovascular Pathology Registry, St. Vincent Hospital, and Nasser, Smith and Pinkerton Cardiology, Inc., Indianapolis, Indiana

---

Current affiliations:
*Department of Biometry/Epidemiology, Medical University of South Carolina, Charleston, South Carolina
[†]Hammot Medical Center, Erie, Pennsylvania

W. Douglas Weaver, M.D.* Department of Medicine, University of Washington School of Medicine, Seattle, Washington

William S. Weintraub, M.D. Department of Medicine, Division of Cardiology, School of Medicine, Emory University, Atlanta, Georgia

Steven W. Werns, M.D. Division of Cardiology, Department of Internal Medicine, University of Michigan Medical Center, Ann Arbor, Michigan

Liwa T. Younis, M.D., Ph.D. Division of Cardiology, St. Louis University Health Sciences Center, St. Louis, Missouri

---

Current affiliation: Division of Cardiovascular Medicine, Henry Ford Healthcare System, Detroit, Michigan

1

Arterial vs. Venous Bypass Graft Surgery

Derek D. Muehrcke, M. Salim Ratnani, and Floyd D. Loop
The Cleveland Clinic Foundation, Cleveland, Ohio

I. INTRODUCTION AND HISTORY

Coronary bypass graft surgery has been subjected to the most intense evaluation any treatment has ever received, yet it has emerged as a common operation. This is a result of its success in treating coronary atherosclerosis. Today, bypass surgery is performed in one of every 1,000 persons in the United States each year. The operation continues to evolve as results documenting the patency rates of different types of grafts are reported. Because it has become clear that certain arterial grafts remain patent longer than venous grafts, the search for new sources of arterial conduits persists in an effort to extend the beneficial effects of bypass surgery. In this review, we examine the current status of the use of different arterial and venous bypass grafts in coronary artery bypass surgery. Special emphasis is placed on the technical aspects of the surgical procedure.

Modern coronary bypass surgery has resulted from technologic advances which extend back to the early years of this century [1]. Alexis Carrel performed the first experimental coronary bypass grafts in 1910. Although bypass grafting was not attempted in patients for several years, several techniques for indirectly increasing myocardial oxygen supply and treating angina pectoris—including cervical sympathectomy, arterialization of the coronary sinus, coronary sinus ligation, pericardial and epicardial scarring operations, and ligation of the internal thoracic (mammary) arteries (ITAs)—were attempted experimentally and clinically [2,3]. The first procedure documented to increase myocardial perfusion was Vineberg's technique of implanting internal thoracic arteries into the myocardium. In a variable number of cases, communications developed with the coronary arteries [4]. If and when these communications developed, patients would experience relief of angina; however, revascularization was inconsistent and was not immediate.

Two important advances set the stage for the development of bypass surgery as a widely used surgical treatment for coronary artery disease. The first was the development of coronary arteriography by Sones [5]. Although his initial coronary angiogram was a serendipitous event, Sones immediately recognized the importance of selective cine coronary arteriography for the diagnosis and treatment of ischemic heart disease and was able to apply it in the examination of large numbers of patients. Also important were the careful follow-up studies, which demonstrated that the probability of complications of coronary atherosclerosis could be predicted by determining the location and severity of coronary artery lesions and left ventricular function [6–8]. Once it became possible to define the anatomy of coronary artery disease and to determine its impact on prognosis, direct anatomic approaches to the treatment of coronary atherosclerosis were inevitable. The second major advance was the development of extracorporeal circulation by Gibbon in 1953. Then, in the 1960s, saphenous veins were used for the first time as bypass conduits for myocardial revascularization.

Surgeons had used saphenous vein grafts to bypass lower-extremity arterial stenoses as early as 1948; and in 1962, Sabiston, at the Johns Hopkins Hospital, extended the application of the concept to the coronary arteries when he performed a saphenous vein graft from the aorta to the right coronary artery [2]. Garrett and DeBakey performed the first successful saphenous vein graft to the left coronary system as an alternative procedure in 1964 when an attempt at an endarterectomy failed [9]. In the Soviet Union, Kolessov, without the benefit of coronary arteriography, performed an ITA graft to the left anterior descending (LAD) coronary artery in 1966 for the treatment of angina [10]. In 1967, Favaloro began a series of aortocoronary saphenous vein grafts [11]. Subsequently, saphenous vein grafting techniques were applied to all coronary arteries. In 1968, Green used the left ITA as a coronary bypass graft [12–14], and thus initiated a second form of bypass grafting.

Angiographic follow-up studies documented that many coronary bypass grafts remained patent, and the effectiveness of bypass surgery in relieving angina was obvious [15,16]. Within a few years, many centers were performing bypass surgery, and by the early 1970s the techniques that form the basis of bypass surgery today—saphenous vein grafting and ITA grafting—were well established. Since then, the fundamental reconstructive techniques used in coronary surgery have changed very little. Conversely, major changes have taken place in techniques for protecting the patient and the myocardium during and after the operation. In addition, the assessment of the long-term results of bypass surgery and the more precise recognition of the subgroups of patients with coronary atherosclerosis who can benefit most from operation have been more fully documented.

Today, controversy centers around selection of the best conduits for initial and subsequent surgical revascularizations. New arterial grafts have been evaluated for their appropriateness in revascularization of the heart, and their long-term patency rates have been compared with the excellent rates of ITA grafts. The advantages and disadvantages of these conduits will be discussed.

II. SURGICAL TECHNIQUE

Many modifications of the basic techniques of coronary bypass grafting have been used successfully. In this section we outline the approach we use at the Cleveland Clinic.

The majority of isolated bypass operations are performed through a median sternotomy. The left ITA graft is prepared by dissection of a thin pedicle from the xyphoid to the left subclavian vein; the pedicle is then wrapped in a dilute papaverine-soaked sponge. If the right ITA is to be used, that graft is prepared next. Simultaneous with ITA dissection, surgical assistants dissect out the greater saphenous vein using interrupted incisions in the leg. The branches of the saphenous vein are tied with 4-0 silk ties rather than clipped. Overdistension of the vein is avoided, and it is stored in a balanced salt solution at room temperature. If the gastroepiploic artery (GEA) is used, it usually can be prepared simultaneously with ITA dissection.

The GEA is exposed by extending the sternal incision 5–8 cm into the epigastrium, entering the peritoneal cavity. Use of a Balfour retractor is helpful. The GEA is removed in a 2- to 3-cm pedicle containing accompanying veins. Depending on the length of conduit required, mobilization can extend from the short gastric branches to the pylorus. Branches can be controlled with clips on the branches to the omentum and ties on the branches to the stomach. A length of 20–22 cm can be obtained, with a proximal diameter of 2.5–4.0 mm and a distal diameter of 1.5–2.0 mm. Greater length can be obtained distally, but the diameter will be correspondingly smaller. After harvesting, the conduit is wrapped in a dilute papaverine-soaked sponge.

After the grafts are prepared, the pericardium is opened, heparin is given, and an arterial cannula is placed in the ascending aorta along with a single two-stage venous cannula in the right atrium (Figure 1). The ITAs are then divided distally, and flow is assessed visually. If the ITA flow appears lower than expected with normal mean pressure, the sternal retractor is closed 6–7 cm because excessive spreading may kink the ITA. If the flow is still not

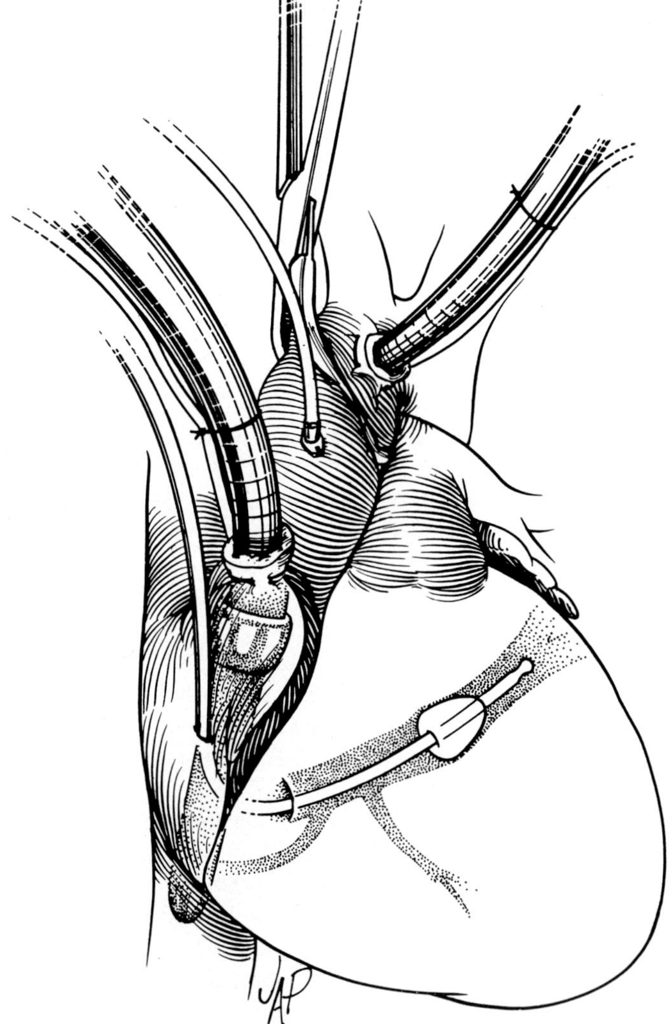

Figure 1 Cannulation for coronary bypass grafting usually includes an arterial cannula in the ascending aorta, a two-stage venous cannula draining the right atrium and extending into the inferior vena cava, a catheter in the ascending aorta for antegrade delivery of cardioplegic solution and for venting of the aorta, and a balloon catheter inserted through a right atrial purse-string suture into the coronary sinus for the retrograde delivery of cardioplegic solution.

adequate, the ITA is examined throughout its course. If flow remains unsatisfactory, the ITA is not used for a graft.

Immediately before cardiopulmonary bypass, a balloon catheter for retrograde delivery of cardiplegic solution is placed into the coronary sinus through a purse-string suture in the right atrium. Cardiopulmonary bypass is then established, and volume is sequestered in the cardiotomy reservoir until the heart stops ejecting. The ascending aorta is cross-clamped, and cardioplegic solution is infused into the aortic root through a needle and then through the coronary sinus catheter. Infusion of cardioplegic solution is repeated after each distal anastomosis. During construction of the distal anastomoses, blood is vented from the aortic root through Y tubing connected to the aortic cardioplegia cannula.

Distal vein grafts to coronary anastomoses are completed first, frequently by use of interrupted 7-0 silk sutures. Although many surgeons use some type of continuous suture technique with excellent results, we have been very pleased with this interrupted technique. We use sequential vein grafts when the amount of vein is limited, when small (<1.25 mm) coronary vessels are to be grafted, or when aortic atherosclerosis limits the sites on the aorta where a proximal anastomosis can be performed. When performing sequential grafting, we attempt to place the most distal anastomosis of the sequential graft to the largest coronary vessel. When aortic atherosclerosis limits the number of sites for proximal vein anastomoses, one may perform one proximal anastomosis and then connect the other vein grafts to that vein ("Y" grafts) (Figure 2). We try to avoid this because of adverse results early in our experience, with occlusion of the secondary limbs of the graft. When we are forced into this situation, we use the largest-diameter segment of the vein for the aortic anastomosis and make the secondary vein anastomoses as proximal as possible.

When all vein anastomoses are completed, the distal arterial graft anastomoses are performed. We use the left ITA to graft the most important left coronary vessel, which usually is the LAD coronary artery (Figure 3). When the right ITA is used as a graft, it may be crossed anterior to the aorta to graft the most important circumflex or diagonal branch (Figure 4). If the right ITA will not reach the target vessel as an in situ graft (left attached to the subclavian artery), it can be divided from its subclavian origin and used as an aorta-to-coronary (free) graft. The proximal anastomoses of free arterial grafts are constructed with an interrupted technique using 6-0 silk. Free arterial grafts are used for two purposes: to avoid crossing the midline, and for extra length to reach distal targets.

The GEA can be brought anteriorly over the stomach or posteriorly through the lesser sac to approach the intended anastomotic site. Care is taken to preserve a parallel orientation between the conduit and the recipient vessel. The left lobe of the liver may be retracted by division of the triangular ligament to

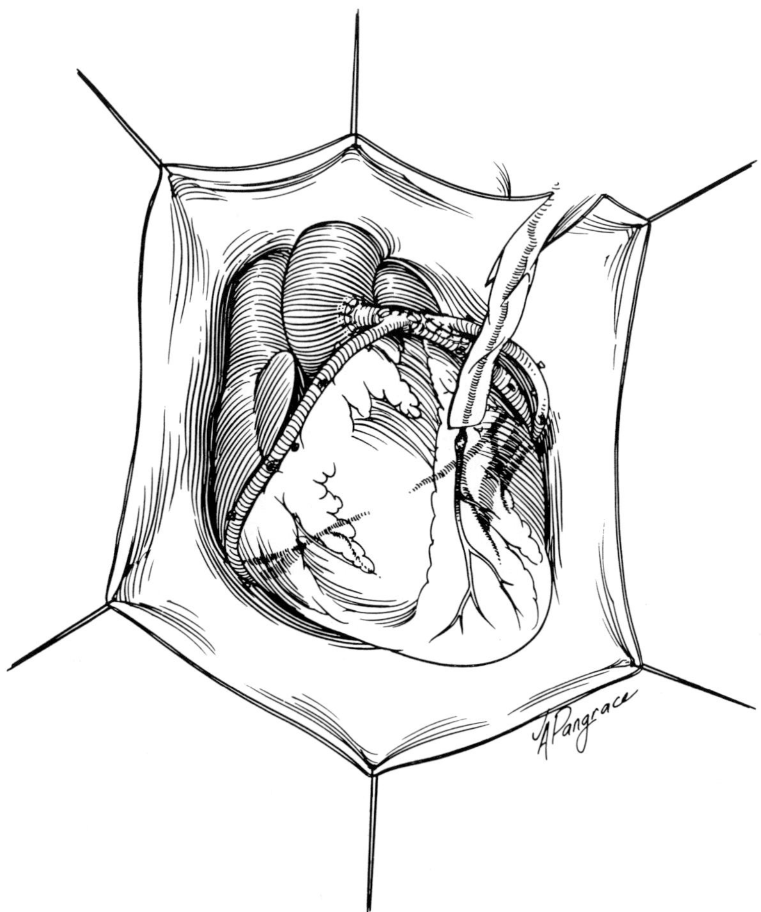

Figure 2   A left ITA graft to the LAD coronary artery and two "Y" grafts off a single proximal vein graft. This technique is very helpful in patients with extensive atherosclerosis of the ascending aorta.

permit optimal positioning of the pedicle in its approach to the anastomotic site. The pedicle is secured to the epicardium after completion of the graft, which is generally performed as the last anastomosis. The anastomosis requires a 3-mm to 4-mm coronary arteriotomy, spatulation of the GEA, and an interrupted 8-0 polypropylene suture technique.

We use a single period of aortic cross-clamping for completion of all anastomoses; once the distal anastomoses are completed, the anastomoses to

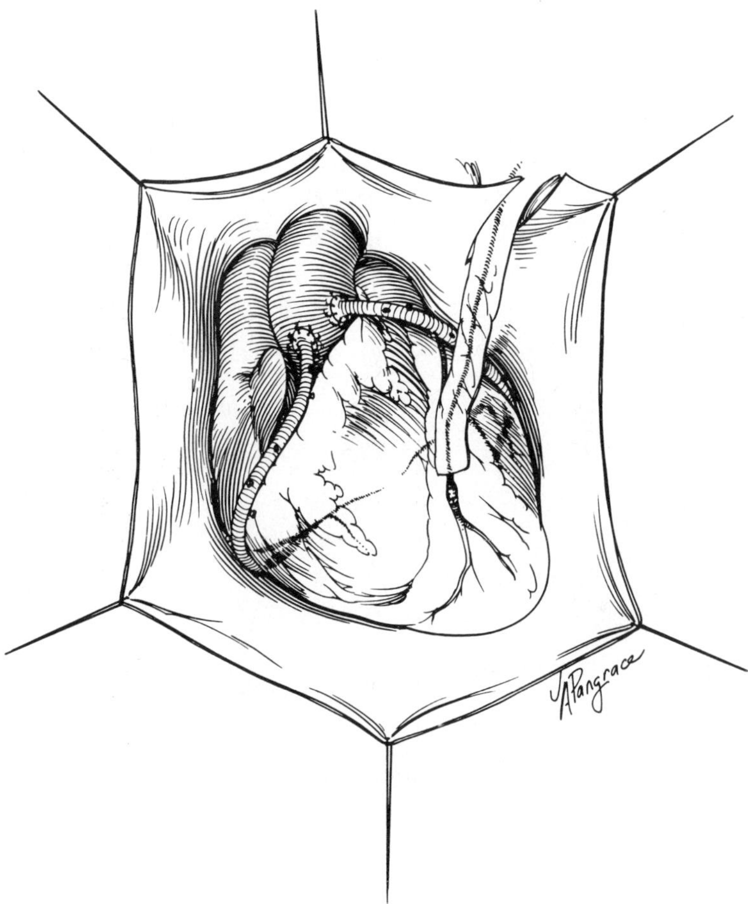

Figure 3   A left ITA graft to the LAD coronary artery and separate vein grafts to the circumflex and right coronary arteries.

the aorta (proximal anastomoses) are done, usually with a continuous technique of 5-0 monofilament suture. After all anastomoses are completed, a warm reperfusion dose of cardioplegic solution containing glutamate and aspartate is given before unclamping. When the heart function has returned and systemic warming is completed, cardiopulmonary bypass is terminated and protamine is given to reverse the heparin. The mediastinal pleura is incised in a posterior direction so that the in situ ITA grafts are routed to the heart through those incisions. The pleuro-pericardial flap is placed over the right

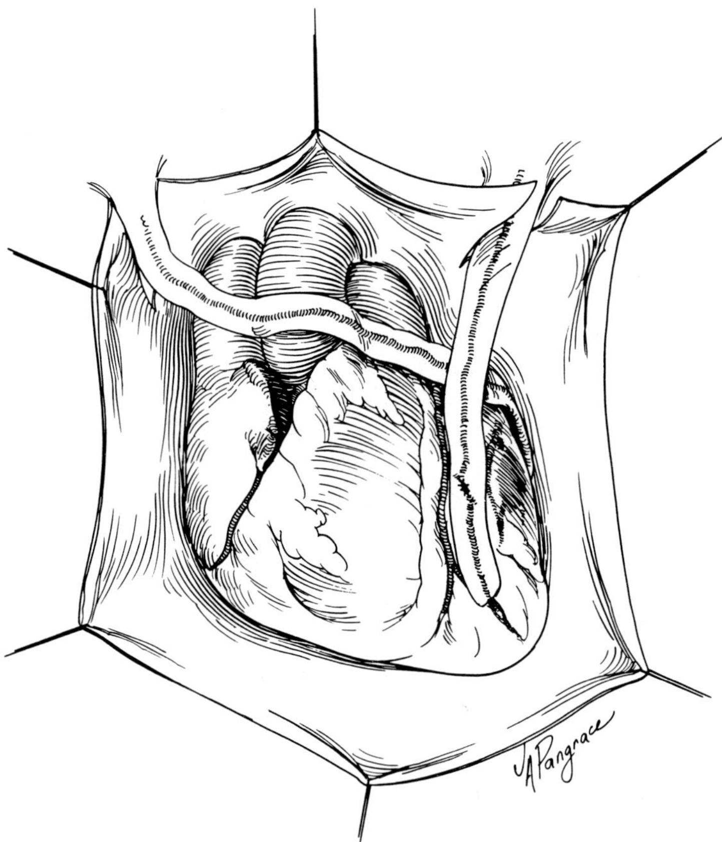

Figure 4   Bilateral ITA grafting, with the left ITA going to the LAD coronary artery and the right ITA to the circumflex as an in situ graft. The posteriorly directed incisions in the pericardium allow the ITAs to take a direct route to the coronary artery and to fall posteriorly so that they do not become adherent to the chest wall after surgery.

ventricle, but the pericardium is not closed nor are pericardial substitutes used. If the pleura has been opened, a chest tube is placed. Mediastinal chest tubes are always used. Sternal closure is accomplished with stainless steel wire, and the subcutaneous and subcuticular layers are closed with absorbable suture.

Throughout the operation, careful attention is paid to blood conservation. An asanguineous pump prime is used. Before heparinization and after reversal with protamine, shed blood is collected with a regionally heparinized collection system and retransfused after surgery.

III. GRAFT PATENCY

A. Vein Graft Patency

The saphenous vein graft has been the mainstay of coronary bypass grafting. Historically this developed as a result of its availability and ease of harvesting. The patency rate of aorta-to-coronary saphenous vein grafts early after operation is good; however, over time, patency decreases significantly. Patency rates from angiographic studies of vein grafts done at a variety of institutions are shown in Table 1. Grafts are classified as either patent or totally occluded and grouped according to the postoperative interval of angiography. Data are from randomized [18,19] and observational studies [17,20], including intermediate and late patency rates from patients who underwent routine postoperative catheterization. It is important to understand that patency rates for patients with symptoms tend to be lower than patency rates for patients studied routinely. The Cleveland Clinic Foundation data in Table 1 refer to all vein grafts studied after surgery from 1971 through 1989, and involve mostly patients who underwent postoperative catheterization because of symptoms or cardiac events [22]. A good rule of thumb is that, at 10 years, about half of vein grafts are closed; and of those that are patent, about half show lumen changes consistent with atherosclerosis [20,22–24].

Most angiographic studies of vein grafts have shown similar patency rates for saphenous vein grafts. Specific factors known to influence early patency rates are the coronary vessel grafted (vein grafts to the LAD coronary artery have better patency rates than grafts to the circumflex and right coronary artery system), the size of the coronary artery grafted, the surgical technique, intraoperative flow through the graft, sex (men have better early vein graft patency than women), and whether the postoperative angiogram was performed routinely or because of symptoms [17,22–24]. Early vein graft patency does not appear to be influenced by risk factors such as diabetes, hyperlipidemia, or smoking [22]. Between 1 and 5 years after operation, the rate of graft occlusion is low; but beyond 5 years, substantial graft occlusion is seen. Late graft occlusion does not appear to be influenced by the vessel grafted but is more frequent in patients with diabetes and hyperlipidemia [22,24].

Additional factors known to affect saphenous vein patency rates include surgical experience, the technique used in preparing the vein grafts, and the perioperative use of platelet inhibitors. Most surgeons agree that decreasing the trauma associated with vein dissection and preparation can decrease endothelial damage to saphenous vein segments. Avoiding vein graft overdistension, as well as avoiding tying side branches too close to the graft, are important in vein graft preparation. In addition, a number of groups have carried out studies to examine the influence of the preparation and storage solution on saphenous vein structure and graft patency. Cantinella and coworkers [25]

Table 1 Patency Rates of Saphenous Vein to Coronary Bypass Grafts According to the Interval Between Surgery and Postoperative Angiography

Author	Early			Intermediate			Late		
	Grafts	Interval	% patent*	Grafts	Interval	% patent*	Grafts	Interval	% patent*
Bourassa et al. [17]	721	<1 mo	87	201	5–7 yr	79	156	10–12 yr	63
ECSS [18]	375	1 yr	79						
		<9 mo	90						
		9–18 mo	77						
CASS [19]	334	<60 days	90	472	60 mo	82			
	292	18 mo	82						
Fitzgibbon et al. [20]	741	1 yr	92	565	5 yr	80	101	>11.5 yr	55
Lawrie et al. [21]	780	0–5 yr	81	606	6–10 yr	68	449	11–15 yr	60
Cleveland Clinic [22]	11,707	<5 yr	76	6,304	5–10 yr	64	2,336	>10 yr	56

*% patent refers to grafts known to be patent 1 year after operation that remained patent at later postoperative intervals.

compared veins stored in heparinized blood at room temperature with those stored in a balanced electrolyte solution (Plasma-lyte; Baxter Healthcare Corp., Deerfield, Ill.) to which heparin and papaverine had been added, and found that veins stored in blood had more contraction, endothelial damage, and microaggregation of fibrin and platelets than those stored in electrolyte solution. These results were confirmed clinically by angiographic studies performed in 40 patients without symptoms between 10 and 14 days after operation, which demonstrated a patency rate of 79% for vein grafts stored in blood compared with 93% for those stored in Plasma-lyte.

Perioperative treatment with platelet inhibitors can also help increase early vein graft patency rates. Platelet deposition and mural thrombus are noted in vein grafts within a few hours of operation, and experimental data have shown that preoperative treatment with platelet inhibitors decreases platelet deposition in canine vein grafts. Most of the initial clinical studies of platelet inhibitors involved preoperative treatment and showed a decreased rate of early vein graft occlusion in the treatment group. Chesebro and coworkers [26] used dipyridamole before surgery and both aspirin and dipyridamole after surgery. Not only was the rate of vein graft occlusion decreased at both 8 days and 1 year after operation, but no increase in postoperative bleeding was found. Data from a Veterans Administration cooperative study in which aspirin was used before surgery also documented a decrease in the vein graft occlusion rate, but an increase in perioperative bleeding was evident [27,28].

B. Internal Thoracic Artery Graft Patency

From the beginning of the bypass surgery era, the left ITA was used for bypass grafting in some centers, almost always as a graft to the LAD coronary artery [14,17,29–34]. Use of the ITA did not become widespread because of the more complex procedure needed to prepare the graft, the increased technical difficulty associated with the anastomosis, concerns about sternal wound complications, increased respiratory morbidity, and uncertainty about adequacy of flow through the ITA. However, once data on long-term patency (≥ 5 years) became available, it was clear that ITA grafts have early patency rates that are slightly superior and late patency rates that are vastly superior to those for vein grafts [22,29,30,34]. Furthermore, the use of the ITA graft has been shown to be associated with a decreased operative mortality rate.

ITA grafts do not seem to be subject to the same pathologic changes, intimal fibroplasia, and atherosclerosis that plague vein grafts. Data on bypass grafts performed at the Cleveland Clinic (Table 2) illustrate that not only are more than 90% of ITA grafts patent early after operation, but almost no attrition of these grafts is seen up to 12 years after surgery [22]. In a report by Grondin and coworkers [34], only 1 of 20 ITA grafts that were patent at 1 year

Table 2 Patency Rates of Internal Thoracic Artery Grafts: The Cleveland Clinic
Foundation 1971–1989

	Number of grafts studied	Number of grafts patent	% Patent
Postoperative interval			
<5 yr	2,835	2,664	94
5–10 yr	1,185	1,102	93
10+ yr	484	462	95
Vessel grafted (in situ ITA graft)			
LAD	4,040	3,826	95
Cx	273	241	88
RCA	72	55	76
Vessel grafts (free ITA graft)			
LAD	76	70	92
Cx	26	24	92
RCA	16	11	69

LAD = left anterior descending coronary artery, ITA = internal thoracic artery; Cx = circumflex
artery; RCA = right coronary artery.

became occluded by 10 postoperative years. Recently, Barner and Barnett [35]
reported on 15 patients who had ITA grafting 15–21 years ago whose grafts
were angiographically proven patent. All patients underwent catheterization
for recurrent angina. Not only were all ITAs widely patent, but they were
without evidence of atherosclerosis.

Patency data from The Cleveland Clinic Foundation Cardiovascular Information Registry concerning postoperative angiography of ITA grafts according to the coronary vessel grafted and postoperative interval are also shown
in Table 2. Appreciation of the favorable patency rates of left ITA grafts to
the LAD coronary artery led to extensions of the use of the ITA, including
right ITA grafts, grafts to the circumflex and right coronary systems, free (aorta-
to-coronary) ITA grafts, and sequential anastomoses with the ITAs [31,32,
36–43]. Our studies with free ITA grafts have documented overall long-term
patency rates slightly lower than those for in situ ITA grafts to the LAD coronary artery, but better than that for saphenous vein grafts. Most of the free
ITA graft occlusions appeared to occur early after surgery and may have been
related to technical difficulties with the proximal anastomosis. Our current
technique for free graft proximal anastomoses involves continuous 6-0 polypropylene sutures. We have documented patency in three free ITA grafts more
than 15 years after operation, indicating that free grafts appear to be protected

from the development of intrinsic pathologic changes. Russo and colleagues [41] restudied 198 distal ITA-to-coronary anastomoses in patients receiving bilateral ITA grafts. Patency was documented in 98.5%; and in 108 distal anastomoses in patients receiving sequential ITA grafts, the patency rate was 98.2%. Rankin and associates [42], in another angiographic study of complex ITA grafting, documented an overall patency rate of 99% for 338 right and left ITA single or sequential grafts. Only 20 ITA grafts to the right coronary artery were studied, with one occlusion being found. Two right ITA grafts routed to the circumflex system through the transverse sinus had poor flow. On the other hand, Dion and coworkers [43] noted a high rate of early patency of right ITA grafts through the transverse sinus to the circumflex artery and an overall patency rate of 97% for sequential ITA grafts. The studies of Russo, Rankin, and Dion and their colleagues involved early postoperative angiograms carried out within a year of operation. In one of the few studies with late patency data, Huddleston and associates [36] noted patency rates of 90% for left ITA grafts versus 79% for right ITA grafts at 5 postoperative years.

Technical factors, including incorrect construction of the anastomosis and kinking of the graft, are probably the prime reasons for ITA graft failure. In addition, we have seen postoperative angiograms in which the ITA appeared to be tented up, probably because of adhesion to extrapericardial structures. The principles of sewing the ITA pedicle to the epicardium, routing the graft in a direct line from its subclavian origin to the anastomotic site, incision of the pericardium posteriorly so that the inflated lung is anterior to the graft, and placing the pericardium anterior to the anastomosis cannot be overemphasized. In addition to improving ITA patency rates, these techniques facilitate future reoperations.

Hemodynamic factors can also play a role in circumstances in which the ITA is used to graft a coronary vessel that is not severely stenotic. In a study of grafts constructed to vessels with a stenosis of less than 50%, Cosgrove and coworkers [44] noted a patency rate of 92% for ITA grafts, compared with a patency rate of 96% for those to vessels with a stenosis of 50% or more. This difference was not significant, but the mean postoperative interval of the angiograms was only 16 months and there was a trend toward decreasing patency with increasing postoperative interval. It is clear that increased flow from the native coronary artery can cause the ITA to become atretic ("string sign"). This atresia may take over a year to occur, and early postoperative angiograms may show patency in ITA grafts that are destined to become attenuated. The lower overall patency rate we noted for ITA grafts to the right coronary artery (see Table 2) may be based on an ITA–coronary flow mismatch, because most of the studies that documented atretic grafts were performed more than a year after operation. Increase in size of atretic ITA grafts associated with progression of the native coronary stenosis has been documented, but we do not know if this phenomenon is predictable [45]. Experimental studies suggest that it may occur [46]. Lust et al. [46], in a dog model, documented the ability of ITA grafts to remain patent despite chronic flow competition from a fully patent native artery. Internal thoracic artery graft flow was maintained above in situ levels, and a recruitable flow reserve from the ITA graft could be demonstrated when the native vessel was later occluded. These data suggest that ITA grafts are dynamic and may remain patent despite significant competitive flow in the native vessel [46].

C. Clinical Impact of Internal Thoracic Artery Bypass Grafts

The superior patency rate of the left ITA graft to the anterior descending coronary artery is reflected in superior clinical results. A study from our center compared the 10-year outcome for patients undergoing elective bypass surgery who received a left ITA graft to the anterior descending coronary artery as part of their operation with the outcome for those who received only vein grafts [29]. Patients with an ITA graft had better survival rates (Figure 5), fewer reoperations, and fewer cardiac events than did patients with only vein grafts. Analysis with multivariate techniques confirmed the positive influence of the ITA-to-LAD coronary artery graft. Sergeant and coworkers [33] also documented improved survival rates for patients with single ITA grafts, as did a report from the CASS study [47]. Work by Gardner and associates [48] demonstrated that the positive impact of the left ITA–LAD coronary artery graft on survival rates, reoperation, and cardiac events extends to the elderly. Studies focusing on perioperative morbidity and mortality have shown that the use of a single ITA graft does not increase perioperative complications [49,50]. Moreover, use of an ITA graft may decrease operative mortality. Recent reports from the Society of Thoracic Surgeons National Cardiac Database, which covers broad multiinstitutional experience with more than 38,000 patients who underwent isolated coronary artery bypass grafting from 1987 through 1991, demonstrated significant improvement in operative mortality rates associated with ITA use compared with bypass grafting using only veins ($p < 0.005$) [51]. Studies performed at the Cleveland Clinic [50] reinforce these data: Cosgrove reviewed the cases of 7,105 patients who underwent primary isolated myocardial revascularization, 49% of whom received vein grafts and 50% of whom received at least one ITA graft. The operative mortality was 1.4% in the vein group and 0.2% in the ITA group. Because the ITA conduit is often not used in patients who are in unstable condition, a multivariate analysis identifying six incremental risk factors for operative mortality was performed. After adjustment for these risk factors, the use of vein grafts was the only incriminating risk factor. Grover et al. [52], in a smaller series, also demonstrated that ITA

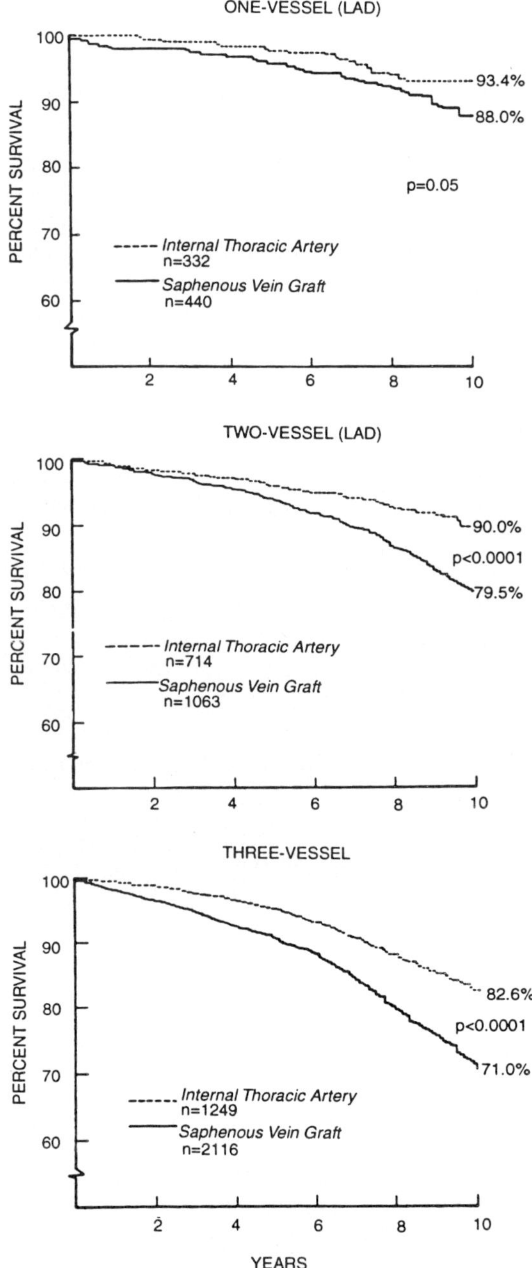

Figure 5 Survival at 10 years, comparing patients who received an internal thoracic (mammary) artery graft to the LAD coronary artery with those who received only vein grafts. In the analysis of patients with one-, two-, and three-vessel disease, survival rates were significantly better for patients with ITA grafts. (Reprinted from Loop et al. [29], with permission.)

grafts, in addition to providing superior long-term patency, decreased operative mortality (after adjusting for patient risk factors).

The reasons for a decreased operative mortality associated with the use of ITA grafts are unclear. The higher earlier patency rates in the ITA grafts may account for this; however, another possibility is that many surgeons perform proximal vein anastomoses with a partial occlusion aortic clamp in place after removal of the aortic cross-clamp and unclamping of the ITA graft. Therefore, during the very important period of reperfusion, while the proximal vein grafts are being performed, the myocardium distal to the coronary occlusions or stenoses in a patient with one or two ITA grafts is perfused through the ITA grafts. Consequently, it is possible that during this reperfusion period, myocardial perfusion is improved, which results in decreased operative mortality. Whenever feasible, use of the left ITA graft to the LAD coronary artery should be a routine part of primary elective operations for coronary bypass grafting.

Although ITA graft use is associated with lower mortality compared with use of only vein grafts in primary bypass cases, the ITA must be used carefully in reoperative coronary artery bypass grafting. ITA grafts need to be used cautiously in patients undergoing reoperative bypass surgery when replacing a stenotic vein graft to a totally occluded LAD. Navia and associates [53] reviewed the Cleveland Clinic experience with 387 patients who underwent surgery to replace a stenotic saphenous vein graft to a totally occluded native LAD coronary artery with an ITA graft, and found an increased mortality rate and increased incidence of hypoperfusion syndrome (Figure 6). The hypoperfusion syndrome was likely a result of the inability of the new ITA graft adequately to replace the blood flow from the replaced stenotic vein graft. Placement of an intraaortic balloon counterpulsation pump did not improve mortality. Hypoperfusion syndrome is best treated with supplemental vein grafting.

Single ITA grafting is better than vein grafting alone, but it is less clear whether bilateral ITA grafting produces better long-term results than a single ITA graft to the LAD coronary artery. The investigation of this question is complicated by three problems. First, results over the first 10 years after surgery are so good for patients receiving a single ITA graft to the LAD coronary artery that improvement in these results will be difficult to demonstrate. Second, in virtually all institutions, patients who receive bilateral ITA grafts are carefully selected and the majority are relatively good-risk patients. Third, large numbers of patients who have received bilateral ITA grafts have not been followed for more than 10 postoperative years. Data reported by Galbut and coworkers [40], Barner and Barnett [35], and our own institution [54] evaluating survival rates after bilateral ITA grafting indicate a 10-year survival rate of 80% to 85% for heterogeneous groups of patients. The use of two ITAs for

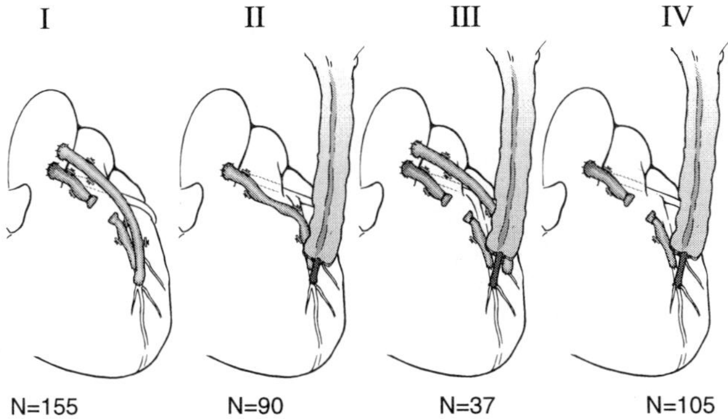

Figure 6 Mortality in patients who underwent a second operation to replace a stenotic vein graft to the LAD artery. There were four methods of managing these patients. In Group I, the atherosclerotic vein graft was divided and replaced with a new saphenous vein graft (SVG) to the left anterior descending coronary artery (LAD); in Group II, the old vein graft was left in place and flow to the LAD was supplemented with a new internal thoracic artery (ITA) graft to the LAD; in Group III, the old SVG was divided and replaced with an ITA graft to the LAD, and an SVG was also placed to the diagonal coronary system; and in Group IV, the old vein graft was divided and replaced with an ITA graft to the LAD. This group had the highest incidence of hypoperfusion syndrome and death. (Reprinted from Navia et al. [53], with permission.)

bypass grafting has been shown to reduce the incidence of ischemic events [39,47,55] without increasing operative mortality rates [55,56]. For patients aged 60 years or younger, this incremental improvement may be more pronounced [55].

It does appear that patients who receive bilateral ITA grafts are less likely to need reoperation. Figure 7 shows data from our institution regarding the cumulative incidence of reoperation after primary surgery for patients receiving none, one, or bilateral ITA grafts. Data reported by Galbut and coworkers [40] and Fiore and associates [39] show a similar decrease in the incidence of reoperation. One group of patients in whom bilateral ITA grafting is specifically indicated is young adults. Young adults with coronary artery disease have a high prevalence of hyperlipidemia and other risk factors and distinctly inferior long-term vein graft patency. Fortunately, ITA graft patency is excellent in these patients [57].

Although there appears to be a benefit associated with using bilateral ITA grafts, especially in young adults with coronary artery disease, controversy surrounds the question of how best to construct bilateral ITA grafts. As mentioned earlier, we frequently use the right ITA as an aortocoronary free graft

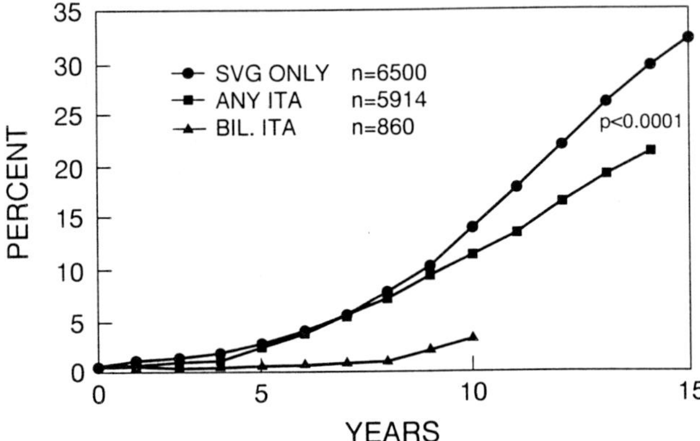

Figure 7 Cumulative risk of reoperation for patients who received, at primary surgery, one ITA graft or saphenous vein grafts (SVG) only (1971 to 1984), compared with patients who received bilateral (BIL) ITA grafts (1971 to 1985). (Reprinted from Lytle BW and Cosgrove DM. Coronary artery bypass surgery. Curr Prob Surg 1992; 29(10):782, with permission.)

to bypass the largest circumflex vessels or as in situ grafts (length allowing) to the circumflex vessels. We have preferred to traverse the midline anterior to the aorta when ITA grafts are used in situ, as opposed to tunneling them through the transverse sinus. However, concerns about the potential danger of injuring an ITA graft crossing the midline during reoperations are very real and have influenced many surgeons to perform free ITA grafts. On occasion, because of a short right ITA graft, a "T" graft may be constructed where the free right ITA is anastomosed to the side of the in situ left ITA, which is anastomosed to the LAD coronary artery. This allows the right ITA to reach coronary arteries it may not have been able to reach otherwise. Many surgeons, however, have concerns about the ability of the ITA to deliver adequate flow to a single coronary vessel, let alone the entire left ventricle. Recently, Tector et al. [58] described their results in 287 patients in whom a "T" graft was constructed by anastomosing the proximal end of the free right ITA to the side of the left ITA. These patients (mean age 64.6 years) received an average of 4.4 ITA distal bypass grafts by liberal use of sequential ITA anastomoses. Every effort was made to revascularize the heart completely using all arterial bypass grafts. Four patients required additional saphenous vein bypass grafts to areas already grafted by an ITA when decreased wall motion was noted on echocardiography before the patient was weaned from cardiopulmonary bypass. All had an uneventful postoperative course. Twenty-six patients underwent postoperative angiography, and 107 of 113 coronary anastomoses (94.7%) were patent. All of the 45 grafts from the left ITA to the LAD and diagonal vessels were patent, but 62 of 68 grafts (91%) from the right ITA were open. One hundred seven patients underwent postoperative stress tests, of which 89.7% were negative. Despite these excellent results, we emphasize the importance of a cautious, individualized approach.

Controversy surrounds the use of ITA grafts in emergencies following failed coronary angioplasty. Many surgeons have expressed concern for the additional time required to mobilize the ITA and the increased need for vasoactive catecholamines in emergency cases, especially when patients present in a hemodynamically unstable condition, which may cause spasm and limit flow in an arterial graft. Caes and Van Nooten [59] demonstrated the safe use of the ITA graft in 27 patients requiring emergency bypass surgery after failed angioplasty. There was no increase in mortality associated with ITA grafting, even when patients were unstable preoperatively. Eighty-four percent of patients requiring emergency bypass grafting were treated with ITA grafts. The Cleveland Clinic experience, however, mirrors that of most other centers. We have used ITA grafts in 22% of our patients requiring emergency bypass grafting [60]. We specifically refrain from using an ITA for grafting if patients have evidence of ongoing ischemia despite intraaortic balloon pumping, have suffered cardiac arrest necessitating cardiopulmonary resuscitation, or have ventricular fibrillation or tachycardia or persistent hypotension of less than 80 mmHg while receiving vasopressors.

As the use of bilateral ITA grafts has increased, so has the need to reoperate on these patients. Although reoperation in patients who have undergone a bilateral ITA bypass is uncommon, it may become necessary if native vessel coronary artery disease progresses, the ITA or vein graft fails, or valvular heart disease develops. We recently reviewed our experience in 36 patients requiring cardiac reoperation following bilateral ITA grafting. There were four early deaths (11%) and two late deaths (average follow-up 4.3 years). Forty-seven ITA grafts were patent preoperatively, and 11 crossed the midline. Two ITA grafts were damaged during reoperation; although both were repaired, one was ultimately replaced. This report demonstrated that the mortality associated with this procedure is relatively high and that these operations are difficult. However, reoperation can be performed at an acceptable risk, and substantial surgical objectives can be achieved with good long-term results.

Several technical maneuvers appeared to be helpful in this difficult group of reoperative patients. It was clear that the safety and ease of reoperative heart procedures can be enhanced by steps taken during the primary operation. Metal clips, used on the ITA pedicle to occlude intercostal side branches, allow the ITA to be easily visualized on the chest roentgenogram and are often spotted quickly during dissection. Opening the pleura, routing the ITA through

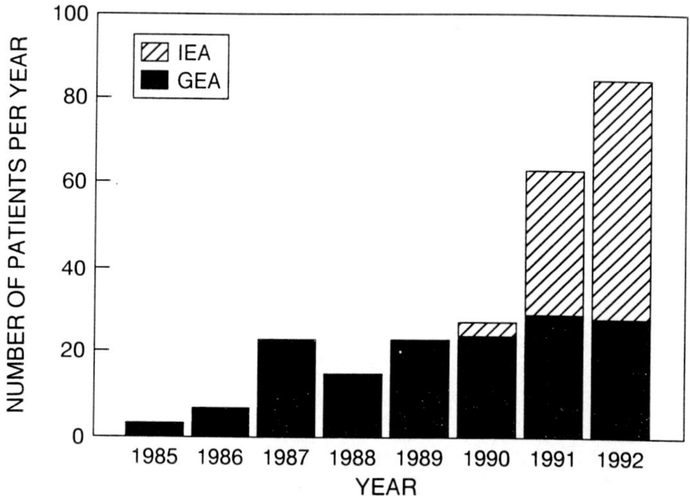

Figure 8 Annual GEA and IEA use. While GEA use has remained relatively constant since first applied in 1985, IEA use has increased since being introduced in November 1990. (Reprinted from Manapat et al. [68], with permission.)

the slit in the mediastinal pleura, and then attaching the ITA pedicle to the heart a few centimeters proximal to the distal anastomosis will keep the graft away from the midline, ensure that the location of the grafts is predictable at reoperation, and prevent kinking. Furthermore, the ITA pedicle should be covered with pericardium whenever possible to prevent injury during resternotomy. The idea of always being prepared to cannulate alternative sites for cardiopulmonary bypass and having adequate conduit to replace damaged grafts is imperative.

IV. ALTERNATIVE BYPASS GRAFTS

The success of ITA grafts and the increase in the number of patients who have limited bypass conduits available (usually because of previous surgery) have led to the use of other arterial grafts. Thus far, the most successful have been the right GEA and the inferior epigastric artery (IEA). Figure 8 demonstrates how GEA and IEA use has increased at The Cleveland Clinic Foundation.

A. Gastroepiploic Artery

The right gastroepiploic artery (GEA) was first used in myocardial revascularization by Bailey and associates [61] for Vineberg-type myocardial implantation. In 1987, Pym and colleagues [62] reported the use of this conduit to bypass the right coronary artery and posterior circumflex branches in nine patients. Carter [63], also in 1987, reported 30 cases using the GEA. Later, Suma [64] extended the use of the GEA to bypass the LAD system. Lytle and associates [65] reported its use as a pedicled graft and as a free graft in 17 patients. Suma [66] documented patency in 88 of 92 grafts, some more than a year after operation; serial angiograms within 1 month of operation and a year later showed late occlusion in only 2 of 35 grafts patent at the first study. Two series demonstrated a 95% patency rate at 5 years [62,67]. We have performed more than 150 GEA grafts, the majority during reoperations [68]. We most often use the GEA as an in situ graft to the right coronary system but have also used in situ grafts to the LAD coronary artery and to the circumflex branches and GEA free grafts to all coronary vessels (Table 3) [65]. Of 30 GEA grafts studied, 16 of 20 in situ grafts and 8 of 10 free (aorta-to-coronary) grafts were patent 6 days to 65 months postoperatively. The incidence of various nonspecific complications is listed in Table 4. Two patients required reoperation for intraabdominal bleeding, one from the spleen and the other from the stomach. Nine patients were identified as having hyperamylasemia (>300 I.U./L) but without clinical signs of pancreatitis. Another patient developed clinical signs of pancreatitis, which resolved with conservative management.

Suma and colleagues [69] found no increase in morbidity associated with the use of the right GEA graft and noted no decrease in gastric mucosal blood flow. Reported complications related to harvesting of the GEA have been rare [65,67,69,70]. Gastric perforation secondary to GEA harvesting has been reported [71]. One patient of 400 undergoing GEA harvesting developed gastric perforation due to gastric ischemia. Herniation through the diaphragmatic defect is also rare. Injury to the in situ conduit associated with laparotomy has

Table 3 Coronary Vessels Grafted with GEA and IEA

Conduit	LAD	Dg	Cx	RCA
GEA				
in situ	7 (6%)	0	11 (9%)	99 (85%)
free	6 (17%)	7 (20%)	12 (34%)	10 (28%)
IEA	10 (8%)	75 (58%)	36 (28%)	9 (7%)

GEA = right gastroepiploic artery; IEA = inferior epigastric artery; LAD = left anterior descending coronary artery; Dg = diagonal artery; Cx = circumflex artery; RCA = right coronary artery and branches.

Table 4 Percentage Postoperative Complications of CABG
Using GEA and IEA*

Complication	GEA (N = 152)	IEA (N = 130)
Death	4%	0.8%
Reoperated for bleeding	4	6
Myocardial infarction	5	3
Low cardiac output	3	3
Arrhythmias	22	23
Neurologic	1	1
Thromboembolic	2	0
Renal	4	2
Respiratory	13	13
Wound	7	4
Sepsis	3	2

*All were statistically not significant.
GEA = right gastroepiploic artery; IEA = inferior epigastric artery.

not been reported but is a concern. We currently use the right GEA graft as an alternative conduit when the ITAs and lower extremity vein have been exhausted, and by choice in young patients, especially those with hyperlipidemia. Figure 9 demonstrates the use of a right GEA graft attached to the posterior descending coronary artery. As evidence increases for favorable patency rates more than a year after operation (particularly in regard to in situ grafts), we are increasing our use of the right GEA graft.

Although recent evidence suggests that the early and late patency rates are comparable for in situ GEA and ITA grafts [72–74], the same is not true of free GEA and ITA grafts. Both arterial grafts appear to have the potential for growth following their placement as coronary artery bypass grafts. Likewise, both vessels have a low incidence of atherosclerosis. These grafts, however, are not equivalent anatomically, which may account for their different responses to vasopressors and patency rates when used as free grafts. The vasa vasora of the GEA penetrates deep into the media, but the ITA vasa vasora enters only the adventitia. The ITA appears to be nourished mostly from the lumen. The GEA media is subject to hypoxic injury when the vasa vasora are divided, as would occur if the vessel were employed as a free graft. Laboratory studies have confirmed that isolated segments of these two arteries have different vasoreactive properties. GEA segments exhibit stronger contractions in response to a depolarizing agent (potassium chloride), to adrenergic stimulation (norepinephrine), and to a product of platelet aggregation (serotonin). Sequential relaxation in response to sodium nitroprusside is not different.

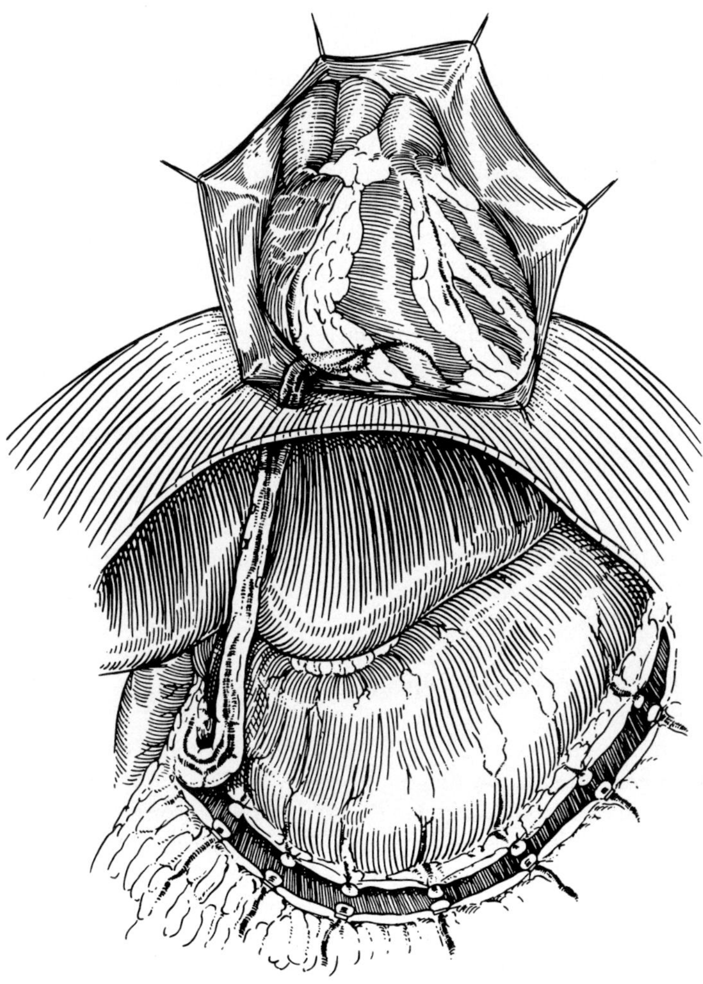

Figure 9 Right GEA anastomosis to the posterior descending coronary artery. (Reprinted from Lytle BW and Cosgrove DM. Coronary artery bypass surgery. Curr Prob Surg 1992; 29(10):783, with permission.)

These anatomical and chemical findings suggest that vasodilators and platelet inhibitors should be employed clinically in the postoperative period, especially in situations in which a free GEA graft is constructed. It is becoming apparent that the late patency rates are less for free GEA grafts than for free ITA grafts [73,74].

B. Inferior Epigastric Artery

The inferior epigastric artery (IEA) graft, which must be used as a free graft, has likewise shown promise as a new arterial conduit [74–77]. The use of alternative arterial grafts such as the IEA graft is predicated on the assumption that arterial conduits are generally better than vein grafts.

The use of the inferior epigastric artery has not been meant to replace the ITA, but rather to serve as an alternative to the use of saphenous veins. The indications for using alternative arterial conduits, therefore, are: (a) reoperations in which the ITAs and saphenous veins have been previously used; (b) patients who have undergone vein stripping; (c) severe peripheral vascular disease of the leg; (d) poor-quality saphenous veins; (e) reoperations due to vein graft failure in young patients; (f) young patients with hyperlipidemia; and (8) patients at high risk for sternal wound problems associated with bilateral ITA usage (obese diabetics).

The IEA was first used as a bypass graft by Puig and coworkers [75] in 1988. Vincent and coworkers [74] successfully used this artery in myocardial revascularization in two patients after noting its potential during kidney transplantations. Buche and coworkers [77] used the IEA in 74 patients, with encouraging early clinical and angiographic results. Limited length results in its placement to the diagonals, ramus marginalis, or first obtuse marginal artery, although distal sites can be reached by making the proximal anastomosis to another arterial conduit.

IEA grafts have been used in 130 patients at the Cleveland Clinic. The IEA was used to bypass mostly the diagonal branch (58%), followed by the circumflex branch, and occasionally the LAD and the right coronary artery or its branches (see Table 3). Of 21 patients studied 5 days to 13 months postoperatively, 18 (85.7%) had patent IEA grafts. In the IEA group of patients, there was no incidence of rectus muscle necrosis, even among 78 patients who had concomitant bilateral ITA grafting. Two patients in this series even had both bilateral IEA and ITA grafts without such a complication. Other potential complications, such as abdominal wall hematoma, injury to the spermatic cord, and testicular necrosis, were not seen in this series.

We harvest the IEA using a midline or paramedian incision from umbilicus to symphysis pubis. The midline approach with lateral retraction of the rectus muscle allows one or both IEAs to be mobilized, but the paramedian incision with medial rectus retraction or splitting of the muscle provides better exposure. A significant percentage of IEAs bifurcate or enter the rectus muscle before reaching the umbilicus, or both, so length is thereby limited, although a bifurcation graft is occasionally useful. Initially, the middle third of the artery is mobilized with a small amount of areolar fatty tissue and its associated veins, followed by proximal dissection, which can usually be carried to within 1 cm of its origin from the external iliac artery. Branches are controlled with small clips and the proximal stump with medium clips or a silk ligature. The two venous comitantes combine into a single trunk before entering the external iliac vein. Distal dissection is continued until the desired length is attained, but this is frequently limited by branching or by the artery entering the rectus muscle, which makes dissection exceedingly tedious. If the artery continues as a single trunk dorsal to the muscle, then the incision can be extended to gain additional length. The mean length is 12 cm, with a range of 9–15 cm, which is significantly less than the 16.5 cm for the ITA and the 20–22 cm for the GEA [78]. The harvested IEA is placed in saline containing 0.5 mg/mL of papaverine. Before it is used it is flushed with 0.5 mg/mL of papaverine. The distal and proximal anastomoses are the same as for the free ITA. Complications associated with use of the IEA graft have been acceptable (Table 4).

C. Radial Artery

In the early years of bypass surgery, a number of groups used the radial artery as an aorta-to-coronary bypass graft [73]. Carpentier and coworkers [79] reported some success; of 40 grafts restudied within a year of operation, 36 were patent. Other investigators did not duplicate that success. Curtis and associates [80] found that 22 (65%) of 34 radial artery grafts restudied within a year of operation were either occluded or stenotic, and Fisk and colleagues [81] reported that 24 (50%) of 48 grafts were patent within 6 months of surgery. Approximately 20 years ago at the Cleveland Clinic, 22 radial artery grafts were performed; 15 were restudied, and only 3 were patent. Early postoperative spasms and subsequent focal intimal hyperplasia were the presumed causes of early graft failure.

Acar et al. [82] recently demonstrated patency in three radial artery grafts 15–18 years after operation, which led to the resumption of use of this conduit combined with calcium channel blocking agents to prevent conduit spasm. At 6–13 months, 29 of 31 grafts were patent, with one having a distal anastomotic stenosis. Thus, this recent experience suggests that the radial artery is an appropriate alternative conduit, and early postoperative spasm may be reduced with the use of calcium channel blockers, thereby improving graft patency.

The reasons for the poor patency of radial artery grafts in early studies in contrast to the recent good results probably relate to our better understanding of the need for atraumatic harvesting of the conduit. In addition, we now recognize the importance of the liberal use of papaverine to overcome graft spasm, avoidance of intergraft saline (which destroys the endothelium), and gentle injection of heparinized blood with papaverine rather than using mechanical dilatation to overcome spasm, all of which may contribute to preventing intimal hyperplasia as a cause of conduit failure [83]. Additionally, calcium channel blockers may be valuable in treating or preventing graft spasm during or after surgery [82].

Of persistent concern is ischemia of the hand or forearm [84], which was not observed in any of the 122 arms from which grafts were taken in the recent experience [82]. Perhaps judicious use of the Allen test combined with Doppler studies and preservation of the origin of the superficial palmar arch can preclude this important complication [82].

D. Conduit Selection

Our current approach to conduit selection for patients undergoing primary bypass grafting is as follows. Essentially all patients receive a left ITA graft to the most important stenotic branch of the left coronary system, usually the LAD coronary artery. Bilateral ITA grafts are used for the majority of patients under 60 years of age and for selected older patients. For patients 30–40 years of age, we attempt extensive arterial revascularization with bilateral ITA grafts, sequential ITA grafts, the right GEA, and the IEA. Young diabetic patients do receive bilateral ITA grafts after a preoperative discussion of the risks of wound complications. If no arterial grafts are available, the greater saphenous vein is used, and the lesser saphenous vein is used if needed. We have not found it necessary to use other bypass conduits. The effect of the extensive or total use of arterial conduits on the long-term clinical results after bypass surgery is an important unanswered question.

Recently, Jegaden et al. [84] reported on the use of bilateral ITA grafts and right GEA grafts in 240 patients whose average age was 60 years. Only 34% had normal left ventricular function. The mean number of distal anastomoses was 3.5 ± 0.7 per patient. The early mortality rate was 0.4%, and complications occurred in 20 patients. Early (postoperative day 15) angiography was performed in 51 asymptomatic patients. The rate of patent anastomosis was 100% for the ITA grafts and 96% for the GEA grafts. The 4-year actuarial survival was 96.5% ± 4.2%; the rate of late cardiac events was 0.6% per patient year. Reports such as these may well direct the future of cardiac bypass surgery as it relates to the use of arterial bypass grafts.

V. CONCLUSION

Coronary artery bypass grafting using arterial conduits is frequently performed. Currently, the ITA graft is used routinely during bypass surgery because of its excellent long-term patency rate and protection from the need for future reoperative bypass procedures. Its use has been extended to the elderly and to emergency bypass procedures following failed angioplasty, as well as to reoperative bypass procedures. Recent reports have suggested that the use of bilateral ITA bypass grafts may be beneficial, especially in younger patients. Newer arterial conduits, such as the GEA and IEA, are suitable alternatives to the use of saphenous vein grafts. Radial artery grafting requires further clinical scrutiny after longer follow-up to determine its usefulness.

REFERENCES

1. Favaloro RG. The present era of myocardial revascularization—some historical landmarks. Int J Cardiol 1983; 4:331–344.
2. Sabiston DC. The William F. Rienhoff, Jr. lecture: The coronary circulation. Johns Hopkins Med J 1974; 134:314–329.
3. McGoon DC. Prologue: from whence. Cardiovasc Clin 1987; 17:1–3.
4. Vineberg DM. Development of anastomoses between coronary vessels and transplanted internal mammary artery. Can Med Assoc J 1946; 55:117–125.
5. Sones FM Jr, Shirey EK. Cine coronary arteriography. Mod Concept Cardiovasc Dis 1962; 31:735–739.
6. Proudfit WL, Shirey EK, Sones FM Jr. Selective cine coronary arteriography: correlation with clinical findings in 1000 patients. Circulation 1966; 33:901–910.
7. Bruschke AVG, Proudfit WL, Sones FM Jr. Progress study of 590 consecutive nonsurgical cases of coronary disease followed 5–9 years. I. Arteriographic correlations. Circulation 1973; 47:1147–1153.
8. Oberman A, Jones WB, Riley CP, et al. Natural history of coronary artery disease. Bull NY Acad Med 1972; 48:1109–1111.
9. Garrett HE, Dennis EW, DeBakey ME. Aortocoronary bypass with saphenous vein graft: seven-year follow-up. JAMA 1973; 223:792–794.
10. Kolessov VI. Mammary artery-coronary artery anastomosis as method of treatment of angina pectoris. J Thorac Cardiovasc Surg 1967; 54:535–544.
11. Favaloro RG. Saphenous vein autograft replacement of severe segmental coronary artery occlusion. Operative technique. Ann Thorac Surg 1968; 5:334–339.
12. Favaloro RG, Effler DB, Groves LK. Severe segmental obstruction of the left main coronary artery and its divisions: surgical treatment by the saphenous vein graft technique. J Thorac Cardiovasc Surg 1970; 60:469–482.
13. Johnson WD, Flemma RJ, Lepley D Jr, Ellison EH. Extended treatment of severe coronary artery disease: a total surgical approach. Ann Surg 1969; 170:460–470.
14. Green GE, Stertzer SH, Reppert EH. Coronary arterial bypass grafts. Ann Thorac Surg 1968; 5:443–450.
15. Green GE, Spencer FC, Tice DA, Stertzer SH. Arterial and venous microsurgical bypass grafts for coronary artery disease. J Thorac Cardiovasc Surg 1970; 60:491–503.
16. Sheldon WC, Favaloro RG, Sones FM Jr, Effler DB. Reconstructive coronary artery surgery: venous autograft technique. JAMA 1970; 213:78–82.

17. Bourassa MG, Campeau L, Lesperance J. Changes in grafts and in coronary arteries after coronary bypass surgery. Cardiovasc Clin 1991; 21:83–100.

18. European Coronary Surgery Study Group. Long-term results of prospective randomized study of coronary artery bypass surgery in stable angina pectoris. Lancet 1982; 2:1173–1179.

19. Bourassa MG, Fisher LD, Campeau L, et al. Long-term fate of bypass grafts: The Coronary Artery Surgery Study (CASS) and Montreal Heart Institute experiences. Circulation 1985; 72:V-71–V-78.

20. Fitzgibbon GM, Leach AJ, Kafka HP, Keon WJ. Coronary bypass graft fate: long-term angiographic study. J Am Coll Cardiol 1991; 17:1075–1080.

21. Lawrie GM, Morris GC Jr, Earle N. Long-term results of coronary artery bypass surgery. Analysis of 1,698 patients followed 15 to 20 years. Ann Surg 1991; 213: 377–385.

22. Lytle BW, Loop FD, Cosgrove DM, et al. Long-term (5 to 12 years) serial studies of internal mammary artery and saphenous vein coronary bypass grafts. J Thorac Cardiovasc Surg 1985; 89:248–258.

23. Roth JA, Cukingnan RA, Brown BG, Gocka E, Carey JS. Factors influencing patency of saphenous vein grafts. Ann Thorac Surg 1979; 28:176–183.

24. Loop FD, Golding LR, MacMillan JP, et al. Coronary artery surgery in women compared with men: analysis of risks and long-term results. J Am Coll Cardiol 1983; 1:383–390.

25. Cantinella FP, Cunningham JN Jr, Srungaram RK, et al. The factors influencing early patency of coronary artery bypass vein grafts: correlation of angiographic and ultrastructural findings. J Thorac Cardiovasc Surg 1982; 83:686–700.

26. Chesebro JH, Fuster V, Elveback LR, et al. Effect of dipyridamole and aspirin on late vein-graft patency after coronary bypass operations. N Engl J Med 1984; 310: 209–214.

27. Goldman S, Copeland J, Moritz T, et al. Saphenous vein graft patency 1 year after coronary artery bypass surgery and effects of antiplatelet therapy. Circulation 1989; 80:1190–1197.

28. Sethi GK, Copeland JG, Goldman S, et al. Implications of preoperative administration of aspirin in patients undergoing coronary artery bypass grafting. J Am Coll Cardiol 1990; 15:15–20.

29. Loop FD, Lytle BW, Cosgrove DM, et al. Influence of the internal mammary artery graft on 10-year survival and other cardiac events. N Engl J Med 1986; 314:1–6.

30. Lytle BW, Loop FD, Thurer RL, et al. Isolated left anterior descending coronary atherosclerosis: long-term comparison of internal mammary artery and venous autografts. Circulation 1980; 61:869–874.

31. Lytle BW, Cosgrove DM, Saltus GL, et al. Multivessel coronary revascularization without saphenous vein: long-term results of bilateral internal mammary artery grafting. Ann Thorac Surg 1983; 36:540–547.

32. Loop FD, Lytle BW, Cosgrove DM, et al. Free (aorto-coronary) internal mammary artery graft: late results. J Thorac Cardiovasc Surg 1986; 92:811–821.

33. Sergeant P, Lesaffre E, Flameng W, et al. Internal mammary artery: methods of use and their effect on survival. Eur J Cardiothorac Surg 1990; 4:72–78.

34. Grondin CM, Campeau L, Lesperance J, et al. Comparison of late changes in internal mammary artery and saphenous vein grafts in two consecutive series of patients 10 years after operation. Circulation 1984; 70(suppl I):I-208–I-212.
35. Barner HB, Barnett MG. Fifteen- to twenty-one-year angiographic assessment of internal thoracic artery as a bypass conduit. Ann Thorac Surg 1994; 57:1526–1528.
36. Huddleston CB, Stoney WS, Alford WC, et al. Internal mammary artery grafts: technical factors influencing patency. Ann Thorac Surg 1986; 42:5–13.
37. Tector AJ, Schmahl TM, Canino VR, et al. The role of the sequential internal mammary artery graft in coronary surgery. Circulation 1984; 70(suppl I):I-222–I-225.
38. Kouchoukos NT, Wareing TH, Murphy SF, et al. Risks of bilateral internal mammary artery grafting. Ann Thorac Surg 1990; 49:210–217.
39. Fiore AC, Naunheim KS, Dean P, et al. Results of internal thoracic artery grafting over 15 years: single vs. double grafts. Ann Thorac Surg 1990; 49:202–209.
40. Galbut DL, Traad EA, Dorman MJ, et al. Seventeen-year experience with bilateral internal mammary artery grafts. Ann Thorac Surg 1990; 49:195–201.
41. Russo P, Orszulak TA, Schaff HV, et al. Use of internal mammary artery grafts for multiple coronary artery bypasses. Circulation 1986; 74(suppl III):III-48–III-52.
42. Rankin JS, Newman GE, Bashore TM, et al. Clinical and angiographic assessment of complex mammary artery bypass grafting. J Thorac Cardiovasc Surg 1986; 92:832–846.
43. Dion R, Verhelst R, Rousseau M, et al. Sequential mammary grafting: clinical, functional and angiographic assessment 6 months postoperatively in 231 consecutive patients. J Thorac Cardiovasc Surg 1989; 98:80–88.
44. Cosgrove DM, Loop FD, Saunders CR, et al. Should coronary arteries with less than fifty percent stenosis be bypassed? J Thorac Cardiovasc Surg 1981; 82:520–530.
45. Dincer B, Barner HB. The "occluded" internal mammary artery graft: restoration of patency after apparent occlusion associated with progression of coronary disease. J Thorac Cardiovasc Surg 1983; 85:318–320.
46. Lust RM, Zeri RS, Spence PA, et al. Effect of chronic native flow competition on internal thoracic artery grafts. Ann Thorac Surg 1994; 57:45–50.
47. Cameron A, Davis KB, Green GE, et al. Clinical implications of internal mammary artery bypass grafts: the Coronary Artery Surgery Study experience. Circulation 1988; 77:815–819.
48. Gardner TJ, Greene PS, Tykiel MF, et al. Internal mammary artery graft in the elderly. Ann Thorac Surg 1990; 49:188–192.
49. Loop FD, Lytle BW, Cosgrove DM, et al. Coronary artery bypass graft surgery in the elderly: indications and outcome. Cleve Clin J Med 1988; 55:23–34.
50. Cosgrove DM, Loop FD, Lytle BW, et al. Does mammary artery grafting increase surgical risk? Circulation 1985; 72(suppl II):170–174.
51. Edwards FH, Clark RE, Schwartz M. Impact of internal mammary artery conduits on operative mortality in coronary revascularization. Ann Thorac Surg 1994; 57:27–32.

52. Grover FL, Johnson RR, Marshall G, Hammermeister KE, and Department of Veterans Affairs Cardiac Surgeons. Impact of mammary grafts on coronary bypass operative mortality and morbidity. Ann Thorac Surg 1994; 57:559–569.

53. Navia D, Cosgrove DM III, Lytle BW, et al. Is the internal thoracic artery the conduit of choice to replace a stenotic vein graft? Ann Thorac Surg 1994; 57:40–44.

54. Lytle BW, Loop FD, Cosgrove DM, et al. Bilateral internal mammary artery grafting: early and late clinical results for 1000 cases (1971–1985) (abstract). In: X World Congress of Cardiology, 1986:1.

55. Cosgrove DM, Lytle BW, Hill AC, et al. Are two internal thoracic arteries better than one? J Thorac Cardiovasc. Surg. In press.

56. Berreklouw E, Schonberger JPAM, Bavinck JH, et al. Similar hospital morbidity with the use of one or two internal thoracic arteries. Ann Thorac Surg 1994; 57:1564–1572.

57. Lytle BW, Kramer JR Jr, Golding LR, et al. Young adults with coronary atherosclerosis: 10-year results of surgical myocardial revascularization. J Am Coll Cardiol 1984; 4:445–453.

58. Tector AJ, Amundsen S, Schmahl TM, Kress DC, Peter M. Total revascularization with "T" grafts. Ann Thorac Surg 1994; 57:33–39.

59. Caes FL, Van Nooten GJ. Use of internal mammary artery for emergency grafting after failed coronary angioplasty. Ann Thorac Surg 1994; 57:1295–1299.

60. Boylan MJ, Lytle BW, Taylor PC, et al. Have PTCA failures requiring emergent bypass operation changed? Ann Thorac Surg 1995; 59:283–287.

61. Bailey CP, Hirose T, Aventura A, et al. Revascularization of the ischemic posterior myocardium. Chest 1967; 52:273–285.

62. Pym J, Brown PM, Charrette EJ, et al. Gastroepiploic-coronary anastomosis: a viable alternative bypass graft. J Thorac Cardiovasc Surg 1987; 94:256–259.

63. Carter MJ. The use of the right gastroepiploic artery in coronary artery bypass grafting. Aust NZ J Surg 1987; 57:317–321.

64. Suma H, Fukumoto H, Takeuchi A. Coronary artery bypass grafting utilizing in situ right gastroepiploic artery: basic study and clinical application. Ann Thorac Surg 1987; 44:394–397.

65. Lytle BW, Cosgrove DM, Ratliff NB, et al. Coronary artery bypass grafting with the right gastroepiploic artery. J Thorac Cardiovasc Surg 1989; 97:826–831.

66. Suma H. Comparative study between the gastroepiploic and the internal thoracic artery as a coronary bypass graft. Eur J Cardiothorac Surg 1991; 5:244–247.

67. Suma H, Wanibuchi T, Terada Y, et al. The right gastroepiploic artery grafts: clinical and angiographic mid-term results in 200 patients. J Thorac Cardiovasc Surg 1993; 105:615–623.

68. Manapat AE, McCarthy PM, Lytle BW, et al. Gastroepiploic and inferior epigastric arteries for coronary artery bypass: early results and evolving applications. Circulation 1994; 90[part 2]:II-144–II-147.

69. Suma H, Wanibuchi Y, Furata S, et al. Does use of gastrepiploic artery graft increase surgical risk? J Thorac Cardiovasc Surg 1991; 101:121–125.

70. Mills NL, Everson CT. Right gastroepiploic artery: a third arterial conduit for coronary bypass. Ann Thorac Surg 1989; 47:706–711.

71. Witkop J, Dillemans BRS, Grandjean JG, Bams JL, Ebels T. Gastric perforation after aortocoronary bypass grafting with the right gastroepiploic artery. Ann Thorac Surg 1994; 58:1170–1171.
72. Dignow RJ, Yeh T Jr, Dyke CM, et al. Reactivity of gastroepiploic and internal mammary arteries—relevance to coronary artery bypass grafting. J Thorac Cardiovasc Surg 1992; 103:116–123.
73. Foster ED, Kranc MAT. Alternative conduits for aortocoronary bypass grafting. Circulation 1989; 79(part 2):134–139.
74. Vincent JG, VanSon JAM, Skofnicki SH. Inferior epigastric artery as a conduit in myocardial revascularization: the alternative free arterial graft. Ann Thorac Surg 1990; 49:323–325.
75. Puig LB, Ciongolli W, Cividanes GUL, et al. Inferior epigastric artery as a free graft for myocardial revascularization. J Thorac Cardiovasc Surg 1990; 99:251–255.
76. Mills NL, Everson CJ. Technique for use of the inferior epigastric artery as a coronary bypass graft. Ann Thorac Surg 1991; 51:208–214.
77. Buche M, Schoevaerdts JC, Louagie Y. Use of the inferior epigastric artery for coronary bypass. J Thorac Cardiovasc Surg 1992; 103:665–670.
78. Barner HB, Naunheim KS, Fiore AC, et al. Use of the inferior epigastric artery as a free graft for myocardial revascularization. Ann Thorac Surg 1991; 52:429–437.
79. Carpentier A, Guermonprez JL, Deloche A, et al. The aorta-to-coronary radial artery bypass graft. Ann Thorac Surg 1973; 16:111–121.
80. Curtis JJ, Stoney WS, Alford WC Jr, et al. Intimal hyperplasia—a cause of radial artery aortocoronary bypass graft failure. Ann Thorac Surg 1975; 20:628–635.
81. Fisk RL, Brooks CH, Callaghan JC, Dvorkin J. Experience with the radial artery graft for coronary artery bypass. Ann Thorac Surg 1976; 21:513–518.
82. Acar C, Jebara VA, Portoghese M, et al. Revival of the radial artery for coronary bypass grafting: revival of an old conduit. Ann Thorac Surg 1992; 54:652–660.
83. Coltharp WA. In: discussion of Acar C, Jebara VA, Portoghese M, et al. Revival of the radial artery for coronary bypass grafting: revival of an old conduit. Ann Thorac Surg 1992; 54:652–660.
84. Jegaden O, Eker A, Montagna P, et al. Risk and results of bypass grafting using bilateral internal mammary and right gastroepiploic arteries. Ann Thorac Surg 1995; 59:955–960.

2

Coronary Artery Bypass Graft Surgery: Postoperative Complications

Steven W. Werns
University of Michigan Medical Center, Ann Arbor, Michigan

While early observational studies and randomized clinical trials demonstrated the efficacy of coronary artery bypass graft (CABG) surgery for relief of angina and prolongation of survival in certain groups of patients, reducing morbidity and mortality after CABG is the major focus of current clinical investigation. Also, the frequency and expense of CABG surgery engenders extensive scrutiny of complication rates by health care policymakers, providers, and consumers. The objective of this chapter is to provide a review of the recent publications pertinent to the major cardiac and noncardiac complications after CABG surgery.

I. MORTALITY

A. Recent Clinical Trials

Contemporary perioperative mortality rates after elective CABG are illustrated by a meta-analysis of eight recently published randomized clinical trials of CABG versus coronary angioplasty (PTCA) [1]. Death during the initial hospitalization occurred in 1.3% (21/1661) of the patients assigned to surgery. The Bypass Angioplasty Revascularization Intervention (BARI) trial [2] randomized 1,829 patients with multivessel coronary artery disease (CAD) to CABG ($n = 914$) or PTCA ($n = 915$). The in-hospital death rate after CABG also was 1.3%. The relatively low mortality rates may reflect the exclusion of high-risk patients, especially by the criterion that all patients had to be suitable for either PTCA or CABG.

The Northern New England Cardiovascular Disease Study Group recently published a study of changes in CABG mortality after a three-component intervention (Figure 1) [3]. The study included all 23 cardiac surgeons performing CABG in Maine, New Hampshire, and Vermont. The preintervention data were collected for 6,638 cases performed between July 1, 1987, and June 30, 1990. On July 1, 1990, a three-component intervention was begun. It consisted of feedback of risk-adjusted outcome data to each surgeon, training in continuous quality improvement techniques, and site visits by teams that included a cardiac surgeon and a perfusionist. The postintervention data were collected for 6,488 cases performed between April 1, 1991, and July 31, 1993. The data collected during the preintervention period were used to develop a multivariate logistic regression model that was used to predict hospital mortality during the postintervention period. The observed number

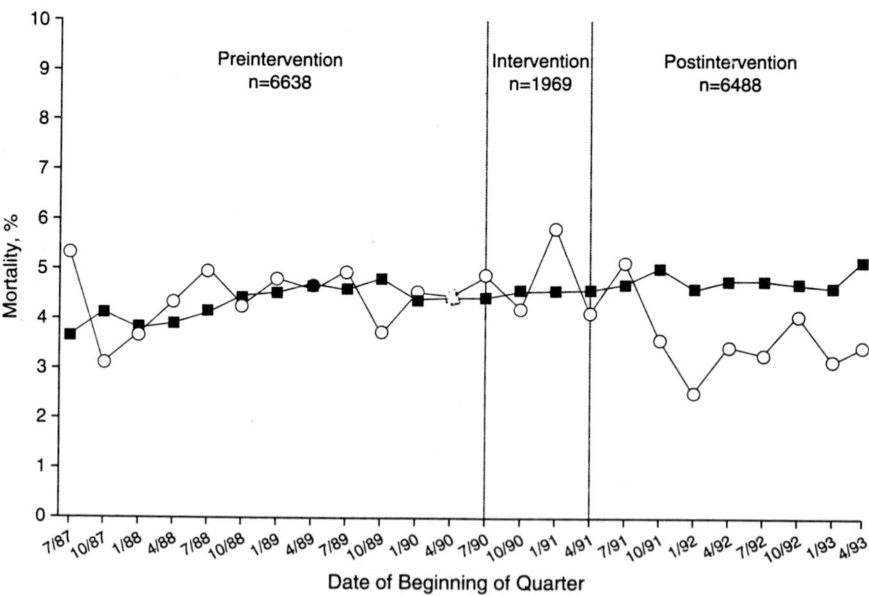

Figure 1 Expected and observed mortality for patients undergoing CABG before and after institution of a three-component intervention aimed at reducing CABG mortality at medical centers participating in the Northern New England Cardiovascular Disease Study Group. ■ = expected mortality; ○ = observed mortality. (Reproduced from Ref. 3.)

of perioperative deaths, 234 (3.61%), was significantly less than the predicted number, 308 (4.75%), yielding a standardized mortality ratio (SMR) of 0.76 (95% CI, 0.67 to 0.90; $p = 0.001$). Analysis of the outcome data for the 18 surgeons who were members of the study from its inception to its completion yielded a nearly identical SMR (0.79; 95% CI, 0.68 to 0.91; $p = 0.002$).

A subsequent analysis of trends in mortality after CABG questioned the conclusion that the reduction in mortality observed in New York State [4] and northern New England [3] are attributable to implementation of statewide outcome studies [5]. Ghali et al. [5] compared the trends in hospital mortality after CABG reported from New York and northern New England with mortality trends in Massachusetts, a state that has not developed a prospective clinical data registry for statewide reporting of CABG outcomes. Mortality after CABG decreased from 4.7% in 1990 to 3.8% in 1994 in Massachusetts, a reduction comparable to the reductions in New York (from 3.5% in 1989 to 2.8% in 1992) and northern New England (from 4.5% in 1987 to 3.6% in 1993).

B. Risk Factors for Perioperative Death

Table 1 lists the risk factors for perioperative death.

Gender

Although the majority of patients enrolled in the randomized trials of CABG have been men, a number of publications have addressed the question of gender as a risk factor for death after CABG. Several authors have suggested that there is a bias against referral of women for coronary angiography and CABG that may account for some reports of higher operative death rates in women [6–8]. Khan et al. [7] analyzed the outcome of 2,297 consecutive patients who had isolated CABG between 1982 and 1987 at Cedars-Sinai Medical Center. The in-hospital mortality rate was significantly higher for women than for men

Table 1 Risk Factors for Perioperative Death

Older age
Left ventricular dysfunction
Left main stenosis
Nonelective surgery
Previous CABG
Comorbidity (renal insufficiency, diabetes, COPD, PVD)
No internal mammary graft

COPD = chronic obstructive pulmonary disease; PVD = peripheral vascular disease.

(4.6% vs. 2.6%; $p = 0.036$; 95% confidence interval 0% to 4.0%). Compared with the men, however, the women were older, and a higher percentage had unstable angina, postmyocardial infarction angina, and congestive heart failure. By multivariate analysis, adjustment for the differences in functional class and age accounted for all of the difference in operative mortality. The authors concluded that women are referred for CABG later in the course of their disease, increasing the risk of operative death [7].

King et al. [9] analyzed age-matched populations of men and women who underwent first-time CABG at the University of Rochester between 1983 and 1988. The in-hospital death rates for women (4.3%; 20/465) and men (3.7%; 17/465; $p = 0.61$) were not significantly different. Mickleborough et al. [10] published a series of 1,487 consecutive patients, 1,132 men and 355 women, who underwent isolated CABG by one surgeon at the Toronto Hospital. The operative mortality was similar for women (1.4%) and men (1.1%).

The Northern New England Cardiovascular Disease Study Group found that gender was not a significant predictor of in-hospital mortality among 3,055 patients who underwent isolated CABG at five medical centers between 1987 and 1989 [11].

A recent study addressed the hypothesis that perioperative mortality may be related to coronary artery diameter, and that coronary artery diameter may be smaller in women [12]. The luminal diameter of the mid-left anterior descending coronary artery at the site of the distal anastomosis was measured intraoperatively with a set of graduated probes. Small vessel size was associated with an increased risk of in-hospital mortality (15.8% for 1.0-mm vessels, 4.6% for 1.5- to 2.0-mm vessels, and 1.5% for 2.5- to 3.5-mm vessels). After controlling for differences in age and body size, gender remained an important predictor of coronary size. Coronary artery diameter in men exceeded that in women within each quartile of four indices of body size: body surface area, body mass index, height, and weight. The findings support the hypothesis that smaller coronary arteries contribute to increased perioperative mortality, and that gender itself may not be an independent risk factor for perioperative mortality after CABG.

Age

Most studies have found that age is an independent predictor of perioperative mortality after CABG. Weintraub et al. [13] described the influence of age on the outcome of CABG among 13,625 patients who underwent isolated first CABG at Emory University or Crawford W. Long Hospitals between 1981 and 1989. Age was found to be a risk factor for neurological events, wound infections, and death. Multivariate analysis revealed that age was an independent correlate of mortality and the most powerful predictor of in-hospital death.

Hannan and Burke [14] analyzed the effect of age on the in-hospital mortality of all 30,972 patients who underwent CABG in the State of New York in 1991 and 1992. The results of multivariate analysis demonstrated that 24 independent preoperative risk factors were related to in-hospital mortality. Age was found to be significantly related to mortality, even after the effect of the other significant risk factors was considered. The odds ratios for in-hospital death increased steeply after age 75. The operative mortality rates were 3.36% for patients aged 70–74, 5.28% for patients aged 75–79, and 8.31% for patients ≥80 years old.

Peterson et al. [15] identified 12 published single-institution case series of outcome after CABG in octogenarians. The composite in-hospital mortality was 10.4% for 1,035 patients, with a range of 5.6% to 24.3%. Also reviewed were national Medicare data for 24,461 patients ≥80 years old who underwent CABG between 1987 and 1990 [15]. The in-hospital mortality was 11.5%, compared with 4.4% for the 147,822 patients 65–70 years old. Increasing age, female gender, preoperative acute myocardial infarction or congestive heart failure [15], and left ventricular ejection fraction <50% [16,17] were found to be independent predictors of 30-day mortality after CABG in octogenarians.

Cedars-Sinai Medical Center reported a series of 15 patients aged ≥90 years who underwent cardiac surgery [18]. One of the seven patients who underwent isolated CABG and one patient who underwent both CABG and mitral valve repair died within 30 days.

Left Ventricular (LV) Function

Perioperative mortality increases as LV systolic function decreases. The CASS perioperative mortality rate was 1.4% for patients with LV ejection fractions >50%, compared with 6.9% for patients with ejection fractions <36% [19]. Christenson et al. [20] reported the outcome after CABG for a series of 91 patients with LV ejection fractions ≤25%. The overall perioperative mortality was 14.3%, compared with 1.2% among a concurrent group of 1,590 patients with ejection fractions >25%. Among the cohort of 91 patients with ejection fractions ≤25%, the perioperative mortality was 20.0% for the 15 patients who underwent both CABG and LV aneurysm resection, compared with 13.2% for the remaining 76 patients, who underwent CABG alone.

Weschler and Junod [21] analyzed 3,848 patients who underwent CABG at Duke University Medical Center to determine the impact of a preoperative clinical diagnosis of congestive heart failure (CHF) on perioperative mortality. Relatively few patients with New York Heart Association class III ($n = 87$) or class IV ($n = 47$) CHF underwent CABG. The perioperative mortality was 14.9% for patients with class IV CHF and 8.0% for patients with class III CHF, compared with 4.2% for 117 patients with class II CHF, 2.5% for 79 patients with class I CHF, and 3.0% for the 3,577 patients with no history of CHF. When a stepwise logistic regression model was computed, however, age, LV ejection fraction, mitral regurgitation, and left main stenosis were significant predictors of increased hospital mortality, but CHF was not identified as a significant incremental risk factor.

Left Main Stenosis

Left main coronary artery stenosis was found to be a significant risk factor for operative mortality among 6,630 patients who had isolated CABG between 1975 and 1978 at the 15 centers that participated in the CASS registry [22]. The operative mortality was 4.2% for patients with ≥50% stenosis of the left main coronary artery, compared with an overall operative mortality of 2.3% among all 6,630 patients who underwent CABG [22,23]. Among the 1,019 patients with left main stenosis, the operative mortality ranged from 1.6% among 432 patients with 50–74% stenosis and a right-dominant system, to 25% among 16 patients with ≥90% stenosis and left dominance, to 40% among 30 patients with ≥90% stenosis who underwent emergency CABG [22]. Discriminant function analysis determined that the best predictors of operative mortality among the patients with left main disease were: urgency of surgery, coronary artery dominance, the duration of anginal symptoms, the percentage of left main stenosis, and left ventricular contraction score [23]. It has been suggested that improvements in preoperative medical management and intraoperative myocardial protection have reduced operative mortality rates among patients with left main stenosis, but the perioperative mortality statistics for 1982–1986 at Toronto General Hospital were significantly greater for patients with left main stenosis (5.8%) than for patients without left main stenosis (3.2%; $p < 0.05$) [24]. One university center in the United States reported a 9.1% perioperative mortality during the period 1981–1986 among 176 patients with ≥50% stenosis of the left main coronary artery [25]. Surgical urgency and gender were the only variables that were significantly related to operative mortality. The authors attributed the relatively high mortality rate to an older population (average age 66 years vs. 57 years in CASS) and to the inclusion of more women (23% vs. 13% in CASS).

Urgency of Surgery

Urgency of surgery influences the risk of perioperative mortality. The Northern New England Cardiovascular Disease Study Group [11] reported that the risk of urgent surgery was twofold greater than that of elective surgery (odds ratio = 2.1), and the risk of emergency surgery was fourfold greater than that of elective surgery (odds ratio = 4.4).

Isolated CABG was performed on 7,334 patients at the three teaching hospitals of the University of Toronto between 1982 and 1986 [24]. Multivariate analysis identified the following risk factors for operative mortality: urgency of surgery, LV ejection fraction, age, female gender, previous CABG, and left main coronary artery stenosis. Urgent surgery for unstable angina was the most significant predictor of outcome during the period 1983–1985.

Reoperation

Previous cardiac surgery increases the risk of in-hospital mortality after CABG. Among a cohort of 3,055 patients analyzed by the Northern New England Cardiovascular Disease Study Group [11], patients with a history of previous CABG had a 3.5-fold greater risk of in-hospital mortality, compared with patients without previous CABG. Weintraub et al. [26] analyzed outcomes after reoperative CABG for a cohort of 2,030 patients who had a first reoperation at Emory University Hospitals between 1975 and 1993. Urgent and emergency surgery, LV ejection fraction <50%, hypertension, older age, and female gender were univariate and multivariate correlates of in-hospital death. The perioperative mortality rates were 5.7% for elective surgery, 10.9% for urgent surgery, and 16.4% for emergency surgery.

The Cleveland Clinic published a series of 1,663 patients who underwent a first reoperation for isolated CABG [27]. There were 62 (3.7%) in-hospital deaths, 41 due to new myocardial infarctions. Four hundred eighty-nine patients had at least one patent mammary artery graft at the time of reoperation. The graft was damaged and replaced in 14, all of whom survived. Multivariate analysis identified no internal mammary artery graft at either primary surgery or reoperation as a variable associated with increased in-hospital mortality. The authors concluded that "the use of internal mammary artery grafts at the primary operation does not increase the risk of a reoperation, and the use of internal mammary artery grafts at reoperation does not increase in-hospital morbidity or mortality."

Savage and Cohn [28] reported the impact of surgical technique on the operative mortality of 131 consecutive patients who underwent reoperative CABG at Brigham and Women's Hospital. The operative approach for the 61 patients during the period 1988–1989 featured dissection of the heart before institution of bypass, the use of antegrade cardioplegia, the use of complete aortic cross-clamp for distal anastomoses, and then a partial occluding cross-clamp during rewarming for proximal anastomoses. During the period 1990–1993, 70 patients underwent reoperative CABG and the following techniques were implemented: "no touch" technique or minimal cardiac dissection before bypass, routine femoral artery and vein exposure, frequent femoral cannulation for cardiopulmonary bypass, antegrade and retrograde blood cardioplegia, and performance of both proximal and distal anastomoses with a single aortic cross-clamp. The operative mortality rates were 16% for the first period and 2% for the later period ($p \leq 0.002$). Multivariate analysis demonstrated that surgery during the later time period was the strongest variable associated with a lower risk of operative mortality.

Comorbid Conditions

Diabetes mellitus, chronic obstructive pulmonary disease, peripheral vascular disease, and renal insufficiency have been identified as comorbid conditions that are associated with increased in-hospital mortality [11]. Logistic regression analysis of 5,051 consecutive patients who underwent CABG at the Cleveland Clinic between 1986 and 1988 identified preexisting renal insufficiency as an independent risk factor for morbidity and mortality after CABG [29]. A preoperative serum creatinine $\geq$1.9 mg/dL was associated with odds ratios of 2.84 for morbidity and 3.69 for mortality after CABG [29].

Risk Stratification

Establishment of the Society of Thoracic Surgeons (STS) National Cardiac Surgery Database has allowed the development of a tool for predicting the probability of operative death, defined as death within 30 days of CABG [30]. The Society of Thoracic Surgeons National Cardiac Surgery Database contains records of 80,881 patients undergoing isolated CABG from January 1980 through December 1990 [30]. A model of operative mortality was developed and validated by dividing the population into two groups of equal size and using a "training-set/test-set" approach. There was excellent agreement between the predicted and observed mortalities of the test group, both for the entire group and for subgroups of the test population.

The cardiac surgery group at the University of Pittsburgh Medical Center compared the outcome predicted by the STS database with their actual surgical results for a group of 728 patients who underwent isolated CABG for the 2-year period ending in October 1993 [31]. The observed mortality and complication rates correlated strongly with the predicted rates. Thus, it appears feasible for institutions to use the model developed by the Society of Thoracic Surgeons as a benchmark to obtain a risk-adjusted comparison of their results against a national standard of care [30].

The Working Group Panel on the Cooperative CABG Database Project [32] analyzed the predictive value of 44 clinical variables for short-term mortality after CABG among 172,184 patients contained in seven databases. The acuteness of CABG, history of previous cardiac surgery, and age were the variables most predictive of mortality after CABG.

C. Surgical Technique

Mammary Artery Grafts

The internal mammary (thoracic) arteries (IMAs) are advocated as the preferred conduits for CABG, primarily because of their demonstrated superiority to vein grafts with respect to long-term patency and long-term survival [33–35]. For example, a recent analysis of the Coronary Artery Surgery Study (CASS) registry revealed that IMA grafts conferred a survival advantage that increased throughout a 15-year follow-up period [35]. In addition, several studies have concluded that IMA grafts decrease operative mortality [36,37]. Grover et al. [36] analyzed the Department of Veterans Affairs Cardiac Surgery Database for two separate time periods, April 1987 through March 1989 and October 1990 through September 1991. With logistic regression analysis used to adjust preoperative risk, the multivariate odds of operative death with use of the IMA for one or more grafts compared with use of vein grafts only was 0.78 for 1987–1989 and 0.72 for 1990–1991 ($p = 0.023$ and 0.013, respectively). The authors concluded that fewer high-risk patients received IMA grafts, but the use of an IMA graft was an independent predictor of a 22%–28% reduction in operative mortality after adjusting for preoperative risk factors. The performance of IMA grafting also was found to be an independent predictor of improved operative survival in patients ≥70 years old [37]. As discussed later, the use of IMA grafts at reoperation does not increase in-hospital morbidity or mortality [27].

Cardioplegia

Mangano et al. [38] performed a meta-analysis of five randomized trials that were conducted to assess the effects of supplementing the cardioplegia solution used for myocardial protection during cardiopulmonary bypass with acadesine, a purine nucleoside. A total of 4,043 patients were randomized to receive either placebo ($n = 2,031$) or acadesine ($n = 2,012$) via the cardioplegia solution and by intravenous infusion for a total of 7 hours starting approximately 15 minutes before induction of anesthesia. The primary measure of efficacy, Q-wave myocardial infarction (MI), was reduced by 27%, from 4.9% in the placebo group to 3.6% in the acadesine group (odds ratio, 0.69; 95% confidence interval, 0.51–0.95; $p = 0.02$). Among the 169 patients with a perioperative MI, the 1-month mortality rate was reduced by 74%, from 21% (21/98) to 6% (4/71) ($p = 0.003$). The favorable results suggest that improvements in myocardial protection during cardiopulmonary bypass have the potential to reduce morbidity and mortality after CABG.

II. MORBIDITY

Table 2 lists complications after CABG. Silber et al. [39] analyzed a database containing 16,673 patients who underwent CABG at 57 U.S. hospitals in 1991 and 1992. The overall complication rate was 43%, and 717 of the 7,173 patients (4.3%) with complications died. The authors emphasized that there was a poor correlation between the rankings of hospitals by mortality statistics and the rankings by complications ($r = 0.07, p = 0.58$). The authors concluded that complication rates should not be used as a substitute for mortality rates to judge hospital quality of care for CABG, a salient point in this era of outcomes research and managed care. Also, variations in the definition and recording of complications make it difficult to compare complication rates.

A. Cardiac Complications

Perioperative Myocardial Infarction

New myocardial infarction (MI) is the most common cause of perioperative death after CABG [40]. Among 1,567 patients who underwent isolated CABG at the Montreal Heart Institute from 1987 to 1988, 34 of the 70 (48.6%) perioperative deaths were caused by a new MI [40]. The presumed causes of perioperative MI include technical factors (e.g., kinking of a graft, graft thrombosis, spasm of an IMA graft), incomplete revascularization, suboptimal myocardial protection, and, for reoperations, embolization of atherosclerotic debris from diseased vein grafts. The true incidence of perioperative MI is uncertain because recognition of perioperative non-Q-wave MI is confounded by the transient occurrence of bundle branch blocks, and the low specificity of ST-T wave abnormalities or release of creatine kinase. Newer enzymatic markers such as troponin may prove to be sensitive markers of perioperative

Table 2   Complications After CABG

Perioperative MI
CHF
Supraventricular arrhythmias
Ventricular arrhythmias
Atrioventricular block
Hemorrhage
Infection
Hypertension
Neurologic (stroke, encephalopathy)
Gastrointestinal

myocardial necrosis, but their prognostic value is unknown [41]. New perioperative Q-wave MI is more readily apparent, and, as discussed later, the prognostic implications of new Q-waves on the postoperative EKG have been studied extensively.

Among 1,340 patients who underwent CABG in 1978 at 10 hospitals participating in the CASS registry, the incidence of perioperative Q-wave infarction was 4.6% [42]. The hospital mortality was 9.7% in the 62 patients who had new postoperative Q-waves vs. 1.0% in the 1,278 patients who did not ($p < 0.001$). In patients who survived to hospital discharge, however, new postoperative Q-waves did not adversely affect 3-year survival. The Cedars-Sinai Medical Center reported the impact of perioperative MI on the 5-year outcome of patients who underwent isolated CABG from 1975 to 1976 [43]. Among the 31 patients with evidence of new Q-wave MI, there was 1 perioperative death, and the 5-year survival of the 30 remaining patients was 96.8%, compared with 94.3% among the 111 patients without electrocardiographic evidence of perioperative MI.

Force et al. [44] reported a series of patients who underwent isolated, first-time CABG at one VA Hospital. Between 1981 and 1985 there were 62 patients (10.6% of patients undergoing CABG) who developed perioperative MIs, defined as new pathological Q-waves that persisted to hospital discharge. Fifty-nine survived to hospital discharge and were followed for 30 months. Their clinical course was compared with 115 patients who had CABG in 1982 and were discharged without new Q-waves. Cardiac events occurred in 31% of the patients with perioperative MI, compared with 12% of the patients without a perioperative MI ($p < 0.01$). Perioperative MI, inadequate revascularization, and postoperative LV ejection fraction <40% were independent predictors of cardiac events and were used to stratify patients into low-, intermediate-, and high-risk subsets. The event-free survival rate was similar for patients without a perioperative MI (87%) and for patients with perioperative MIs who were adequately revascularized and had a postoperative ejection fraction >40%. Event-free survival was 13% for patients with all three negative prognostic variables and 68% for patients with perioperative MI and only one of the other two variables. The Seattle Heart Watch registry also concluded that late survival was adversely affected by perioperative infarction [45]. Thus, it is generally accepted that perioperative MI is associated with an increased in-hospital mortality, but there has been disagreement regarding the impact of perioperative MI on the long-term outcome of patients who survive to hospital discharge.

Congestive Heart Failure

Congestive heart failure is the second most common cause of perioperative death after CABG [40]. Among 1,567 patients who underwent isolated CABG at the Montreal Heart Institute from 1987 to 1988, postoperative CHF occurred in only 2.4% of the patients, but 23 of the 70 (32.9%) perioperative deaths were related to postoperative CHF [40]. There is an increased incidence of low cardiac output, however, among patients who undergo CABG after acute MI. The cardiac surgery team at Georgetown University reported that inotropic support and/or intraaortic balloon pumping was required by 38/145 (26%) of patients who underwent isolated CABG within 4 weeks of an acute MI [46]. The time interval between the MI and CABG was not a predictor of postoperative cardiac failure.

Arrhythmias

Cardiac arrhythmias are the most common complication after CABG. The incidence of all cardiac arrhythmias was 13.6% among 1,567 patients who underwent CABG at the Montreal Heart Institute between 1987 and 1988 [40]. Although most postoperative arrhythmias are responsive to medical therapy and/or electrical cardioversion, rare fatalities occur; two of the 70 deaths in the Montreal Heart series were directly related to cardiac arrhythmias. The epidemiology, management, and prognosis of arrhythmias and conduction disturbances after CABG were reviewed recently by Pires et al. [47].

Supraventricular Arrhythmias. An excellent review of atrial arrhythmias after cardiothoracic surgery was published recently [48]. The reported incidence of supraventricular arrhythmias post-CABG has varied. Among 100 patients in one study [49], supraventricular arrhythmias were documented in 23 patients, with a mean time of 52.3 ± 3.4 hours between the surgery and the onset of the arrhythmia. The arrhythmia was atrial fibrillation (AF) in 34 of the 37 observed episodes. Postoperative AF occurred in 189 of 570 consecutive patients (33%) who underwent isolated CABG at the Brigham and Women's Hospital between September 1993 and July 1994 [50]. The incidence of postoperative AF was 28.4% in another series of 1,666 patients undergoing isolated CABG, with a peak occurrence (43.1% of episodes) 2 days after surgery. The strongest correlate of the risk of AF was age, but the mean age of patients with AF, 61 ± 7 years, was only slightly greater than the age of patients without AF, 57 ± 9 years. The overall incidence of AF after CABG was 27% among 2,265 patients enrolled in the Multicenter Study of Perioperative Ischemia, a prospective observational study conducted at 24 university-affiliated hospitals in the United States [51]. A history of AF doubled the risk of postoperative AF, and 158 of 332 (48%) patients with preoperative AF developed AF after CABG.

Concomitant valvular surgery is associated with an increased likelihood of AF after cardiac surgery. At Barnes Hospital between 1986 and 1991, 3,983 patients who were in normal sinus rhythm preoperatively underwent continuous electrocardiographic monitoring from the end of cardiac surgery to the time of discharge from the hospital [52]. Excluding transient, nonsustained arrhythmias that required no treatment or only supplemental oxygen or potassium, the incidence of atrial arrhythmias was 31.9% after isolated CABG, 60.1% after CABG and aortic valve replacement, and 63.6% after CABG and mitral valve replacement [52]. A severe ($\geq70\%$) stenosis of the proximal or mid-right coronary artery also may increase the risk of AF [53]. The incidence of AF was 43% among 45 patients with severe RCA stenosis and 19% among 64 patients without severe RCA disease ($p = 0.001$).

The adjusted length of hospital stay attributable to AF was 4.9 days, resulting in >\$10,055 in hospital charges at the Brigham and Women's Hospital [50]. Because postoperative atrial arrhythmias are associated with longer intensive care unit and hospital stays and with an increased risk of stroke, prophylactic pharmacologic therapy is employed by many cardiac surgeons, and numerous clinical trials have been conducted to test the effects of a variety of drugs. A survey of 75 U.S. chiefs of cardiothoracic surgery revealed that 25 use digoxin and 42 use a beta-blocker for prophylaxis of supraventricular arrhythmias after CABG [54]. Randomized trials of preoperative administration of digoxin have produced conflicting results, yielding both lower and higher frequencies of supraventricular arrhythmias and AF in the dixogin groups compared with the control groups [55–57].

In contrast to the digoxin trials, studies of several beta-blockers have demonstrated beneficial effects. White et al. [58] evaluated the effect of timolol on supraventricular arrhythmias after CABG. Forty-one patients were randomly assigned to treatment with timolol or placebo beginning 3–7 hours after surgery. Timolol decreased both the frequency of supraventricular tachycardia and AF and the number of patients with severe arrhythmias requiring treatment.

Several studies of prophylactic calcium channel antagonists have been published [49,59]. One double-blind, randomized trial evaluated verapamil 80 mg every 8 hours beginning immediately after CABG [59]. Atrial arrhythmias, primarily atrial fibrillation, occurred in 29% (20/70) of the patients who received verapamil and in 28% (19/71) of the patients who received placebo. Another double-blind, randomized study assigned patients to either placebo or verapamil 80 mg every 6 hours beginning within 36 hours after surgery [49]. There were 37 episodes of supraventricular arrhythmias, 34 of which were AF, occurring in 23 of the 100 control patients and in 14 of the 100 verapamil-treated patients. Hypotension, pulmonary edema, or both developed in 13 of the verapamil-treated patients, compared to only 1 control patient. Thus, verapamil reduced the incidence of supraventricular arrhythmias, but its hemodynamic side effects were unacceptable.

Andrews et al. [57] performed a meta-analysis of randomzied trials to determine the efficacy of digoxin, verapamil, and beta-blockers as prophylactic agents against supraventricular arrhythmias after CABG (Figure 2). Their literature search identified 69 manuscripts that addressed the topic. After exclusion of studies because of inadequate randomization techniques or confounding drug therapy, there were 24 randomized, controlled trials suitable for analysis. For the three verapamil trials, neither the individual odds ratios nor the summary odds ratio for the pooled results reached statistical significance. For the five digoxin trials, one trial showed a significant favorable treatment effect and one showed a significant detrimental effect. The summary odds ratio for the digoxin trials was 0.97 (95% confidence interval 0.62–1.49). Thirteen of the 19 beta-blocker trials demonstrated a significant beneficial effect, and none found a significant detrimental effect. The summary odds ratio for the beta-blocker trials indicated a markedly decreased likelihood of supraventricular arrhythmias in patients treated with beta-blockers (odds ratio = 0.28, confidence interval 0.21–0.36). Similar conclusions were drawn by Kowey et al. [60], who performed a meta-analysis of nine beta-blocker trials and seven digoxin trials. Prophylactic administration of beta-blockers, but not digoxin, was found to reduce significantly the incidence of supraventricular arrhythmias after CABG. In patients who did develop supraventricular arrhythmias despite prophylactic beta-blockade, the ventricular rate was significantly slower than in patients who did not receive prophylactic beta-blockers [57]. Thus, perioperative treatment with beta-blockers has been recommended in patients without contraindications to beta-blocker use [57].

Several studies have examined pharmacologic conversion of atrial fibrillation or flutter after CABG. One study randomized 40 patients with post-

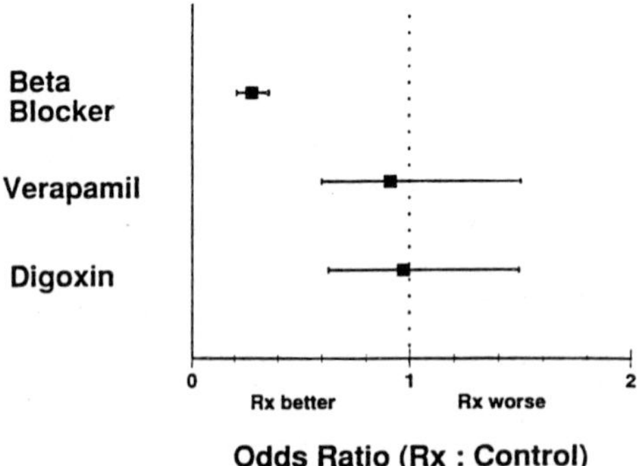

Figure 2 Summary odds ratios for the development of supraventricular arrhythmias for perioperative treatment with digoxin, with verapamil, and with beta-blockers. The length of each horizontal line indicates the 95% confidence interval for each estimate of the odds ratios. (Reproduced from Ref. 57.)

operative atrial arrhythmias to either intravenous sotalol or intravenous digoxin and disopyramide [61]. Conversion to sinus or junctional rhythm occurred within 12 hours in 17 of 20 patients in each group. Although 12 sotalol patients converted within 1 hour, compared to only five patients in the digoxin/disopyramide group, disopyramide was not administered until 2 hours after the first dose of digoxin. Hypotension, defined as a systolic blood pressure ≤90 mm Hg or a decrease by at least 20 mm Hg, occurred during the loading dose of sotalol in 17 of 20 patients, but only two patients required withdrawal of the drug because of hypotension. Four patients were withdrawn from disopyramide because of urinary retention.

Another study compared amiodarone with quinidine in 80 patients who had cardiac surgery (41 had CABG) and developed atrial fibrillation or flutter that persisted 2 hours after treatment with dixogin [62]. The patients were randomized to intravenous amiodarone, given as a 5-mg/kg bolus, or oral quinidine, 400 mg initially and then an additional 400 mg 4 hours later. Reversion to sinus rhythm occurred within 8 hours after treatment in 25 of the 39 patients (64%) who received quinidine compared with 17 of 41 (41%) who received amiodarone ($p = 0.04$).

In conclusion, atrial fibrillation and flutter are common after CABG and are associated with an increased length and cost of hospitalization and with increased risk of stroke. Prophylactic beta-blockade reduces the occurrence of atrial arrhythmias and slows the ventricular rate in patients who develop an atrial arrhythmia. Antiarrhythmic drugs, such as ibutilide, quinidine, disopyramide, and sotalol, are effective for conversion of atrial fibrillation or flutter to sinus rhythm.

Ventricular Arrhythmias. Ventricular premature beats (PVC) and non-sustained ventricular tachycardia (VT) are very common after CABG. Smith et al. [63] analyzed continuous ambulatory electrocardiographic recordings for 7 days after CABG in 50 patients. While only 6% of patients had >30 PVCs/hr preoperatively, 34% had >30 PVCs/hr postoperatively. VT, defined as ≥3 beats, was recorded in only 6% of patients preoperatively, but during the postoperative period 54% of patients had VT. Although 48% of the patients developed transient periods of ST segment changes indicative of ischemia after CABG, only 3 of 68 postoperative episodes of VT occurred during ischemic ST segment changes, and only 5 occurred within 3 hours of ischemic episodes.

Recurrent sustained VT or ventricular fibrillation (VF) are relatively uncommon after CABG. Refractory, de novo ventricular arrhythmias occurred in 12 of 1,675 patients who underwent CABG during a 2.5-year period at Johns Hopkins Hospital [64]. The number of arrhythmic events ranged between 4 and 50 per patient, and their onset occurred between 2 days and 5 months after CABG.

An ongoing study known as the CABG Patch Trial is evaluating the benefits of prophylactic implantable cardioverter-defibrillator implantation in patients at high risk of ventricular arrhythmias after CABG.

Atrioventricular (AV) Block

A prospective study of conduction defects after isolated CABG was performed at the University of Michigan [64]. New bundle branch block or fascicular block developed in 42 of 93 consecutive patients, and third-degree AV block occurred in four patients. The conduction defects were still present at the time of hospital discharge in 46% of patients. Right bundle branch block accounted for 65% of all new conduction defects. The cardiopulmonary bypass pump and aortic cross-clamping times were significantly longer in patients who developed new conduction defects.

The cardiac surgery program at the University of Massachusetts reviewed the incidence of bradyarrhythmias among 1,614 consecutive patients who underwent isolated CABG from 1988 to 1990 [66]. Only 13 patients received permanent pacemakers before discharge, because of postoperative bradyarrhythmias. Eight of the 13 patients had persistent complete heart block; seven of the eight patients had preoperative conduction disturbances: five had left bundle branch block, one had right bundle branch block, and one had left anterior fascicular block. Five of the 13 patients who received pacemakers had severe bradycardia due to sick sinus syndrome.

A restrospective analysis of 233 consecutive patients who underwent isolated CABG performed by a single surgeon identified a marked decrease in the incidence of conduction disturbances after the operative technique was changed from hypothermic to normothermic perfusion and cardioplegia [67]. The incidence of new postoperative conduction disturbances in the cold cardioplegia group was 57.6% immediately after surgery, 19.6% at the time of hospital discharge, and 17.4% at the time of late follow-up. For the normothermic cardioplegia group, the incidence of new conduction disturbances was 27.5% immediately after surgery and 1.7% at the time of discharge and late follow-up.

B. Noncardiac Complications

Hemorrhage

A number of factors increase the risk of postoperative bleeding: "redo" CABG, preoperative administration of antiplatelet or thrombolytic drugs, and deficiency of plasma coagulation factors due to hepatic dysfunction or incomplete neutralization of heparin. The Veterans Administration Cooperative Study of antiplatelet agents in the prevention of early thrombotic vein graft closure revealed that preoperative treatment with aspirin increased the frequency of graft patency but was associated with more bleeding and a greater reoperation rate (6.5% for aspirin-treated patients, compared with 1.7% for patients not treated with aspirin) [68]. Urgent CABG was performed after PTCA in 33 patients who were treated with c7E3, an antagonist of the platelet glycoprotein IIb/IIIa receptor, as part of the EPIC study [69]. Major blood loss, defined as >5 g/dL decrease in hemoglobin, occurred in 27 of 33 patients treated with c7E3 (82%), compared with 18 of 25 patients treated with placebo (72%).

Aprotinin, a serine protease inhibitor, is one of several agents that have been tested to determine efficacy in the prevention of postoperative bleeding after CABG. Levy et al. [70] published the results of a multicenter, double-blind, placebo-controlled trial to evaluate the safety and efficacy of aprotinin in adult patients undergoing repeat CABG. A total of 287 patients were randomly assigned to one of four treatment groups: high-dose aprotinin, low-dose aprotinin, pump-prime aprotinin only, and placebo. The percentage of patients who required donor erythrocyte transfusions was reduced from 75% in the placebo group to 54% and 46% in the high-dose and low-dose aprotinin groups, respectively. Despite concerns about an increased risk of thrombotic complications associated with aprotinin treatment, there were no significant differences among treatment groups in the incidence of MI.

Fremes et al. [71] published a meta-analysis of the trials conducted to evaluate desmopressin, ε-aminocaproic acid, tranexamic acid, and aprotinin. Although only aprotinin reduced the proportion of patients who required blood transfusions, both aprotinin and ε-aminocaproic acid decreased reoperation for bleeding, and each of the drugs significantly reduced postoperative chest tube blood loss. Mortality was not affected by any of the therapies.

Infection

Mediastinitis after CABG is a severe complication that increases perioperative mortality and reduces long-term survival after hospital discharge [72]. The cardiac surgery program at Duke University Medical Center analyzed the risk factors for mediastinitis among a cohort of 6,459 consecutive patients who underwent CABG over a 7-year period [72]. Eighty-three patients (1.3%) developed postoperative mediastinitis. By univariate analysis seven variables were associated with an increased risk of mediastinitis: obesity, CHF class, diabetes mellitus, previous CABG, duration of cardiopulmonary bypass, presence of comorbid conditions, and poor hemostasis. In descending order of significance, obesity, CHF class, previous CABG, and duration of bypass were the four independent predictors of mediastinitis identified by multivariate analysis. Neither bilateral IMA grafting nor the combination of diabetes and bilateral IMA grafting were significant predictors of mediastinitis. The Cleveland

Clinic also reported that bilateral IMA grafting was not a risk factor for mediastinitis [34]. Multivariate analysis of the VA Cardiac Surgery Database, however, identified bilateral IMA grafts as a significant risk factor for mediastinitis [36]. Nevertheless, after adjustment for preoperative risk factors, analysis of the VA database [36] and of series reported from the Cleveland Clinic [73] and Johns Hopkins [37] revealed a reduced operative mortality with use of the IMA.

Hypertension

Several antihypertensive agents have been studied to determine their effects on myocardial function in the post-CABG period. Mullen et al. [74] conducted a prospective, randomized trial that compared intravenous sodium nitroprusside, intravenous diltiazem, and intranasal nifedipine. Among 95 patients who underwent elective CABG and agreed to participate in the study, postoperative hypertension, defined as mean arterial pressure >95 mm Hg, developed in 62 (63%). The hemodynamic and myocardial effects of volume loading and atrial pacing were assessed before and after institution of the antihypertensive agents. The three drugs equally reduced blood pressure, while heart rate decreased during diltiazem infusion and increased during administration of nitroprusside and nifedipine. Myocardial performance (the relation between stroke work index and end-diastolic volume index) was unchanged by nitroprusside, while diltiazem and nifedipine depressed myocardial performance. Compared with nitroprusside, which has been shown to cause coronary steal, diltiazem and nifedipine had favorable effects on myocardial oxygen and lactate metabolism during atrial pacing. Also, fatal cyanide and thiocyanate poisoning can occur during prolonged nitroprusside infusion [75]. Thus, alternative vasodilator agents, such as nitroglycerin and diltiazem, may be preferable to sodium nitroprusside for treatment of hypertension post-CABG.

Neurologic

Neurologic complications after CABG have been studied extensively, as evidenced by a recent review article that cited 106 pertinent references [76]. The types of cerebral injury are categorized as stroke, diffuse encephalopathy, and ophthalmological complications. Perioperative cerebral deficits are attributed to two general mechanisms: (1) cerebral hypoperfusion caused by hypotension, and (2) embolization of air, thrombus (e.g., from the left ventricle), or atheromatous debris (e.g., from the ascending aorta).

Stroke. Gardner et al. [77] performed a retrospective analysis of 3,279 consecutive patients who underwent isolated CABG at the Johns Hopkins Hospital between 1974 and 1983. Stroke occurred in 56 patients (1.7%). A case-control study was conducted by identifying the two patients without a stroke who immediately preceded each stroke patient. By univariate analysis five factors were identified as significant risk factors for stroke: age, previous cerebrovascular disease, severe atherosclerosis of the ascending aorta, protracted cardiopulmonary bypass time, and severe perioperative hypotension.

More recent data on the incidence of stroke after CABG were provided by the Multicenter Study of Perioperative Ischemia, a prospective observational study of patients who underwent elective CABG in 24 U.S. medical institutions between September 1991 and September 1993 [78]. Among the 2,108 patients, there were eight deaths attributed to cerebral injury (0.38%), and a nonfatal stroke occurred in 55 of the 2,108 patients (2.6%). Proximal aortic atherosclerosis identified intraoperatively by the cardiac surgeon was the strongest independent predictor of so-called type I cerebral outcomes (including nonfatal stroke and death due to stroke or hypoxic encephalopathy). The hospital mortality rate among all patients with type I cerebral outcome was 21% (14/66).

Carotid bruits also have been reported to increase the risk of stroke post-CABG. Among a cohort of 5,915 consecutive patients who underwent isolated CABG at the Massachusetts General Hospital from 1970 to 1984, carotid bruits were noted preoperatively in 13 of 54 patients who had postoperative stroke or transient ischemic attacks, compared with 4 of 54 randomly selected control patients [79]. With multiple logistic regression used to adjust for confounding factors, carotid bruits conferred a 3.8-fold increase in the risk of postoperative neurologic deficits.

The approach to the patient who had asymptomatic carotid artery disease remains controversial. The Cleveland Clinic published a small randomized trial that compared isolated CABG with combined CABG and carotid endarterectomy in patients with at least 70% stenosis of one carotid artery, no neurologic symptoms, and unstable CAD [80]. The stroke risk was 6.9% in the patients who underwent isolated CABG, compared with 2.8% in the patients who underwent combined CABG and carotid surgery. Nevertheless, a conservative approach has been advocated based on the view that the stroke risk of carotid endarterectomy may equal the risk of stroke after CABG without carotid surgery.

Encephalopathy.   Among 2,108 patients in the Multicenter Study of Perioperative Ischemia, 63 patients (3.0%) suffered type II cerebral outcomes, defined as a new deterioration in intellectual function, confusion, agitation, disorientation, memory deficit, or seizure without evidence of focal injury [78]. The hospital mortality rate among patients with type II cerebral outcome was 10% (6/63).

Several prospective studies have been performed to investigate the pathophysiology of cognitive impairment after CABG. Newman et al. [81]

measured cognitive function the day before surgery and the day before discharge. There was a significant decline in six of nine measures of cognitive function. Both preoperative cognitive function and the postoperative decline in cognitive function were significantly associated with increased age. During cardiopulmonary bypass, autoregulation of cerebral blood flow was measured using the xenon-133 clearance method. The changes in cognition were not associated with the measures of cerebral autoregulation, and there was no effect of age on the slope of the cerebral blood flow response to changes in mean arterial pressure.

McLean et al. [82] measured neurological function before CABG, 5 days after CABG, and 3 months after CABG in 201 patients randomized to normothermic or moderate hypothermic cardiopulmonary bypass (CPB). Forty-eight patients were not included in the final analysis, for various reasons, including incomplete data (18 patients) and refusal to continue the study (17 patients). The test scores of psychomotor speed and coordination showed deterioration 5 days postoperatively in 74 of the 153 patients (48%) who completed the entire series of test batteries. Repeat testing 3 months after CABG revealed that the deterioration of test scores had resolved in all but 15 of the patients (10%). The tests of memory did not show deterioration after CABG, unlike Newman's study, which showed an age-related decline in short-term memory [81]. McLean et al. [82] found no neuroprotective effect of moderate hypothermia.

Pulmonary

Pumonary complications after CABG include bronchospasm, pneumonia, noncardiogenic pulmonary edema, pneumothorax, pleural effusion, postperiocardiotomy syndrome, and phrenic nerve damage. Chronic obstructive pulmonary disease was found to be an independent risk factor for morbidity and mortality after CABG in a series of 5,051 patients who underwent CABG at the Cleveland Clinic [29].

Renal

Although preexisting renal insufficiency is an independent risk factor for morbidity and mortality after CABG [29], acute renal failure (ARF) after CABG is uncommon in patients with normal preoperative renal function. The overall risk of ARF requiring dialysis was 0.9% among 34,874 patients who underwent isolated CABG at 43 Veterans Administration medical centers between April 1987 and March 1994 [83]. Independent risk factors for ARF requiring dialysis included preoperative renal insufficiency or CHF, and preoperative placement of an intraaortic balloon pump. The operative mortality was 63.7% among patients with ARF requiring dialysis.

Gastrointestinal

Gastrointestinal (GI) complications after CABG include bleeding from the upper or lower GI tracts, intestinal or hepatic ischemia, cholecystitis, pancreatitis, and paralytic ileus. Christenson et al. [84] reported a GI complication rate of 2.3% among 3,129 undergoing CABG between 1984 and 1993. The most common GI complications were cholecystitis (17/3129 = 23%) and intestinal ischemia (17/3129 = 23%). The mortality rate was 16.4% among the 73 patients with GI complications, compared with 3.4% for the entire series. The highest mortality rates were associated with fulminant liver failure (75%), intestinal ischemia (29%), and cholecystitis (18%). Postoperative low cardiac output and hypovolemic hypotension were independent predictors for the development of GI complications, suggesting that splanchnic hypoperfusion is a major factor in the pathogenesis of GI complications after CABG.

III. CONCLUSION

CABG is more effective than medical therapy for relief of symptoms in patients with stable or unstable angina. Compared with medical therapy, CABG improves survival only among patients with significant stenosis of the left main coronary artery or three-vessel CAD with left ventricular dysfunction. Among patients eligible for randomization to either CABG or PTCA, survival after CABG or PTCA is similar for patients with either single-vessel or multivessel CAD, excluding patients with left main stenosis. Therefore, among patients without left main stenosis or left ventricular dysfunction, the frequency and severity of complications after CABG should be important determinants of the choice between medical therapy, PTCA, or CABG. Complications after CABG are associated with increased costs and mortality, and occur among approximately 40% of patients. Therefore, the development of surgical techniques that reduce complication rates would have a major impact on both resource utilization and survival after CABG.

REFERENCES

1. Pocock SJ, Henderson RA, Rickards AF, Hampton JR, King SB III, Hamm C, Puel J, Hueb W, Goy J, Rodriguez A. Meta-analysis of randomized trials comparing coronary angioplasty by bypass surgery. Lancet 1995; 346:1184–1189.
2. The Bypass Angioplasty Revascularization Investigation (BARI) Investigators. Comparison of coronary bypass surgery with angioplasty in patients with multivessel disease. N Engl J Med 1996; 335:217–225.

3. O'Connor G, Plume S, Olmstead E, Morton J, Maloney C, Nugent W, Hernandez F, Clough R, Leavitt B, Coffin L, Marrin C, Wennberg D, Birkmeyer J, Charlesworth D, Malenka D, Quinton H, Kasper J. A regional intervention to improve the hospital mortality associated with coronary artery bypass graft surgery. JAMA 1996; 275:841–846.

4. Hannan E, Kilburn H, Racz M, Shields E, Chasson M. Improving the outcomes of coronary artery bypass surgery in New York State. JAMA 1994; 271:761–766.

5. Ghali W, Ash A, Hall R, Moskowitz M. Statewide quality improvement initiatives and mortality after cardiac surgery. JAMA 1997; 277:379–382.

6. Ayanian JZ, Epstein AM. Differences in the use of procedures between women and men hospitalized for coronary heart disease. N Engl J Med 1991; 325:221–225.

7. Khan SS, Nessim S, Gray R, Czer LS, Chaux A, Matloff J. Increased mortality of women in coronary artery bypass surgery: evidence for referral bias. Ann Intern Med 1990; 112:561–567.

8. Steingart RM, Packer M, Hamm P, Coglianese ME, Gersh B, Geltman EM, Sollano J, Katz S, Moye L, Basta LL, Lewis SJ, Gottlieb SS, Bernstein V, McEwan P, Jacobson K, Brown EJ, Kukin ML, Kantrowitz NE, Pfeffer MA. Sex differences in the management of coronary artery disease. N Engl J Med 1991; 325:226–230.

9. King KB, Clark PC, Hicks GL. Patterns of referral and recovery in women and men undergoing coronary artery bypass grafting. Am J Cardiol 1992; 69:179–182.

10. Mickleborough LL, Takagi Y, Maruyama H, Sun Z, Mohamed S. Is sex a factor in determining operative risk for aortocoronary bypass graft surgery? Circulation 1995; 92(suppl II):II-80–II-84.

11. O'Connor G, Plume S, Olmstead E, Coffin L, Morton J, Maloney C, Nowicki E, Levy D, Tryzelaar J, Hernandez F, Adrian L, Casey K, Bundy D, Soule D, Marrin C, Nugent W, Charlesworth D, Clough R, Katz S, Leavitt B, Wennberg J. Multivariate prediction of in-hospital mortality associated with coronary artery bypass graft surgery. Circulation 1992; 85:2110–2118.

12. O'Connor N, Morton J, Birkmeyer J, Olmstead E, O'Connor G. Effect of coronary artery diameter in patients undergoing coronary bypass surgery. Circulation 1996; 93:652–655.

13. Weintraub WS, Craver JM, Cohen CL, Jones EL, Guyton RA. Influence of age on results of coronary artery surgery. Circulation 1991; 84(suppl III):III-226–III-235.

14. Hannan EL, Burke J. Effect of age on mortality in coronary artery bypass surgery in New York, 1991–1992. Am Heart J 1994; 128:1184–1192.

15. Peterson ED, Cowper PA, Jollis JG, Bebchuk JD, DeLong ER, Muhlbaier LH, Mark DB, Pryor DB. Outcomes of coronary artery bypass graft surgery in 24,461 patients aged 80 years or older. Circulation 1995; 92(suppl II):II-85–II-91.

16. Weintraub WS, Clements SD, Ware J, Craver JM, Cohen CL, Jones EL, Guyton RA. Coronary artery surgery in octogenarians. Am J Cardiol 1991; 68:1530–1534.

17. Mullany C, Darling G, Pluth J, Orszulak T, Schaff H, Ilstrup D, Gersh B. Early and late results after isolated coronary artery bypass surgery in 159 patients aged 80 years and older. Circulation 1990; 82(suppl IV):IV-229–IV-236.

18. Tsai TP, Denton TA, Chaux A, Matloff JM, Kass RM, Blanche C, Khan SS. Results of coronary artery bypass grafting and/or aortic or mitral valve operation in patients $\geq$90 years of age. Am J Cardiol 1994; 74:960–962.

19. Alderman E, Fisher L, Litwin P, Kaiser G, Myers W, Maynard C, Levine F, Schloss M. Results of coronary artery surgery in patients with poor left ventricular function (CASS). Circulation 1983; 68:785–795.

20. Christenson JT, Maurice J, Simonet F, Bloch A, Fournet PC, Velebit V, Schmuziger M. Effect of low left ventricular ejection fractions on the outcome of primary coronary bypass grafting in end-stage coronary artery disease. J Cardiovasc Surg 1995; 36:45–51.

21. Wechsler A, Junod F. Coronary bypass grafting in patients with chronic congestive heart failure. Circulation 1989; 79(suppl I):I-92–I-96.

22. Kennedy JW, Kaiser GC, Fisher LD, Fritz JK, Myers W, Mudd JG, Ryan TJ. Clinical and angiographic predictors of operative mortality from the collaborative study in coronary artery surgery (CASS). Circulation 1981; 63:793–802.

23. Chaitman BR, Rogers WJ, Davis K, Tyras DH, Berger R, Bourassa MG, Fisher L, Stover-Hertzberg V, Judkins MP, Mock MB, Killip T. Operative risk factors in patients with left main coronary-artery disease. N Engl J Med 1980; 303:953–957.

24. Christakis GT, Ivanov J, Weisel RD, Birnbaum PL, David TE, Salerno TA. The changing pattern of coronary artery bypass surgery. Circulation 1989; 80(suppl I):I-151–I-161.

25. Gomberg J, Klein LW, Seelaus P, Parr GVS, Agarwal JB, Helfant RH. Surgical revascularization of left main coronary artery stenosis: determinants of perioperative and long-term outcome in the 1980s. Am Heart J 1988; 116:440–446.

26. Weintraub WS, Jones EL, Craver JM, Grosswald R, Guyton RA. In-hospital and long-term outcome after reoperative coronary artery bypass graft surgery. Circulation 1995; 92(suppl II):II-50–II-57.

27. Lytle BW, McElroy D, McCarthy P, Loop FD, Taylor PC, Goormastic M, Stewart RW, Cosgrove DM. Influence of arterial coronary bypass grafts on the mortality in coronary reoperations. J Thorac Cardiovasc Surg 1994; 107:675–683.

28. Savage E, Cohn L. "No touch" dissection, antegrade–retrograde blood cardioplegia, and single aortic cross-clamp significantly reduce operative mortality of reoperative CABG. Circulation 1994; 90(part 2):II-140–II-143.

29. Higgins TL, Estafanous FG, Loop FD, Beck GJ, Blum JM, Paranandi L. Stratification of morbidity and mortality outcome by preoperative risk factors in coronary artery bypass patients. JAMA 1992; 267:2344–2348.

30. Edwards FH, Clark RE, Schwartz M. Coronary artery bypass grafting: the Society of Thoracic Surgeons national database experience. Ann Thorac Surg 1994; 57:12–19.

31. Hattler BG, Madia C, Johnson C, Armitage JM, Hardesty RL, Kormos RL, Pham SM, Payne DN, Griffith BP. Risk stratification using the Society of Thoracic Surgeons Program. Ann Thorac Surg 1994; 58:1348–1352.

32. Jones R, Hannan E, Hammermeister K, DeLong E, O'Connor G, Luepker R, Parsonnet V, Pryor D. Identification of preoperative variables needed for risk adjustment of short-term mortality after coronary artery bypass graft surgery. J Am Coll Cardiol 1996; 28:1478–1487.

33. Cameron AA, Green GE, Brogno DA, Thornton J. Internal thoracic artery grafts: 20-year clinical follow-up. J Am Coll Cardiol 1995; 25:188–192.

34. Loop F. Internal-thoracic-artery grafts. Biologically better coronary arteries. N Engl J Med 1996; 334:263–265.

35. Cameron A, Davis KB, Green G, Schaff HV. Coronary bypass surgery with internal-thoracic-artery grafts—effects on survival over a 15-year period. N Engl J Med 1996; 334:216–219.

36. Grover FL, Johnson RR, Marshall G, Hammermeister KE. Impact of mammary grafts on coronary bypass operative mortality and morbidity. Department of Veterans Affairs Cardiac Surgeons. Ann Thorac Surg 1994; 57:559–568.

37. Gardner TJ, Greene PS, Rykiel MF. Routine use of the left internal mammary artery graft in the elderly. Ann Thorac Surg 1990; 49:188–194.

38. Mangano D. Effects of acadesine on myocardial infarction, stroke, and death following surgery. A meta-analysis of the 5 international randomized trials. JAMA 1996; 277:325–332.

39. Silber JH, Rosenbaum PR, Schwartz JS, Ross RN, Williams SV. Evaluation of the complication rate as a measure of quality of care in coronary artery bypass graft surgery. JAMA 1995; 274:317–323.

40. Pelletier L, Carrier M. Early postoperative care and complications. In: Waters D, Bourassa M, eds. Care of the Patient with Previous Coronary Bypass Surgery. Philadelphia: F.A. Davis Company, 1991:3–24 (Brest A, ed. Cardiovascular Clinics; vol 21).

41. Etievent JP, Chocron S, Toubin G, Taberlet C, Alwan K, Clement F, Cordier A, Schipman N, Kantelip JP. Use of cardiac troponin I as a marker of perioperative myocardial ischemia. Ann Thorac Surg 1995; 59:1192–1194.

42. Chaitman BR, Alderman EL, Sheffield LT, Tong T, Fisher L, Mock MB, Weins RD, Kaiser GC, Roitman D, Berger R, Gersh B, Schaff H, Bourassa MG, Killip T. Use of survival analysis to determine the clinical significance of new Q waves after coronary bypass surgery. Circulation 1983; 67:302–308.

43. Gray RJ, Matloff JM, Conklin CM, Ganz W, Charuizi Y, Wolfstein R, Swan HJC. Perioperative myocardial infarction: late clinical course after coronary artery bypass surgery. Circulation 1982; 66:1185–1189.

44. Force T, Hibberd P, Weeks G, Kemper AJ, Bloomfield P, Tow D, Josa M, Khuri S, Parisi AF. Perioperative myocardial infarction after coronary artery bypass surgery. Circulation 1990; 82:903–912.

45. Namay DL, Hammermeister KE, Zia MS, DeRouen TA, Dodge HT, Namay K. Effect of perioperative myocardial infarction on late survival in patients undergoing coronary artery bypass surgery. Circulation 1982; 65:1066–1071.

46. Katz NM, Kubanick BA, Ahmed SW, Green CE, Pearle DL, Satler LF, Rackley CE, Wallace RB. Determinants of cardiac failure after coronary bypass surgery within 30 days of acute myocardial infarction. Ann Thorac Surg 1986; 42:658–663.

47. Pires LA, Wagshal AB, Lancey R, Huang SK. Arrhythmias and conduction disturbances after coronary artery bypass graft surgery: epidemiology, management, and prognosis. Am Heart J 1995; 129:799–808.

48. Ommen S, Odell J, Stanton M. Atrial arrhythmias after cardiothoracic surgery. N Engl J Med 1997; 336:1429–1434.

49. Davison R, Hartz R, Kaplan K, Parker M, Feiereisel P, Michaelis L. Prophylaxis of supraventricular tachyarrhythmia after coronary bypass surgery with oral verapamil: a randomized, double-blind trial. Ann Thorac Surg 1985; 39:336–339.

50. Aranki S, Shaw D, Adams D, Rizzo R, Couper G, VanderVliet M, Collins J, Cohn L, Burstin H. Predictors of atrial fibrillation after coronary artery surgery. Current trends and impact on hospital resources. Circulation 1996; 94:390–397.

51. Mathew J, Parks R, Savino J, Friedman A, Koch C, Mangano D, Browner W. Atrial fibrillation following coronary artery bypass graft surgery. Predictors, outcomes, and resource utilization. JAMA 1996; 276:300–306.

52. Creswell LL, Schuessler RB, Rosenbloom M, Cox JL. Hazards of postoperative atrial arrhythmias. Ann Thorac Surg 1993; 56:539–549.

53. Mendes LA, Connelly GP, McKenney PA, Podrid PJ, Cupples LA, Shemin RJ, Ryan TJ, Davidoff R. Right coronary artery stenosis: an independent predictor of atrial fibrillation after coronary artery bypass surgery. J Am Coll Cardiol 1995; 25:198–202.

54. Lauer MS, Eagle KA, Buckley MJ, DeSanctis RW. Atrial fibrillation following coronary artery bypass surgery. Prog Cardiovasc Dis 1989; XXXI:367–378.

55. Johnson L, Dickstein R, Freuhan C. Prophylactic digitilization for coronary artery bypass surgery. Circulation 1976; 53:819–822.

56. Tyras DH, Stothert JC, Kaiser GC, Barner HB, Codd JE, Willman VL. Supraventricular tachyarrhythmias after myocardial revascularization: a randomized trial of prophylactic digitalization. J Thorac Cardiovasc Surg 1979; 77:310–314.

57. Andrews TC, Reimold SC, Berlin JA, Antman EM. Prevention of supraventricular arrhythmias after coronary artery bypass surgery. Circulation 1991; 84(suppl III): III-236–III-244.

58. White HD, Antman EM, Glynn MA, Collins JJ, Cohn LH, Shemin RJ, Friedman PL. Efficacy and safety of timolol for prevention of supraventricular tachyarrhythmias after coronary artery bypass surgery. Circulation 1984; 70:479–484.

59. Williams DB, Misbach GA, Kruse AP, Ivey TD. Oral verapamil for prophylaxis of supraventricular tachycardia after myocardial revascularization. J Thorac Cardiovasc Surg 1985; 90:592–596.

60. Kowey PR, Taylor JE, Rials SJ, Marinchak RA. Meta-analysis of the effectiveness of prophylactic drug therapy in preventing supraventricular arrhythmia early after coronary artery bypass grafting. Am J Cardiol 1992; 69:963–965.

61. Campbell TJ, Gavaghan TP, Morgan JJ. Intravenous sotalol for the treatment of atrial fibrillation and flutter after cardiopulmonary bypass. Br Heart J 1985; 54:86–90.

62. McAlister HF, Luke RA, Whitlock RM, Smith WM. Intravenous amiodarone bolus versus oral quinidine for atrial flutter and fibrillation after cardiac operations. J Thorac Cardiovasc Surg 1990; 99:911–918.

63. Smith RC, Leung JM, Keith FM, Merrick S, Mangano DT. Ventricular dysrhythmias in patients undergoing coronary artery bypass graft surgery: incidence, characteristics, and prognostic importance. Am Heart J 1992; 123:73–81.

64. Topol EJ, Lerman BB, Baughman KL, Platia EV, Griffith LSC. De novo refractory ventricular tachyarrhythmias after coronary revascularization. Am J Cardiol 1986; 57:57–59.

65. Baerman JM, Kirsh MM, de Buitleir M, Hyatt L, Juni JE, Pitt B, Morady F. Natural history and determinants of conduction defects following coronary artery bypass surgery. Ann Thorac Surg 1987; 44:150–153.

66. Emlein G, Huang SKS, Pires LA, Rofino K, Okike ON, VanderSalm TJ. Prolonged bradyarrhythmias after isolated coronary artery bypass graft surgery. Am Heart J 1993; 126:1084–1090.

67. Flack J, Hafer J, Engelman R, Rousou J, Deaton D, Pekow P. Effect of normothermic blood cardioplegia on postoperative conduction abnormalities and supraventricular arrhythmias. Circulation 1992; 86(suppl II):II-385–II-392.

68. Goldman S, Copeland J, Moritz T, Henderson W, Zadina K. Improvement in early saphenous vein graft patency after coronary artery bypass surgery with antiplatelet therapy: results of a Veterans Administration cooperative study. Circulation 1988; 77:1324–1332.

69. Boehrer JD, Kereiakes DJ, Navetta FI, Califf RM, Topol EJ. Effects of profound platelet inhibition with c7E3 before coronary angioplasty on complications of coronary bypass surgery. Am J Cardiol 1994; 74:1166–1170.

70. Levy JH, Pifarre R, Schaff HV, Horrow JC, Albus R, Spiess B, Rosengart TK, Murray J, Clark RE, Smith P, Nadel A, Bonney SL, Kleinfield R. A multicenter, double-blind, placebo-controlled trial of aprotinin for reducing blood loss and the requirement for donor-blood transfusion in patients undergoing repeat coronary artery bypass grafting. Circulation 1995; 92:2236–2244.

71. Fremes SE, Wong BI, Lee E, Mai R, Christakis GT, McLean RF, Goldman BS, Naylor CD. Meta-analysis of prophylactic drug treatment in the prevention of postoperative bleeding. Ann Thorac Surg 1994; 58:1580–1588.

72. Milano CA, Kesler K, Archibald N, Sexton DJ, Jones RH. Mediastinitis after coronary artery bypass graft surgery. Circulation 1995; 92:2245–2251.

73. Cosgrove D, Loop F, Lytle B. Does mammary artery grafting increase surgical risk? Circulation 1985; 72(suppl 2):170–174.

74. Mullen JC, Miller DR, Weisel RD, Birnbaum PL, Teoh KH, Madonik M, Ivanov J, Laidley DT, Liu P, Teasdale SJ. Postoperative hypertension: a comparison of diltiazem, nifedipine, and nitroprusside. J Thorac Cardiovasc Surg 1988; 96:122–132.

75. Patel C, Laboy V, Venus B, Mathru M, Wier D. Use of sodium nitroprusside in post-coronary bypass surgery: a plea for conservation. Chest 1986; 89:663–667.

76. Hornick P, Smith PL, Taylor KM. Cerebral complications after coronary bypass grafting. Curr Opin Cardiol 1994; 9:670–679.

77. Gardner TJ, Horneffer PJ, Manolio TA, Pearson TA, Gott VL, Baumgartner WA, Borkon AM, Watkins L, Reitz BA. Stroke following coronary artery bypass grafting: a ten-year study. Ann Thorac Surg 1985; 40:574–581.

78. Roach G, Kanchuger M, Mangano C, Newman M, Nussmeier N, Wolman R, Aggarwal A, Marschall K, Graham S, Ley C, Ozanne G, Mangano D. Adverse cerebral outcomes after coronary bypass surgery. N Engl J Med 1996; 335:1857–1863.

79. Reed GL, Singer DE, Picard EH, DeSanctis RW. Stroke following coronary-artery bypass surgery. N Engl J Med 1988; 319:1246–1250.

80. Hertzer N, Loop F, Beven E, O'Hara P, Krajewski L. Surgical staging for simultaneous coronary and carotid disease: a study including prospective randomization. J Vasc Surg 1989; 9:455–463.

81. Newman MF, Croughwell ND, Blumenthal JA, White WD, Lewis JB, Smith LR, Frasco P, Towner EA, Schell RM, Hurwitz BJ, Reeves JG. Effect of aging on cerebral autoregulation during cardiopulmonary bypass. Association with postoperative cognitive dysfunction. Circulation 1994; 90[part 2]:II-243–II-249.
82. McLean RF, Wong BI, Naylor CD, Snow WG, Harrington EM, Gawel M, Fremes SE. Cardiopulmonary bypass, temperature, and central nervous system dysfunction. Circulation 1994; 90[part 2]:II-250–II-255.
83. Chertow G, Lazarus M, Christiansen C, Cook E, Hammermeister K, Grover F, Daley J. Preoperative renal risk stratification. Circulation 1997; 95:878–884.
84. Christenson JT, Schmuziger M, Maurice J, Simonet F, Velebit V. Gastrointestinal complications after coronary artery bypass grafting. J Thorac Cardiovasc Surg 1994; 108:899–906.

3

The Natural History of Saphenous Vein Bypass Graft Disease

Martial G. Bourassa
Montreal Heart Institute, Montreal, Quebec, Canada

The large prospective randomized surgical trials of the late 1970s and early 1980s have established the role of coronary artery bypass surgery as a therapeutic option in several subsets of patients with coronary artery disease [1–4]. Because of the high prevalence of severe coronary artery disease in developed countries, coronary artery bypass surgery is the most frequently performed cardiac surgical procedure. Patient selection, better surgical techniques, and refinements in postoperative management have contributed to reduce the morbidity and mortality of the procedure, in spite of the fact that in the current area of interventional cardiology, patients referred to surgery often are older and have more diffuse triple vessel disease and more left ventricular dysfunction [5–7].

Because of its relative immunity to atherosclerosis, the ability to enlarge with increased flow demands, and higher patency rates resulting in higher rates of survival and event-free survival compared to saphenous vein grafts, the internal mammary artery is recognized as the conduit of choice for surgical revascularization [8–18]. Limitations to the use of the internal mammary artery as a bypass graft include increased operating time, increased bleeding, the possibility of sternal wound infection (especially when bilateral internal mammary artery grafts are used), and increased susceptibility to injury at reoperation. The internal mammary artery graft is unsuitable in patients undergoing urgent bypass surgery because of unstable angina or cardiogenic shock. Other arterial conduits, such as the right gastroepiploic artery, the radial artery, and the inferior epigastric artery, have also been advocated for coronary artery bypass grafting, but their mid- and long-term patency rates have not yet been adequately documented [19–21].

Saphenous vein bypass grafts (SVBGs) have been shown to have relatively high early and late attrition rates after surgery, mainly because of graft thrombosis and because of the development of late atherosclerosis, which makes them less suitable than arterial conduits for coronary artery bypass grafting [22–38]. Nevertheless, autologous saphenous vein grafts still remain the most widely used conduits for bypass surgery, mainly because of their ready availability and ease of removal and because of the insufficient number of arterial grafts available to achieve complete revascularization in most patients with multivessel coronary disease. Thus, improvement of long-term patency of saphenous vein grafts remains a major objective. With this objective in mind, this chapter will briefly review the incidence and severity, the mechanisms, and the main predictors of saphenous vein bypass graft disease.

I. INCIDENCE AND SEVERITY OF SVBG CHANGES

A. The Montreal Heart Institute Experience [22–33]

Coronary angiography and graft opacification were performed in consecutive patients who underwent CABG at our institution between September 1969 and August 1972. Four hundred patients had repeat angiography at approximately 1 month, 237 at 1 year, 107 between 5 and 7 years, and 82 between 10 and 12 years postoperatively. Among these cases, serial angiographic examinations were performed at 2 weeks, 1 year, 5–7 years and 10–12 years after aorto-coronary saphenous vein bypass grafting in 147 grafts from 82 patients [27,28, 31]. Reasons for exclusion from the follow-up studies included death, patient or physician refusal, medical problems, occluded grafts, and reoperation.

Early Graft Changes

Graft Patency Rates.   Cumulative SVBG patency rates were 87% at 1 month and 79% at 1 year after bypass surgery (Table 1). In the 82 patients who underwent consecutive angiographic examinations, patency rates were higher, i.e., 96% early and 90% at 1 year (Table 2). These rates are probably overestimated, however, since only patients with at least one patent graft at these earlier examinations were restudied late after bypass surgery.

Stenosis at Anastomotic Site.   Greater than 50% diameter stenosis at the site of the distal coronary anastomosis was observed at the early postoperative angiographic examination in 7% of grafts (Table 3). These constricted anastomoses were attributed primarily to faulty surgical techniques, and they tended to increase as a result of turbulent flow and secondary intimal fibromuscular

Table 1 Cumulative SVBG Patency Rates

Source	Year of report	No. of patients	No. of distal anastomoses	Graft patency rates (%)				
				<1 month	~1 year	~5 years	~10 years	~15 years
MHI [32]	1984	400	721	87				
		237	395		79			
		107	201			78		
		82	147				63	
CASS [33]	1985	129	334	90				
		121	309		82			
		197	507			82		
NDMC [38]	1996	1,388	5,065	88				
		—	3,993		81			
		—	1,978			75		
			856				60	
			353					50

MHI: Montreal Heart Institute; CASS: Coronary Artery Surgery Study; NDMC: National Defense Medical Center (Ottawa)

hyperplasia. Approximately half of the grafts with early anastomotic narrowings were occluded at 1 year, and half of the remainder occluded during the subsequent 10 years.

Diffuse and Localized Graft Narrowing. Two-thirds of patent grafts showed an angiographically detectable (≥20%) reduction in caliber between 1 month and 1 year after bypass surgery. This reduction in internal diameter varied widely, even in individual patients, from 20% to 80%, with an average reduction of 30% at 1 year. In general, reduction in caliber of the graft was directly related to the initial size of the vein and inversely related to graft flow. Finally,

Table 2 SVBG Patency Rates in Consecutive Patients

Authors	Year of report	No. of patients	No. of distal anastomoses	Graft patency rates (%)			
				<1 month	~1 year	~5 years	~10 years
Campeau et al. [31]	1983	82	147	96	90	81	63
Lytle et al. [34]	1985	501	786	—	87	73	—
FitzGibbon et al. [37]	1991	222	741	92	87	80	41

Table 3 SVBG Narrowings (≥50%) Early After CABG

| | | No. of distal anastomoses | | ≥50% narrowings (%) | |
Source	Year of report	At 1 month	At 1 year	At 1 month	At 1 year
MHI [27]	1975	624	278	7	11
CASS [33]	1985	—	240	—	10
NDMC [36]	1986	—	1,179	—	11

MHI: Montreal Heart Institute; CASS: Coronary Artery Surgery Study; NDMC: National Defense Medical Center (Ottawa)

diffuse narrowing of the graft did not increase after the first postoperative year and did not appear to lead to late graft closure.

Localized narrowings were observed at the distal anastomosis or on the main body of grafts in 11% of these conduits at the 1-year evaluation (Table 3). Localized narrowings on the body of the graft were characterized angiographically by smooth vessel walls with areas of tubular narrowing of variable length. These segmental stenoses were attributed to mechanical and or ischemic injury of the vein during operation. Like constrictions at the coronary anastomoses, significant localized narrowings (≥50%) on the main body of grafts often led to late graft occlusion.

Late Graft Changes

Late Graft Patency Rates.   Cumulative graft patency rates were 78% between 5 and 7 years after bypass surgery (Table 1). Thus, grafts that were patent at 1 year usually remained open 5 years later. In contrast to the low attrition rate between 1 and 5–7 years, the incidence of graft occlusion increased strikingly between 5 and 7 and 10 and 12 years after operation. Cumulative graft patency rates dropped from 79% between 5 and 7 years to 63% between 10 and 12 years after surgery (Table 1). In the 82 patients undergoing consecutive angiographic examinations, late patency rates were similar to those observed in our pooled data, i.e., 81% between 5 and 7 years and 63% between 10 and 12 years after bypass surgery (Table 2).

Late Graft Narrowing.   Major late changes in patient SVBGs were observed both at the 5- to 7- and 10- to 12-year evaluations. These changes consisted of wall irregularities and localized narrowings of various shapes. Multiple graft lesions were also observed. The incidence and severity of these graft modifications, which apparently were produced by atherosclerosis, were circumscribed during the first 7 years after bypass surgery. At 5–7 years, only 17% of vein grafts showed irregularities of outline at angiography and only

Table 4 SVBG Disease Late After CABG

| Source | Year of report | No. of distal anastomoses | | Graft atherosclerosis (%) | | | |
| | | At 5 years | At 10 years | Irregularities of outline | | Narrowing ≥50% | |
				At 5 years	At 10 years	At 5 years	At 10 years
MHI [31]	1983	142	93	17	46	5.6	32
CASS [33]	1985	386	—	—	—	7.8	—
NDMC [37]	1991	565	403	38	75	5.0	26

MHI: Montreal Heart Institute; CASS: Coronary Artery Surgery Study; NDMC: National Defense Medical Center (Ottawa)

approximately 6% had localized stenoses that were greater than 50% (Table 4). However, these atherosclerotic changes increased markedly as time elapsed postoperatively, and at 10–12 years almost half of the vein grafts that remained patent showed wall irregularities, and one-third had localized narrowings of 50% or more (Table 4). Thus, at follow-up angiography between 10 and 12 years after operation, approximately one-third of saphenous bypass grafts were occluded, one-third showed angiographic evidence of atherosclerosis, and the remaining one-third were apparently free of atherosclerotic changes. The development of atherosclerosis appeared to be the most significant cause of late graft closure.

B. The Coronary Artery Surgery Study Experience [33]

In the Coronary Artery Surgery Study (CASS), 129 patients with a total of 334 distal anastomoses underwent postoperative angiography within 60 days of the surgical procedure; 121 patients with 309 distal anastomoses underwent repeat angiography at 18 months after operation; finally, 197 patients with 507 distal anastomoses underwent repeat angiography 60 months after surgery (Table 1).

Approximately 10% of the surgically treated patients at each of the 11 clinical sites in CASS were randomly selected for early postoperative angiography. In addition, although this was not a requirement of the study protocol, investigators at the clinical sites were encouraged to invite all their surviving patients to undergo angiography at 18 months and 5 years after surgery. Between 70% and 75% of patients were angina-free at the time of angiography at 18 months and at 5 years after surgery in CASS.

Within 60 days of surgery, 90% of distal anastomoses were patent. At 18 months, 82% of distal anastomoses were patent; and again, at 5 years, 82% of distal anastomoses were patent (Table 1). Approximately 10% of patent SVBGs had ≥50% localized narrowings at 18 months, as a result of technical problems at surgery or progressive intimal hyperplasia postoperatively (Table 3). Approximately 8% had significant (≥50%) stenoses at 5 years, presumably related to atherosclerosis (Table 4).

C. The Cleveland Clinic Experience [34]

Lytle et al. obtained serial angiograms in 501 patients after CABG. Study 1 was obtained at a mean interval of 15 months after surgery. At that time, 87% of the SVBGs were patent, of which 5% were stenotic or irregular. Study 2 was performed at a mean interval of 7.3 years, at which time 73% of the grafts were patent, of which 18% were stenotic or irregular (Table 2).

D. The National Defense Medical Center Experience [35–38]

FitzGibbon et al. reported on several series of patients undergoing repeat angiography after bypass surgery. In 1978, they reported on graft patency prior to hospital discharge and at 1 year after surgery in 409 patients and 1,400 SVBGs. Graft patency rates were 89% and 81%, respectively. In 1986, they described angiographic findings at less than 1 month, at 1 year, and at 5 years after surgery in 353 patients and 1,179 grafts. Graft patency rates were 90%, 83%, and 74%, respectively. In addition, ≥50% stenoses were present in 11% of SVBGs at 1 year (Table 3) and in 20% at 5 years. In 1991, they described consecutive postoperative angiographic examinations on 741 SVBGs in 222 patients (Table 2). All grafts were evaluated early (at less than 1 month), at 1 year, at 5 years, and more than 6.5 (mean 9.6) years after operation. At the late examination, 237 grafts were restudied an average of 7.5 years, 403 an average of 10 years, and 101 over 11.5 years after operation. Graft patency rates in these consecutive studies decreased from 92% early, to 87% at 1 year, and to 80% at 5 years. Late patency rates were 59% at 7.5 years, 59% at 10 years, and 55% after 11.5 years. Early after operation, no patent graft showed irregularities of outline. However, 7% showed a stenosis reducing the graft lumen to a diameter ≤50% of the grafted artery's diameter. Most of these narrowings were at the distal anastomosis between the graft and the coronary artery and were presumably related to faulty surgical technique. At 1 year, 8% of patent grafts had at least some irregularities of outline. Six percent of them showed a narrowing that reduced the graft lumen by ≥50%. By 5 years, 38% of patent grafts had irregularities of outline and were considered to have developed atherosclerosis. However, only 5% of patent grafts showed a 50% or more reduction of the graft lumen (Table 4).

In 1996, FitzGibbon et al. reported cumulative long-term angiographic follow-ups in 1,388 patients (Table 1). Angiograms were performed on 5,065 grafts early, on 3,993 grafts at 1 year, and on 1,978 grafts at 5 years after operation, and 353 grafts were examined after 15 or more years. Vein graft patency rates were 88% early, 81% at 1 year, 75% at 5 years, and 50% at 15 or more years. When suboptimal grafts were excluded, the proportion of excellent grafts decreased to 40% after 12.5 or more years. SVBG disease appeared by 1 year, and the rate accelerated by >2.5 years, involving 48% of grafts at 5 years and 81% at 15 or more years; 44% of the latter grafts were narrowed 50% or more.

E. Long-Term Attrition of SVBGs

As shown in Table 1, repeat angiographic evaluation of SVBGs in large nonconsecutive series of patients after bypass surgery show quite consistent data. Roughly speaking, 90% of saphenous vein grafts are patent at 1 month and 80% are patent at 1 year after operation. Therefore, there is a steep attrition of these grafts during the first year after surgery, of which half occurs during the first month. In consecutive patients, as shown in Table 2, early graft patency rates are higher, and roughly 90% of grafts are patent at 1 year. This may represent an overestimation, however, since only patients with at least one patent graft at these early stages are systematically restudied late after operation. At 5–7 years, patency rates of saphenous vein grafts range from 75% to 80% in both consecutive and nonconsecutive studies. Thus, the attrition rate decreases to a mere 1% or 2% per year between 1 and 7 years after operation. There is a subsequent sharp drop in patency rates to 60% or less at 10–12 years after operation, representing a 3%–4% yearly attrition rate between 7 and 12 years after operation. Finally, at 15 years or more, 50% of saphenous vein grafts have become occluded.

Depending upon surgical skill and technique, some patent SVBGs show significant narrowings (≥50%) of the coronary anastomotic site at the early postoperative angiographic examination. Approximately half of the grafts with these early anastomotic narrowings become occluded during the first year after operation, and the other half occlude during the next 10 years. At 1 year, approximately 10% of patent SVBGs have 50% or more diameter stenosis at the distal anastomotic site or on the body of the graft as a result of progressive intimal fibromuscular hyperplasia (Table 3). Like constrictions at the site of anastomosis, significant localized narrowings on the body of the graft often lead to late graft occlusion.

Luminal irregularities that are presumed to be caused by atherosclerosis are observed at angiography in 20%–40% of patent SVBGs between 5 and 7 years after bypass surgery. However, only 5%–8% of grafts with these atherosclerotic changes show a ≥50% diameter stenosis at 5–7 years (Table 4). There is a marked progression in the incidence and severity of these angiographic findings at 10–12 years after bypass surgery, where 50%–75% of patent SVBGs show irregularities of outline and roughly one-fourth to one-third of them have ≥50% diameter stenoses (Table 4). At 15 years, most patent grafts show some irregularities of outline, and almost half of them are narrowed 50% or more [38]. Graft closure was noted between 10 and 12 years after operation in 43% of grafts with 50% or more stenosis at 5–7 years, as compared with only 20% of "normal" grafts or grafts with only luminal irregularities at 5–7 years [31,38,39].

II. MECHANISMS OF GRAFT FAILURE

A. Early Graft Thrombosis [40,41]

Some acellular fibrosis and modest thickening of intima are frequently present when unused saphenous vein remnants are examined histologically. However, a 50% or more preexisting luminal narrowing is seen in 1% or less of saphenous veins selected for bypass grafting. Depending upon the harvesting technique, denudation of endothelial cells is frequent in freshly harvested veins before their insertion. In grafts of patients who died early postoperatively, the endothelium often appears disrupted and the intimal surface is usually covered, partially or completely, by fibrin. Thrombosis appears to be the main cause of graft occlusion within 1 month of operation. Early thrombosis is precipitated by local factors related to problems of graft preparation, to technical difficulties of operation (kinking, compression, dissection), or to anastomotic stenoses that cause poor blood flow in the graft.

Endothelial injury exposes the thrombogenic subendothelium and media to circulating blood. Platelets become activated at the site of injury and play a central role in the initiation and progression of mural platelet thrombosis, which may eventually lead to graft occlusion. Accumulation of platelet thrombi is particularly marked at the suture points of the distal anastomotic site. In addition to releasing mitogenic substances that can affect the vessel wall, the adherent platelets also release thromboxane A_2, ADP, and other substances that contribute to activation and recruitment of other platelets in the vicinity. During these processes, the coagulation pathway is activated and thrombin is generated. Thrombin causes further platelet aggregation and also catalyzes the polymerization of fibrin, which stabilizes the platelet thrombus on the vessel wall. Endothelial cell loss and vessel injury may result in inactivation of antithrombotic defense mechanisms that are synthesized or secreted by endothelial cells and in decreased activity of adenosine diphosphate, prostacyclin, and EDRF.

B. Intimal Hyperplasia and Fibrosis [40,41]

Intimal proliferative hyperplasia and fibrosis cause intimal thickening and reduction of lumen diameter. Hyperplasia is characterized by a large amount of fibroblasts in the intima, surrounded by ground substance and only sparce collagen fibers, whereas fibrosis is made up almost entirely of acellular connective tissue and abundant collagen fibers. Intimal hyperplasia becomes a prominent feature beyond 1 month after surgery. This phenomenon occurs in almost all grafts, tends to be diffuse and homogeneous, and leads to a reduction of about 30% of the luminal diameter by 1 year after surgery. Chronic exposure of the vein graft to the high-pressure pulsatile arterial flow, for which the vein is not suited, probably contributes to chronic endothelial dysfunction, leading to platelet activation and platelet-dependent proliferation of smooth muscle cells in the intima. Even a monolayer of platelets that adheres to the exposed subendothelium can release enough mitogenic factors to stimulate the slow and gradual process of primary intimal smooth muscle proliferation. The organization of subocclusive mural thrombi formed within the first year after operation also may contribute to luminal vein graft narrowing and to secondary smooth muscle cell proliferation. Platelet-derived growth factors released by activated platelets, as well as mitogenic factors derived from other cells, have chemotactic properties that can cause the migration of smooth muscle cells from the media to the intima and the proliferation of smooth muscle cells in the intima at the sites of endothelial injury.

C. Late Graft Atherosclerosis [21,40]

SVBGs can develop atherosclerotic changes that are almost identical to those seen in the coronary arteries [40]. The basic lesion, atheroma or fibrofatty plaque, consists of a raised focal plaque within the intima, having a core of lipid and a covering fibrous cap. The earliest macroscopic alteration is the development of fatty streaks; later, increasingly more complex calcified atheromas develop. Rupture of these atherosclerotic plaques in SVBGs often leads to late vein graft thrombosis.

Some important morphological differences have been described between SVBG and native coronary atherosclerosis [21]. The atherosclerotic process in SVBGs appears to be more diffuse and concentric, and the fibrous cap tends to be weaker and thinner, leading to a greater risk of exposing cellular elements and lipid debris to the bloodstream. Finally, the lesion in SVBGs shows a more prominent infiltrate of inflammatory cells and may be more friable and fragile and, therefore, more prone to embolism of atherosclerotic debris, especially during reoperation or angioplasty.

True atherosclerosis is almost always absent in vein grafts examined histologically during the first 12 months after bypass surgery. Approximately 10% of SVBGs show evidence of atherosclerosis between 1 and 3 years after operation. Atherosclerosis is documented histologically in 65%–70% of SVBGs between 6 and 12 years after surgery. The atherosclerotic process progressively increases in severity late after surgery and is primarily responsible for late graft closure [40].

III. FACTORS INFLUENCING PATENCY OF SVBGs

A. Early SVBG Patency

As shown in Table 5, the major determinants of early SVBG patency rates are endothelial injury, low SVBG flow, technical errors, and lack of antiplatelet therapy peri- and postoperatively. Endothelial injury to the saphenous vein results mainly from surgical manipulation during harvesting and preparation for grafting. First, interruption of the nutritive blood supply of the vein wall and exposure of the vein to arterial blood flow and pressure cause unavoidable ischemia and reperfusion injury. Second, surgical manipulation can result in indirect trauma to the endothelium during rinsing, distention, and storage prior to implantation of the graft. These phenomena may be responsible for structural and biochemical damage to the endothelium and to the vessel wall. Loss of endothelium exposes subintimal tissues to the blood, leads to local deposition of platelets and fibrin, and thus predisposes to early vein graft closure.

The critical role of low SVBG flow caused by poor distal runoff and/or small caliber of the recipient coronary arteries ($\leq$1.5 mm in diameter) as a determinant of graft patency rates during the first year after bypass surgery was demonstrated almost 25 years ago [22–25]. Several recent reports have confirmed the critical importance of this factor [31,32,42,43–46].

Table 5 Factors Influencing Patency of SVBGs

	Early SVBG patency	Late SVBG patency
Major determinants	Endothelial injury	Elevated blood lipids
	Low SVBG flow	Plaque rupture and late thrombosis
	Technical errors	
	Lack of antiaggregant therapy	Lack of or inadequate lipid-lowering therapy
Secondary contributors	Bypass of circumflex or right coronary artery	Cigarette smoking
		Diabetes mellitus
	Nonsequential grafting	

SVBG patency rates were higher in the second than in the first series of patients who underwent bypass surgery at our institution in the early 1970s, as a result of improved surgical technique [27,28,31]. Technical errors usually consist of significant constrictions at the distal anastomotic site, kinking of the graft because of excessive length, or linear tension on the graft and coronary artery because of insufficient length. These technical problems are probably infrequent nowadays but, when they occur, may lead to graft closure within the first year after bypass surgery.

The beneficial effect of antiplatelet therapy on prevention of SVBG occlusion after bypass surgery has been firmly established in several recent clinical trials [40–44,47–52]. Drug regimens such as aspirin in low (50-mg or 100-mg) or moderate (325-mg) doses begun early postoperatively (≥6 hours), dipyridamole started preoperatively and aspirin given postoperatively, and ticlopidine begun early postoperatively and administered daily thereafter have all been shown to reduce saphenous vein graft occlusion rates markedly early and, in most instances, through the first year after bypass surgery. Thus, lack of antiplatelet therapy during the early postoperative period is a major determinant of early graft thrombosis.

Other factors that have been shown to predict graft occlusion during the first years after operation include the specific artery grafted and the use of nonsequential bypass grafts [37,45,46,50]. The occlusion rate of SVBGs to the right and circumflex coronary arteries is higher than that for left anterior descending grafts. Single-bypass grafts also tend to occlude more often than grafts with sequential anastomoses. In both instances, however, the presence of higher blood rates in the grafts may contribute significantly to their improved patency rates.

B. Late SVBG Patency (Table 5)

Several studies published in the last 15 years have shown a close correlation between SVBG atherosclerosis and plasma lipid levels [53–58]. Two recent clinical trials have conclusively shown that aggressive lipid-lowering therapy can significantly reduce the long-term progression of atherosclerosis in SVBGs [59,60]. The Post Coronary Artery Bypass Graft Trial investigators have compared moderate to aggressive treatment of blood lipids on obstructive changes in SVBGs and have concluded that aggressive lowering of LDL cholesterol levels to below 100 mg per deciliters was very effective to reduce the progression of atherosclerosis in SVBGs [60]. Thus aggressive lipid-lowering therapy can be considered as a major determinant of late graft patency in hypercholesterolemic patients who have undergone coronary artery bypass surgery.

Because of its weak fibrous cap and high lipid content, the atherosclerotic lesion in SVBGs has a high tendency to rupture late after bypass surgery. Thus thrombosis superimposed on plaque rupture frequently contributes to late SVBG obstruction [40].

Finally, cigarette smoking and diabetes mellitus have been implicated as risk factors, often in association with hypercholesterolemia, for graft atherosclerosis and occlusion [56–58].

REFERENCES

1. Veterans Administration Coronary Artery Bypass Surgery Cooperative Study Group. Eleven-year survival in the Veterans Administration randomized trial of coronary bypass surgery for stable angina. N Engl J Med 1984; 311:1333–1339.
2. Varnauskas E, European Coronary Surgery Study Group. Twelve-year follow-up of survival in the randomized European Coronary Surgery Study. N Engl J Med 1988; 319:332–337.
3. Alderman EL, Bourassa MG, Cohen LS, Davis KB, Kaiser GC, Mock MB, Pettinger M, Robertson TL, CASS Investigators. Ten-year follow-up of survival and myocardial infarction in the randomized Coronary Artery Surgery Study. Circulation 1990; 82:1629–1646.
4. Yusuf S, Zucker D, Peduzzi P, Fisher LD, Takaro T, Kennedy JW, Davis K, Killis T, Passamani E, Norris R, Morris C, Mathur V, Varnauskas E, Chalmers TC. Effect of coronary artery bypass graft surgery on survival: overview of 10-year results from randomized trials by the Coronary Artery Bypass Graft Surgery Trialists Collaboration. Lancet 1994; 344:563–570.
5. Naunheim KS, Fiore AC, Wadley JJ, McBride LR, Kanter KR, Pennington DG, Barner HB, Kaiser GC, Willman VL. The changing profile of the patient undergoing coronary artery bypass surgery. J Am Coll Cardiol 1988; 11:494–498.
6. Christakis GT, Ivanov J, Weisel RD, Birnbaum PL, David TE, Salerno TA. The changing pattern of coronary artery bypass grafting. Circulation 1989; 80:I-151–I-161.
7. Parsonnet V, Dean D, Bernstein AD. A method of uniform stratification of risk for evaluating the results of surgery in acquired adult heart disease. Circulation 1989; 79:I-3–I-12.
8. Grondin CM, Campeau L, Lespérance J, Enjalbert M, Bourassa MG. Comparison of late changes in internal mammary artery and saphenous vein grafts in two consecutive series of patients 10 years after operation. Circulation 1984; 70(suppl I): 208–212.
9. Barner HB, Standeven JW, Reese J. Twelve-year experience with internal mammary artery for coronary artery bypass. J Thorac Cardiovasc Surg 1985; 9:668–675.
10. Lytle BW, Loop FD, Cosgrove DM, Ratliff NB, Easley K, Taylor PC. Long-term (5 to 12 years) serial studies of internal mammary artery and saphenous vein coronary bypass grafts. J Thorac Cardiovasc Surg 1985; 89:248–258.

11. Loop FD, Lytle BW, Cosgrove DM, Stewart RW, Goormatic M, Williams GW, Golding LAR, Gill CC, Taylor PC, Sheldon WC, Proudfit WL. Influence of the internal-mammary-artery graft on 10-year survival and other cardiac events. N Engl J Med 1986; 314:1–6.

12. Cameron A, Kemp HG Jr, Green GE. Bypass surgery with the internal mammary artery graft; 15 year follow-up. Circulation 1986; 74(suppl III):30–36.

13. Ivert T, Huttunen K, Landou C, Bjork VO. Angiographic studies of internal mammary artery grafts 11 years after coronary artery bypass grafting. J Thorac Cardiovasc Surg 1988; 96:1–12.

14. Galbut DL, Traad EA, Dorman MJ, DeWitt PL, Larsen PB, Kurlansky PA, Button JH, Ally JM, Gentach TO. Seventeen-year experience with bilateral internal mammary artery grafts. Ann Thorac Surg 1990; 49:195–201.

15. Fiore AC, Naunheim KS, Dean P, Kaiser GC, Pennington DG, Willman VL, McBride LR, Barner HB. Results of internal thoracic artery grafting over 15 years. Single versus double grafts. Ann Thorac Surg 1990; 49:202–209.

16. Barner HB, Barnett MG. Fifteen- to twenty-one-year angiographic assessment of internal thoracic artery as a bypass conduit. Ann Thorac Surg 1994; 57:1526–1528.

17. Cameron AA, Green GE, Brogno DA, Thornton J. Internal thoracic artery grafts: 20-year clinical follow-up. J Am Coll Cardiol 1995; 25:188–192.

18. Boylan ML, Lytle BW, Loop FD, Taylor PC, Borsh JA, Goormatic M, Cosgrove DM. Surgical treatment of isolated left anterior descending coronary stenosis. Comparison of left internal mammary artery and venous autograft at 18 to 20 years of follow-up. J Thorac Cardiovasc Surg 1994; 107:657–662.

19. Acar C, Jebara VA, Porroghese M, Beyssen B, Pagny JY, Grare P, Chachques K, Fabiani JN, Deloche A, Guermonprez JL, Carpentier AF. Revival of the radial artery for coronary artery bypass grafting. Ann Thorac Surg 1992; 54:652–660.

20. Morgenstern DA, Mills NL. New conduits for coronary artery bypass. Coronary Artery Dis 1993; 4:677–681.

21. Nwasokwa ON. Coronary artery bypass graft disease. Ann Intern Med 1995; 123: 528–454.

22. Bourassa MG, Lespérance J, Campeau L, Simard P. Factors influencing patency of aortocoronary vein grafts. Circulation 1972; 45(suppl I):I-79–I-85.

23. Lespérance J, Bourassa MG, Saltiel J, Grondin C. Late changes in aortocoronary vein grafts. Angiographic features. Am J Roentgenol Rad Ther Nucl Med 1972; 116:74–81.

24. Lespérance J, Bourassa MG, Biron P, Campeau L, Saltiel J. Aorta to coronary artery saphenous vein grafts. Preoperative angiographic criteria for successful surgery. Am J Cardiol 1972; 30:459–465.

25. Grondin C, Castonguay Y, Lespérance J, Bourassa MG, Campeau L, Grondin P. Attrition rate of aorta-to-coronary artery saphenous vein grafts after one year. A study in a consecutive series of 96 patients. Ann Thorac Surg 1972; 14:223–231.

26. Lespérance J, Bourassa MG, Saltiel J, Campeau L, Grondin CM. Angiographic changes in aortocoronary vein grafts. Lack of progression beyond the first year. Circulation 1973; 48:633–643.

27. Campeau L, Crochet D, Lespérance J, Bourassa MG, Grondin CM. Postoperative changes in aortocoronary saphenous vein grafts revisited. Angiographic studies at

2 weeks and at one year in two series of consecutive patients. Circulation 1975; 52:369–377.

28. Campeau L, Lespérance J, Corbara F, Hermann J, Bourassa MG. Aortocoronary saphenous vein bypass graft changes 5 to 7 years after surgery. Circulation 1978; 59(suppl I):I-70–I-75.

29. Grondin C, Campeau L, Lespérance J, Solymoss BC, Vouhé P, Castonguay YR, Meere C, Bourassa MG. Atherosclerotic changes in coronary vein grafts six years after operation. Angiographic aspect in 110 patients. J Thorac Cardiovasc Surg 1979; 77:24–31.

30. Bourassa MG, Campeau L, Lespérance J, Grondin CM. Changes in grafts and in coronary arteries after saphenous vein aortocoronary bypass surgery. Results at repeat angiography. Circulation 1982; 65(suppl II):II-90–II-97.

31. Campeau L, Enjalbert M, Lespérance J, Vaislic C, Grondin CM, Bourassa MG. Atherosclerosis and late closure of aortocoronary saphenous vein grafts. Sequential angiographic studies at 2 weeks, 1 year, 5 to 7 years, and 10 to 12 years after surgery. Circulation 1983; 68(suppl II):II-1–II-7.

32. Bourassa MG, Enjalbert M, Campeau L, Lespérance J. Progression of atherosclerosis in coronary arteries and bypass grafts: Ten years later. Am J Cardiol 1984; 53:102C–107C.

33. Bourassa MG, Fisher LD, Campeau L, Gillespie MJ, McConney M, Lespérance J. Long-term fate of bypass grafts: the Coronary Artery Surgery Study (CASS) and Montreal Heart Institute experiences. Circulation 1985; 72(suppl V):71–78.

34. Lytle BW, Loop FD, Cosgrove DM, Ratliff NB, Eastley K, Taylor PC. Long-term (5–12 years) serial studies of internal mammary artery and saphenous vein coronary artery bypass grafts. J Thorac Cardiovasc Surg 1990; 15:15–20.

35. FitzGibbon GM, Burton JR, Leach AJ. Coronary bypass graft fate. Angiographic grading of 1400 consecutive grafts early after operation and of 1132 after one year. Circulation 1978; 5:1070–1074.

36. FitzGibbon GM, Leach AJ, Keon WJ, Burton JR, Kafka HP. Coronary bypass graft fate. Angiographic study of 1179 vein grafts early, one year, and five years after operation. J Thorac Cardiovasc Surg 1986; 91:773–778.

37. FitzGibbon GM, Leach AJ, Kafka HP, Keon WJ. Coronary bypass graft fate: long-term angiographic study. J Am Coll Cardiol 1991; 17:1075–1080.

38. FitzGibbon GM, Kafka HP, Leach AJ, Keon WJ, Hooper GD, Burton JR. Coronary bypass graft fate and patient outcome: Angiographic follow-up of 5065 grafts related to survival and reoperation in 1388 patients during 25 years. J Am Coll Cardiol 1996; 28:616–626.

39. Campos EE, Cinderella JA, Farhi ER. Long-term angiographic follow-up of normal and minimally diseased saphenous vein grafts. J Am Coll Cardiol 1993; 21: 1175–1180.

40. Solymoss BC, Leung TK, Pelletier LC, Campeau L. Pathologic changes in coronary artery saphenous vein grafts and related etiologic factors. In: Waters DD, Bourassa MG, eds. Care of the Patient with Previous Coronary Bypass Surgery: Cardiovascular Clinics. Philadelphia: F.A. Davis Company, 1991:45–65.

41. Lam JYT, Solymoss BC, Campeau L. Platelets and thrombosis in vein graft occlusion: Role of the patient. In: Waters DD, Bourassa MG, eds. Care of the Patient

with Previous Coronary Bypass Surgery: Cardiovascular Clinics. Philadelphia: F.A. Davis Company, 1991:67–81.

42. Chesebro JH, Clement IP, Fuster V, Elveback LR, Smith HC, Bardsley WT, Frye RL, Holmes DR Jr, Vlietstra RE, Pluth JR, Wallace RB, Puga FJ, Orszulak TA, Piehler JM, Schaff HV, Danielson K. A platelet-inhibitor drug trial in coronary-artery bypass operations: Benefit of perioperative dipyridamole and aspirin therapy on early postoperative vein-graft patency. N Engl J Med 1982; 307:73–78.

43. Goldman S, Copeland J, Moritz T, Henderson W, Zadina K, Ovitt T, Doherty J, Read R, Chesler E, Sako Y, Lancaster L, Emery R, Sharma GVRK, Josa M, Pacold I, Montoya A, Parikh D, Sethi G, Holt J, Kirklin J, Shabetai R, Moores W, Aldridge J, Masud Z, Demota H, Floten S, Haakenson C, Harker LA. Improvement in early saphenous vein graft patency after coronary artery bypass surgery with antiplatelet therapy. Circulation 1988; 77:1324–1332.

44. Goldman S, Copeland J, Moritz T, Henderson W, Zadina K, Ovitt T, Doherty J, Read R, Chesler E, Sako Y, Lancaster L, Emery R, Sharma GVRK, Josa M, Pacold I, Montoya A, Parikh D, Sethi G, Holt J, Kirklin J, Shabetai R, Moores W, Aldridge J, Masud Z, DeMots H, Floten S, Haakenson C. Saphenous vein graft patency 1 year after coronary artery bypass surgery and effects of antiplatelet therapy. Results of a Veterans Administration Cooperative Study. Circulation 1989; 80:1190–1197.

45. Paz MA, Lupon J, Bosch X, Pomar JL, Sanz G, and the GESIC Study Group. Predictors of early saphenous vein aortocoronary bypass graft occlusion. Ann Thorac Surg 1993; 56:1101–1106.

46. Cataldo G, Braga M, Pirotta N, Lavezzari M, Rovelli F, Marubini E, on behalf of Studio Indobufene Nell Bypass Aortocoronarico (SINBA). Factors influencing 1-year patency of coronary artery saphenous vein grafts. Circulation 1993; 88: 93–98.

47. Chesebro JH, Fuster V, Elveback LR, Clements IP, Smith HC, Holmes DR, Bardsley WR, Pluth JR, Wallace RB, Puga FJ, Orszulak TA, Piehler JM, Danielson GK, Schaff HV, Frye RL. Effect of dipyridamole and aspirin on late vein-graft patency after coronary bypass operations. N Engl J Med 1984; 310:209–214.

48. Brown BG, Cukingnan RA, De Rouen T, Goede LV, Wong M, Fee HJ, Roth JA, Carey JS. Improved graft patency in patients treated with platelet-inhibiting therapy after coronary bypass surgery. Circulation 1985; 72:138–146.

49. Pfisterer M, Jockers G, Regenass S. Trial of low-dose aspirin plus dipyridamole versus anticoagulants for prevention of aortocoronary vein graft occlusion. Lancet 1989; ii:1–7.

50. Sanz G, Pajaron A, Alegria E, Coello I, Cardona M, Fournier JA, Gomez-Recio M, Ruano J, Hidalgo R, Medina A, Oller G, Colman T, Malpartida F, Bosch X, and the Grupo Espanol para el Seguimiento del Injerto Coronario (GESIC). Prevention of early aortocoronary bypass occlusion by low-dose aspirin and dipyridamole. Circulation 1990; 82:765–773.

51. Limet R, David JL, Magotteaux J, Larock M, Rigo P. Prevention of aorta-coronary bypass graft occlusion. Beneficial effect of ticlopidine on early and late patency rates of venous coronary bypass grafts: a double-blind study. J Thorac Cardiovasc Surg 1987; 94:773–783.

52. Van der Meer J, Hillege HL, Kootstra GJ, Ascoop CAPL, Mulder BJM, Pfisterer M, van Gilst WH, Lie KL. Prevention of one-year vein-graft occlusion after aortocoronary-bypass surgery; a comparison of low-dose aspirin, low-dose aspirin plus dipyridamole, and oral anticoagulants. Lancet 1993; 342:257–264.
53. Lie JT, Lawrie GM, Morris GC Jr. Aortocoronary bypass saphenous vein graft atherosclerosis: Anatomic study of 99 vein grafts from normal and hyperlipoproteinemic patients up to 75 months postoperatively. Am J Cardiol 1977; 40:906–914.
54. Atkinson JB, Forman MB, Perry JM, Virmani R. Correlation of saphenous vein bypass graft angiograms with histologic changes at necropsy. Am J Cardiol 1985; 55:952–955.
55. Atkinson JB, Forman MB, Vaughn WK, Robinowitz M, McAllister HA, Virmani R. Morphologic changes in long-term saphenous vein bypass grafts. Chest 1985; 88:341–348.
56. Neitzel GF, Barboriak JS, Pintar K, Qureshi I. Atherosclerosis in aortocoronary bypass grafts: morphologic study and risk factor analysis 6 to 12 years after surgery. Arteriosclerosis 1986; 6:594–600.
57. Palac RT, Meadows WR, Hwang MH, Loeb HS, Pifarre R, Gunnar RM. Risk factors related to progressive narrowing of aortocoronary vein grafts studied 1 and 5 years after surgery. Circulation 1982; 66(suppl I):40–44.
58. Campeau L, Enjalbert M, Lespérance J, Bourassa MG, Kwiterovich P Jr, Wacholder S, Sniderman A. The relation of risk factors to the development of atherosclerosis in saphenous vein bypass grafts and the progression of disease in the native circulation: a study 10 years after aortocoronary bypass surgery. N Engl J Med 1984; 311:1329–1332.
59. Blankenhorn DH, Nessim SA, Johnson RL, Sanmarco ME, Azen SP, Cashin-Hemphill L. Beneficial effects of combined colestipol-niacin therapy on coronary atherosclerosis and coronary venous bypass grafts. JAMA 1987; 257:3233–3240.
60. The Post Coronary Artery Bypass Graft Trial Investigators. The effect of aggressive lowering of low-density lipoprotein cholesterol levels and low-dose anticoagulation on obstructive changes in saphenous-vein coronary-artery bypass grafts. N Engl J Med 1997; 336:153–162.

4
Changes in Venous Autografts Used as Aortocoronary Conduits

William C. Roberts
Baylor University Medical Center, Dallas, Texas

Since its introduction 30 years ago, numerous patients have benefited from coronary artery bypass grafting. Despite its benefits to most patients, coronary bypass is not free of complications. Stenosis or complete occlusion of venous grafts used as aortocoronary conduits still occurs. While all venous grafts develop some morphologic changes, the degree and functional significance of the changes vary widely. This chapter describes structural changes observed early and late in saphenous veins used as aortocoronary conduits.

I. DEGREES OF NARROWING OF THE NATIVE EPICARDIAL CORONARY ARTERIES IN SYMPTOMATIC MYOCARDIAL ISCHEMIA

Before focusing on the changes in saphenous veins used as aortocoronary conduits, a brief discussion on the status of the native epicardial coronary arteries in patients likely to undergo aortocoronary bypass grafting appears appropriate. Examination at necropsy or examination of coronary endarterectomy specimens during life of the four major (right, left main, left anterior descending, and left circumflex) epicardial coronary arteries in patients over 30 years of age with symptomatic myocardial ischemia and angiographic narrowing >50% in diameter of one or more major coronary arteries discloses that atherosclerotic plaques are present in virtually every 5-mm segment of the entire lengths of the arteries [1,2]. In patients with angiographically so-called "single-vessel disease," approximately 40% of the lumen of each 5-mm segment of the four major arteries (average of 54 segments per patient) is obliterated by plaque; in patients with angiographically "double-vessel disease," approximately 50% of the total lumen is obliterated by plaque; in patients with "triple-vessel disease," approximately 60% of the total lumen is filled with plaque; and in patients with "quadruple-vessel disease," approximately 70% of the total lumen is filled with plaque. Thus, the greater the number of major coronary arteries significantly narrowed at angiography, the greater the total amount of atherosclerotic plaque in the major epicardial coronary arteries.

II. THE NORMAL SAPHENOUS VEIN

The normal human saphenous vein contains a thin *intima* consisting of relatively acellular fibrous tissue covered by a single layer of endothelial cells separated from the media by a rudimentary internal elastic membrane. The *media* consists of multiple layers of smooth muscle cells separated by bundles of collagen, ground substance, and occasional short elastic fibers. Most medial smooth muscle layers have a circular orientation; in areas near the venous valves, however, the middle circular layers have a more longitudinal arrangement. Frequently, longitudinally oriented smooth muscle fascicles make up the innermost layers of the media. The *adventitia* is composed of bundles of collagen with scattered fascicles of longitudinally oriented smooth muscle cells. Broad, loose bands of elastic fibers are present in abundance. Vasa vasorum are present and may extend into the outermost portion of the media.

III. FINDINGS IN REMNANT SAPHENOUS VEINS EXCISED FOR AORTOCORONARY CONDUITS BUT NEVER USED

Some degree of intimal fibrous thickening occurs commonly in saphenous veins excised for aortocoronary bypass but never used. Waller and Roberts [3] examined nearly 3,500 cm of unused but excised saphenous vein from 402 patients having coronary bypass surgery. The length of the unused saphenous veins ranged from 0.5 to 52 cm per patient (mean 8.5). A histologic section was examined from each of the 6,788 5-mm-long segments: The lumen in 0.4% of the sections was narrowed 76–100% in cross-sectional area by fibrous tissue; 0.6% were narrowed 51–75% in cross-sectional area; 12% were narrowed 26–50%; and 87% were narrowed 25% or more in cross-sectional area. The percentage of 5-mm segments of unused vein narrowed more than 75% in cross-sectional area was similar in men and women, and it was similar in each of five decades (31–40, 41–50, 51–60, 61–70, and 71–80 years). Thus, approximately 1% of saphenous veins excised for coronary bypass are narrowed more than 50% in cross-sectional area by fibrous tissue before they are used as aortocoronary conduits.

IV. NUMBER OF AORTIC ANASTOMOTIC SITES, NUMBERS OF CONDUITS, AND NUMBERS OF CORONARY ANASTOMOTIC SITES

I doubt if any two surgeons perform the bypass operation in quite the same manner, and such individual variations may affect patient outcome and graft outcome. The phrases "two bypasses" and "three bypasses" and "four bypasses" are commonly used, but their meaning is not always precise. I suspect that most users of the phrase "three bypasses" are referring to the number of coronary anastomoses. A patient may have three coronary anastomotic sites and only one conduit ("round-the-world" bypass) or two conduits or three conduits with similar numbers of aortic anastomotic sites. To prevent confusion, it might be best always to state the number of aortic anastomosis sites, the number of conduits, and the number of coronary anastomotic sites. To me it seems most reasonable for each of these three to be the same: If a patient is to have three coronary anastomotic sites, it might be ideal to have three conduits and three separate aortic anastomitic sites. If only one conduit is used with a single aortic anastomotic site and the single conduit is anastomosed to seven different coronary arteries, the outcome is not ideal if the single aortic anastomosis closes or the single conduit closes proximally. With similar numbers of aortic anastomotic sites, conduits, and coronary anastomotic sites, this circumstance is less likely to occur.

The location of the coronary anastomotic site appears to be relatively similar with most surgeons. The distal 1 cm of the right coronary artery is probably ideal, because the most severe narrowing of this artery tends to be its distal third rather than the proximal or middle third [4]. The most common anastomotic site of the left anterior descending artery is probably about two-thirds down its length, and this location, of course, is logical, because this artery tends to be more severely narrowed in its proximal third than in either its middle or its distal third [4]. The same situation also appears reasonable for the first diagonal artery. Anastomoses in the obtuse marginal arteries are usually within 3 cm of their origin from the left circumflex.

Tension on the conduit is one of the various technical factors that can affect flow in aortocoronary conduits [5]. Abnormal tension is indicated by grooving or indentation into the right atrial wall or right atrioventricular sulcus or by flattening of the graft passing anterior to the pulmonary trunk. If the graft is under tension, leakage at the bypass anastomosis is probably more likely than without tension. *Twisting of a conduit* may prevent successful bypass grafting [6].

V. EARLY CHANGES IN SAPHENOUS VEINS USED AS AORTOCORONARY CONDUITS

In 1906, Carrel and Guthrie [7] described intimal thickening of veins implanted into the arterial system in dogs, and concluded that veins placed in the arterial circulation had a strong tendency to assume the character of an artery. In further vein transplantation experiments in 1908, Carrel [8] described four characteristic changes in veins used as arteries in the peripheral circulation: (a) intimal thickening, (b) adventitial thickening (from fibrosis), (c) loss of the inner one-third of the media, and (d) loss of elastic fibers producing a fibrous tube. In addition, medial hypertrophy was observed in some grafts. These changes have subsequently been confirmed in humans in saphenous veins used for femoral–popliteal and aortocoronary bypass.

Spray and Roberts [9,10] studied a large number of saphenous vein grafts from patients dying within a year after aortocoronary bypass. Vein grafts from patients dying intraoperatively showed minimal medial edema (clear spaces between layers of smooth muscle) and disrupted adventitia (occurring during excision of the vein before grafting). By two weeks, mural edema was more pronounced, some medial smooth muscle cells were necrotic, and inflammatory infiltrates were present. The endothelium often was disrupted, and the intimal surface usually was covered, either partially or completely, by fibrin. By three weeks, cells with characteristics of smooth muscle appeared in the subendothelial portion of the intima. The cells generally were oriented such that their longest diameter was parallel to the direction of blood flow. Thereafter, the subendothelial intimal lesions became more generalized, less cellular ground substance appeared in abundance, and short elastic fibers and vascular channels occasionally were present. The smooth muscle fibers of the media gradually diminished in number and were replaced, in part or in whole, by fibrous tissue. Fibrous tissue also increased in the adventitia, and its elastic fibers became severely disrupted or disappeared completely. Organizing fibrin on the external surface of the grafts probably contributed to the adventitial fibrosis. Capillaries were present in the adventitia, and they often extended into the fibrotic media. Thus, the saphenous vein used as an artery becomes a fibrous-tissue conduit.

VI. LATE CHANGES IN SAPHENOUS VEINS USED AS AORTOCORONARY CONDUITS

Kalan and Roberts [11] described at necropsy findings in 123 saphenous vein grafts and in 1,865 5-mm segments of the grafts in 53 patients who had had a single aortocoronary bypass operation 13–185 months (mean 58) before death. Of the 53 patients, 32 (60%) died from a cardiac cause, and of their 73 saphenous vein aortocoronary conduits, 36 (49%) were narrowed at some point more than 75% in cross-sectional area by atherosclerotic plaque. The remaining 21 patients (40%) died from a noncardiac cause, and of their 50 saphenous vein conduits, 10 (20%) were narrowed at some point more than 75% in cross-sectional area by plaque. Of the 53 patients, 31 (58%) had at least one bypass graft maximally narrowed greater than 75% in cross-sectional area at some point by fibromuscular tissue with or without lipid; 12 patients (23%) had maximal graft narrowing of 51–75%; 8 patients (15%), 26–50%; and 2 patients (4%), 0–25%. The percentage of patients with a graft narrowed over 75% at necropsy did not increase as the interval from bypass surgery to death increased.

Of the 123 saphenous vein grafts, 47 (38%) were maximally narrowed greater than 75% in cross-sectional area; 44 (36%), 51–75%; 22 (18%), 26–50%; and 10 (8%), 0–25%. Of the 47 grafts narrowed over 75% in cross-sectional area, 29 actually were narrowed greater than 95% in cross-sectional area by fibrous tissue. The percentage of saphenous veins narrowed greater than 75% at necropsy was not affected by gender (men 38%, women 36%), presence or absence of systemic hypertension (40% vs. 33%), or presence or absence of diabetes mellitus (30% vs. 48%). The percentage of grafts narrowed over 75% in cross-sectional area did not correlate with the interval between bypass surgery and death or with the coronary artery to which the graft was connected.

The degree of narrowing of the saphenous vein graft was related to the degree of luminal narrowing of the native coronary artery at, or within 2 cm distal to, the saphenous vein–coronary artery anastomosis. Of the 49 grafts attached to a coronary artery that was narrowed greater than 75% at or distal to the anastomosis, 33 (67%) were significantly narrowed; of the 74 grafts attached to a coronary artery narrowed less than 75% distal to the anastomotic site, 14 (19%) were severely narrowed.

Analysis of the 1,865 5-mm-long saphenous vein segments disclosed that 209 segments (11%) were narrowed 96–100% in cross-sectional area; 172 (5%), 76–95%; 407 (22%), 51–675%; 685 (37%), 26–50%; and 392 (21%), 0–25%. Similar percentages of segments were narrowed greater than 75% in men and women (22% vs. 15%); in diabetics and nondiabetics (18% vs. 26%), and in hypertensives and nonhypertensives (21% vs. 20%). Further, the interval from coronary bypass to death did not correlate with the percentage of segments severely narrowed.

Although the percentage of saphenous vein segments narrowed greater than 75% in cross-sectional area at necropsy did not correlate with the interval from bypass grafting to death, it did relate to the mode of death. Of the 32 patients dying from a cardiac cause, 295 (27%) of 1,104 saphenous vein segments were narrowed greater than 75%, whereas of the 21 patients dying from a noncardiac cause, 86 (11%) of 761 saphenous vein segments were so narrowed. The percentage of segments of native coronary artery narrowed greater than 75% was similar in patients with cardiac and noncardiac modes of death [673 of 1,441 (47%) vs. 333 of 895 (37%)].

VII. COMPOSITION OF TISSUE CAUSING LUMINAL NARROWING LATE IN THE SAPHENOUS VEINS USED AS AORTOCORONARY CONDUITS

Lipid was present in the wall of a graft (Figure 1) in 39 of the 53 patients (74%). Fifteen had intracellular lipid alone (foam cells), and 24 had both foam cells and extracellular lipid. Extracellular lipid was not found in a saphenous vein graft until 26 months after bypass. Lipid was present in 69 (56%) of the 123 saphenous vein grafts from the 39 patients. Intracellular lipid was present in all 69 grafts, either alone (33 grafts) or along with extracellular lipid (36 grafts). The amount of lipid present appeared to increase as the interval from coronary bypass to death increased. Foam cells were located near the luminal surfaces of the intimal fibrous tissue, and they did not narrow the lumen appreciably. Extracellular lipid deposits were located deeper in the plaque, separated from the lumen by a layer of fibrous tissue, and they often contributed significantly to luminal narrowing.

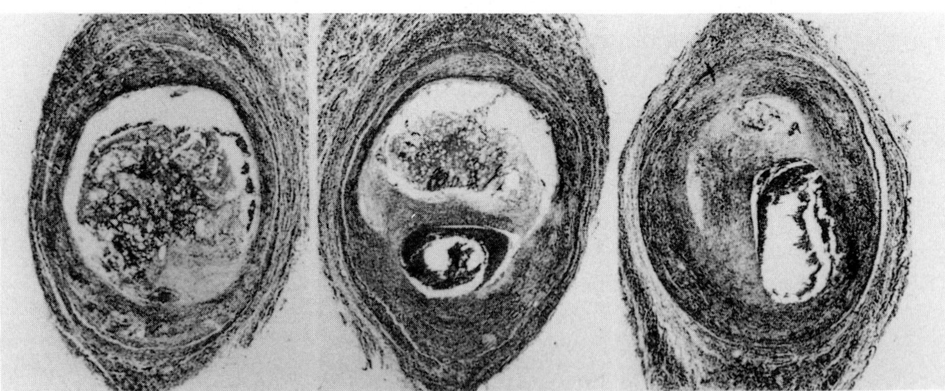

Figure 1 Saphenous vein to right coronary artery in a 44-year-old woman (NNMC No. A83-104) who died of chronic congestive heart failure 43 months after four-vessel bypass. This graft was the only graft severely narrowed. Left, at this site, graft is totally occluded by combination of fibrous tissue and pultaceous debris that contains both extravasated erythrocytes and fibrin. Open space in this section is an artifact of sectioning. Center, narrowing at this site is due primarily to extracellular lipid. Right, narrowing at this site is due mainly to fibrous tissue. Residual lumen (middle and right) contain postmortem clot. (Movat stains. Each 20×.) (From Ref. 27.)

Hemorrhage into plaque (into the lipid portion only) was found in 26 (21%) of the saphenous vein grafts from 17 (32%) of the patients (Figure 2). It was seen as early as 24 months after bypass, and it did not increase in frequency thereafter as the interval from bypass to death increased. Luminal narrowing greater than 75% in cross-sectional area was significantly more common in grafts with plaque hemorrhage than in those without.

Luminal thrombus was present in 16 (13%) of the saphenous vein grafts from 14 (26%) of the patients. Thrombus was not seen until 32 months after bypass, and its frequency did not increase thereafter as the interval from bypass to death increased. Thrombus within the graft lumen was present in 16 of 69 grafts that had deposits of lipid in their walls (Figure 3), and was present in none of 54 grafts devoid of lipid. In 14 of these 16 grafts, hemorrhage into plaque also was found.

Calcific deposits were present in 13 (11%) of the 123 saphenous vein grafts from 11 patients, and they were first seen 34 months after coronary bypass. All the deposits were small. They were present in 18 (1%) of the 1,865 5-mm saphenous vein segments.

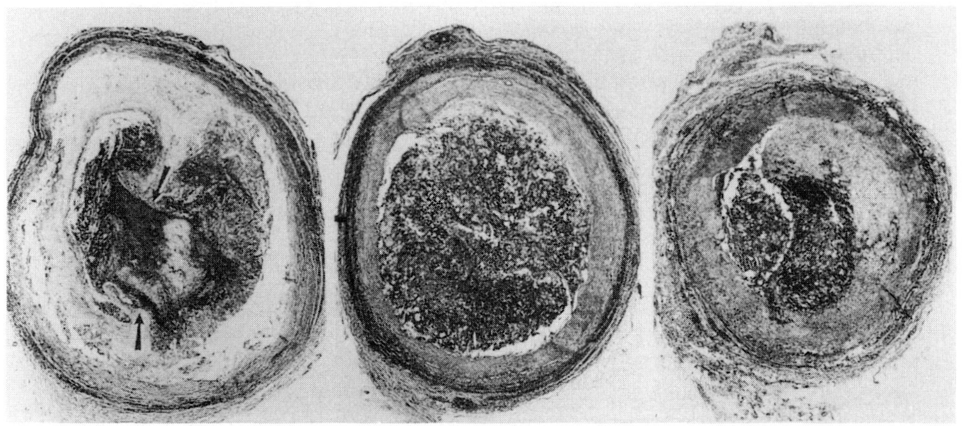

Figure 2 Saphenous vein to left anterior descending coronary artery in a 69-year-old man (NNMC No. A84-122) who died of acute myocardial infarction 34 months after three-vessel bypass. Two of the three conduits, one of which is shown here, were severely narrowed. Left, in the section shown here, fibrous capsule over extracellular lipid has ruptured (between arrows) with thrombus in residual lumen and hemorrhage into pultaceous debris. Center, lumen at this site is occluded by organizing fibrous tissue and hemorrhage into pultaceous debris. Right, at this level there is fibrous tissue, organizing thrombus, and hemorrhage into plaque. Each 5-mm segment of the saphenous vein conduits is different. (Movat stains. Each 20×.) (From Ref. 27.)

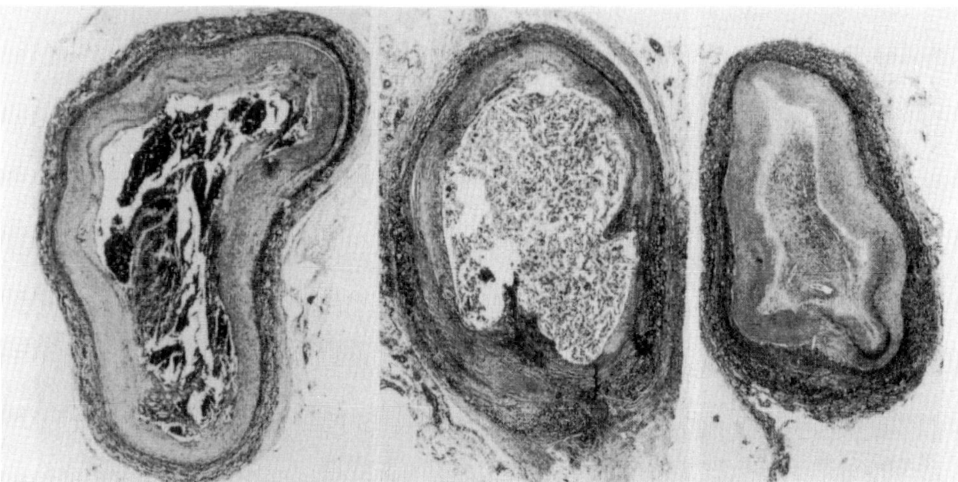

Figure 3 Saphenous vein graft to right coronary artery at three different sites in a
63-year-old man (GT No. 84A-137) who died of cancer (malignant mesothelioma) 144
months after insertion of saphenous vein graft coronary artery and internal mammary
artery to left anterior descending coronary artery. He never had evidence of myocardial
ischemia postoperatively. Saphenous vein graft was occluded and internal mammary
artery graft was wide open. Left, at this site, thrombus is present in the graft. Center,
at this site, lumen is obliterated, mainly by pultaceous debris. Right, at this site, graft
is occluded by fibrous tissue except for a few revascularized channels. (Movat stains.
Each 20×.) (From Ref. 27.)

The aforementioned data indicate that virtually all saphenous veins used
as aortocoronary conduits for longer than a year develop atherosclerotic plaques
in each 5-mm segment of their entire lengths. Thus, the late atherosclerotic
plaquing in saphenous veins used as aortocoronary conduits is diffuse, just as
it is in native coronary arteries in patients with fatal myocardial ischemia [1,2].
The amounts of luminal narrowing in the saphenous veins used as aortocoronary conduits were significantly greater in those patients who died from
a cardiac cause than in those who died from a noncardiac cause. Surprisingly,
the interval from coronary bypass to death did not correlate with either the
percentage of vein conduits or the percentage of 5-mm segments of vein conduit narrowed over 75% in cross-sectional area by plaque. Moreover, the percentage of 5-mm segments of saphenous vein conduit severely narrowed was
similar in the 35 patients surviving up to 5 years compared to the 18 patients
surviving over 5 years.

The composition of the plaques in the saphenous vein conduits is similar to that in the native coronary arteries. Fibrous tissue or fibromuscular tissue was the dominant component of the plaques in the saphenous vein conduits, just as it is the dominant component of plaques in the native coronary arteries in patients with fatal coronary artery disease without coronary bypass [12,13].

The frequency of the various modes of death among the patients dying late after coronary bypass is a bit different from that of patients with symptomatic myocardial ischemia without coronary bypass [14]. Of the 53 coronary bypass patients studied, only 32 (60%) died from a cardiac cause; therefore, 21 (40%) died from a noncardiac cause. Among patients with symptomatic myocardial ischemia who do not have coronary bypass, approximately 95% die from a cardiac cause. The fact that 40% of the bypass cases studied died from a noncardiac cause supports the view that the bypass operation in many patients prolongs life, long enough in many to develop various fatal noncardiac conditions. Of the 53 bypass patients reported by Kalan and Roberts [11], 10 (19%) died from cancer, a percentage far higher than for patients with symptomatic myocardial ischemia not having coronary surgery.

The study by Kalan and Roberts [11] reemphasizes that coronary bypass is useful but that it does not deter progression of the underlying atherosclerotic process. In a slight way, the bypass operation might even cause acceleration of the atherosclerotic process, because in about 25% of persons having coronary bypass the serum total cholesterol increases and the body weight increases substantially during the first year after operation. Because lowering the serum (or plasma) total cholesterol level (and specifically the low-density lipoprotein [LDL] cholesterol) decreases the chances of "heart attack" and may cause some portion of atherosclerotic plaques to regress and other portions to at least not progress, a strong case can be advanced for combined simultaneous initiation of both low-fat, low-cholesterol diet therapy and lipid-lowering drug therapy as soon as is reasonably feasible after a coronary bypass operation [15].

In January 1997, the Post Coronary Artery Bypass Graft Trial Investigators [16] reported results of studying 1,351 patients who had undergone aortocoronary bypass grafting 1–11 years earlier and who had LDL cholesterol levels between 130 and 175 mg/dL, triglyceride levels <300 mg/dL, and at least one patent vein graft on coronary angiography. The study divided the patients into those in whom an "aggressive" treatment plan was employed, with the goal of lowering LDL cholesterol to 60–85 mg/dL, and those in whom a "moderate" treatment plan was employed, with the goal of lowering LDL cholesterol to 130–140 mg/dL. In the aggressive treatment group a mean of 76 ± 13 mg of lovastatin was employed, and 30% also received 8 g/day of cholestyramine; in the moderate treatment group a mean of 4 ± 1 mg of lovastatin was employed, and 5% also received 8 g/day of cholestyramine. Coronary angiography was repeated an average of 4.3 years after the baseline angiogram. The primary angiographic outcome was the mean percentage per patient of grafts with a decrease of 0.6 mm or more in lumen diameter. As measured annually during the study, the mean LDL cholesterol level of patients who received aggressive treatment ranged from 93 to 97 mg/dL; with moderate treatment, the range was from 132 to 136 mg/dL. The mean percentage of grafts with progression of atherosclerosis was 27% for patients whose LDL cholesterol level was lowered with aggressive treatment and 39% for those who received moderate treatment. There was no significant difference in angiographic outcome between the patients receiving warfarin and those who did not receive warfarin. The rate of revascularization over the four years of study was 29% lower in the group whose LDL cholesterol level was lowered aggressively compared to the group receiving moderate treatment (6.5% vs. 9.2%). Thus, aggressive lowering of LDL cholesterol levels to <100 mg/dL reduced the progression of atherosclerosis in aortocoronary bypass grafts. This recent study, therefore, gives strong support to the use of lipid-lowering agents, particularly the statin drugs, after aortocoronary bypass operations to lower the LDL cholesterol to <100 mg/dL.

VIII. CAUSES OF MORPHOLOGIC CHANGES IN SAPHENOUS VEINS USED AS AORTOCORONARY CONDUITS

Although the causes of the changes in saphenous vein grafts are in many ways similar to the causes leading to atherosclerotic plaques in native coronary arteries [17], additional mechanisms almost surely play a role when a vein is switched to an arterial location. The early changes in the saphenous veins are similar to the phlebosclerotic lesions in venous varicosities, changes presumably caused by the response of the vein to increases in hydrostatic pressure. Arteriovenous shunts of any origin (congenital, traumatic, or iatrogenic) show intimal thickening, presumably the result of increased pressure and flow. Subendothelial proliferative lesions in the pulmonary arteries of patients with pulmonary hypertension and in vena cava and portal veins in patients with chronic right-sided congestive cardiac failure or portal hypertension also are seen in the saphenous veins transferred to the aortocoronary position. Brody and colleagues [18,19] attempted to differentiate the effects of pressure and ischemia on femoral vein grafts in dogs. Vein segments were either left intact or dissected free from their adventitia, thereby severing the vasa vasora and producing medial ischemia. Next, the vein segments either were left in the venous system or were arterialized by creation of an arteriovenous fistula. The presence of medial ischemia in the absence of elevated pressure and flow produced medial fibrosis in the vein without subendothelial intimal proliferative lesions. Elevated intravascular pressure alone, however, without alterations in blood supply to the media by the vasa vasorum produced intimal lesions without evidence of medial fibrosis. The combination of elevated intraluminal pressure and medial ischemia resulted in medial and intimal changes similar to the changes seen in human saphenous veins used as aortocoronary conduits.

The intimal process in saphenous veins, and specifically the degree of luminal narrowing in saphenous veins in the aortocoronary position, is almost certainly accelerated when flow through the conduit is relatively poor. The major cause of poor flow is severe narrowing in the native coronary artery (to which the vein is attached) at or just distal to the site of anastomosis [9–11,20]. The smaller the native coronary arteries to which the graft is to be connected, the less the amount of atherosclerotic plaque necessary to cause significant luminal narrowing. Smaller-sized hearts have smaller coronary arteries than larger-sized hearts [21]. Small patients tend to have smaller hearts than larger patients. Thus, similar amounts of plaque cause more luminal narrowing in small patients than in large patients. Women, on average, are smaller than men, and, therefore, on average they have smaller hearts and smaller coronary arteries. Coronary bypass might be expected therefore to have poorer results in women than in men because the smaller arteries might cause poor flow through the conduits by plaque in the native coronary arteries.

Kalan and Roberts [22] found this very scenario to be probably the case. Their 121 necropsy patients dying within 60 days of a coronary bypass operation had significantly lower mean heart weights than did the 90 patients dying late, and this fact held true for both sexes. Most patients with normal-sized hearts were in the early-death group; conversely, most patients in the late-death group had hearts of increased weight. These findings suggest that patients with normal- or near-normal-sized hearts have a higher early mortality after coronary bypass than do persons with hearts of increased weight. Furthermore, more changes leading to luminal narrowing of bypass conduits might be expected in persons with small native coronary arteries (small hearts), because the runoff through the graft may not be as good as in patients with larger native coronary arteries (larger hearts).

IX. COMPARISON OF MORPHOLOGIC CHANGES IN SAPHENOUS VEINS TO THOSE IN INTERNAL MAMMARY ARTERIES USED AS AORTOCORONARY CONDUITS

For practical purposes, none of the aforedescribed changes in saphenous veins used as aortocoronary conduits are found in internal mammary arteries used in the coronary position. As pointed out by others clinically [23,24], the patency rate both early and late is splendid with the mammary artery but much less with the saphenous vein. Although the internal mammary artery late after bypass remains much smaller than the saphenous vein when each is utilized in the same patient, the internal mammary artery remains virtually devoid of intimal deposits, whereas the saphenous vain (in the same patient), although much larger, may develop severe atherosclerotic plaque in its lumen [25,26].

REFERENCES

1. Roberts WC. Qualitative and quantitative comparison of amounts of narrowing by atherosclerotic plaques in the major epicardial coronary arteries at necropsy in sudden coronary death, transmural acute myocardial infarction, transmural healed myocardial infarction and unstable angina pectoris. Am J Cardiol 1989; 64: 324–328.
2. Roberts WC. Coronary "lesion," coronary "disease," "single-vessel disease," "two-vessel disease": word and phrase misnomers providing false impressions of the extent of coronary atherosclerosis in symptomatic myocardial ischemia. Am J Cardiol 1990; 66:
3. Waller BF, Roberts WC. Remnant saphenous veins after aortocoronary bypass grafting: analysis of 3,394 centimeters of unused vein from 402 patients. Am J Cardiol 1985; 55:65–71.
4. Vlodaver Z, Edwards JE. Pathology of coronary atherosclerosis. Progr Cardiovasc Dis 1971; 14:256–274.
5. Spray TL, Roberts WC. Tension on coronary bypass conduits. A neglected cause of real or potential obstruction of saphenous vein grafts. J Thorac Cardiovasc Surg 1976; 72:282–287.
6. Roberts WC, Lachman AS, Virmani R. Twisting of an aortocoronary bypass conduit. A complication of coronary surgery. J Thorac Cardiovasc Surg 1978; 75: 772–776.
7. Carrel A, Guthrie CC. Results of biterminal transplantation of veins. Am J Med Sci 1906; 132:415–422.
8. Carrel A. Results of transplantation of blood vessels, organs, and limbs. JAMA 1908; 51:1662–1667.
9. Spray TL, Roberts WC. Status of the grafts and the native coronary arteries proximal and distal to coronary anastomotic sites of aortocoronary bypass grafts. Circulation 1977; 55:741–749.
10. Spray TL, Roberts WC. Changes in saphenous veins used as aortocoronary bypass grafts. Am Heart J 1977; 94:500–516.
11. Kalan JM, Roberts WC. Morphologic findings in saphenous veins used as coronary arterial bypass conduits for longer than 1 year: necropsy analysis of 53 patients, 123 saphenous veins, and 1,865 five-millimeter segments of veins. Am Heart J 1990; 119:1164–1184.
12. Kragel AH, Reddy SG, Wittes JT, Roberts WC. Morphometric analysis of the composition of atherosclerotic plaques in the four major epicardial coronary arteries in acute myocardial infarction and in sudden coronary death. Circulation 1989; 80:1747–1756.

13. Kragel AH, Reddy SG, Wittes JT, Roberts WC. Morphometric analysis of the composition of coronary arterial plaques in isolated unstable angina pectoris with pain at rest. Am J Cardiol 1990; 66:

14. Roberts WC, Potkin BN, Solus DE, Reddy SG. Mode of death, frequency of healed and acute myocardial infarction, number of major epicardial coronary arteries severely narrowed by atherosclerotic plaque, and heart weight in fatal atherosclerotic coronary artery disease: analysis of 889 patients studied at necropsy. J Am Coll Cardiol 1990; 15:196–203.

15. Roberts WC. Lipid-lowering after an atherosclerotic event. Am J Cardiol 1989; 64:693–695.

16. The Post Coronary Artery Bypass Graft Trial Investigators. The effect of aggressive lowering of low-density lipoprotein cholesterol levels and low-dose anticoagulation on obstructive changes in saphenous-vein coronary-artery bypass grafts. N Engl J Med 1997; 336(3):153–162.

17. Roberts WC. Preventing and arresting coronary atherosclerosis. Am Heart J 1995; 130:580–600.

18. Brody WR, Kosek JC, Angell WW. Changes in vein grafts following aortocoronary bypass induced by pressure and ischemia. J Thorac Cardiovasc Surg 1972; 64: 847–854.

19. Brody WR, Angell WW, Kosek JC. Histologic fate of the venous coronary artery bypass in dogs. Am J Pathol 1972; 66:111–130.

20. Waller BF, Roberts WC. Amount of narrowing by atherosclerotic plaque in 44 nonbypassed and 52 bypassed major epicardial coronary arteries in 32 necropsy patients who died within 1 month of aortocoronary bypass grafting. Am J Cardiol 1980; 46:956–962.

21. Roberts CS, Roberts WC. Cross-sectional area of the proximal portions of the three major epicardial coronary arteries in 98 necropsy patients with different coronary events. Relationship to heart weight, age, and sex. Circulation 1980; 62: 953–959.

22. Kalan JM, Roberts WC. Significance of cardiac weight in patients having coronary artery bypass grafting for angina pectoris. Am J Cardiol 1988; 62:36–40.

23. Grondin CM, Campeau L, Lesperance J, Enjalbert M, Bourassa MG. Comparison of late changes in internal mammary artery and saphenous vein grafts in two consecutive series of patients 10 years after operation. Circulation 1984; 70(suppl I): I-208-I-212.

24. Loop FD, Lytle BW, Cosgrove DM, Stewart RW, Goormastic M, Williams GW, Golding LAR, Gill CC, Taylor PC, Sheldon WC, Proudfit WL. Influence of the internal-mammary-artery graft on 10-year survival and other cardiac events. N Engl J Med 1986; 314:1–6.

25. Barbour DJ, Roberts WC. Additional evidence for relative resistance to atherosclerosis of the internal mammary artery compared to saphenous vein when used to increase myocardial blood flow. Am J Cardiol 1985; 56:488.

26. Kalan JM, Roberts WC. Comparison of morphologic changes and luminal sizes of saphenous vein and internal mammary artery after simultaneous implantation for coronary arterial bypass grafting. Am J Cardiol 1987; 60:193–196.

5

Molecular and Cellular Biology of Saphenous Vein Bypass Graft Disease

Mark J. Ricciardi
University of Michigan Medical Center, Ann Arbor, Michigan

David W. M. Muller
St. Vincent's Hospital, Darlinghurst, New South Wales, Australia

In the late 1800s, the first attempts to transplant segments of artery and vein into the canine carotid arterial circulation failed because of acute graft thrombosis. Using improved surgical techniques, Carrel, in 1908, successfully achieved graft patency [1] and noted that while the interposed artery "does not undergo marked modification," the jugular vein "quickly undergoes structural changes, consisting chiefly of the thickening of its wall" [1]. The advent of coronary artery bypass grafting some 60 years later made this and many subsequent studies highly relevant for the large proportion of patients who ultimately experience early postoperative graft failure or late graft atherosclerosis and occlusion. Complementary angiographic studies performed over the past two decades have quantified the extent of the problem. One month after arterialized vein grafting, approximately 10% of grafts are already occluded; at 1 year, 17% are occluded, and 9% are diseased; at 5 years, 26% are occluded, and 42% are diseased; and at 10 years, 50% are occluded, with half of the remaining vein grafts severely atherosclerotic [2–4]. Graft failure occurs by three major, time-dependent mechanisms. Early failure occurs predominantly because of thrombotic closure. Intimal thickening, particularly at the proximal and distal anastomoses, causes recurrent ischemia in the intermediate term, and late failure occurs as a result of progressive atherosclerosis. The strong correlation between graft patency and long-term clinical outcome [5] makes an understanding of these processes, and of the potential for molecular and genetic therapies to improve vascular graft patency, of great relevance and considerable clinical importance.

I. HISTOPATHOLOGY OF VEIN GRAFT DISEASE

A. The Normal Saphenous Vein

The normal saphenous vein has a thin intima of acellular fibrous tissue covered by a single layer of endothelial cells. The intima is separated by the internal elastic membrane from the media, which consists of multiple layers of smooth muscle cells surrounded by collagen, ground substance, and elastic fibers. Smooth muscle cell orientation in the media is circular, except at the level of the venous valves, where the muscle fibers are arranged longitudinally. The adventitia consists mostly of bundles of collagen with some longitudinally oriented smooth muscle cells. The vasa vasorum lies within the adventitia and extends to the interface with the media. When compared with a similarly sized artery, the vein has a thinner media and lower overall wall thickness.

B. Human Histologic Studies

Studies of explanted human saphenous vein grafts have documented a series of events that ultimately lead to graft failure. An almost universal finding in these studies is a substantial degree of endothelial damage [6,7]. Analyses of unused vein graft segments, harvested at the time of operation, showed focal endothelial denudation throughout the length of the harvested vein segments [8]. This suggests that even before exposure to the shear forces of the arterial circulation, the venous endothelium is injured by surgical handling and loss of its vasa vasorum. These immediate changes are followed rapidly by infiltration of the subendothelial tissues and media by inflammatory cells [9,10], and by the formation of a fibrinous coating over the graft surface. Within 4 days of implantation, macrophages can be detected in the intima and media by monoclonal antibody staining [9].

Following these early changes, intimal and medial thickening occurs [11–14]. Proliferation of fibroblasts, smooth muscle cells, and capillaries occurs early [14], and within 2 months of implantation, smooth muscle cells are detectable in the neointima; intimal and medial cellularity subsequently diminish, with an increase in fibrous tissue and collagen content in all three cell layers. Such findings led Spray and Roberts to conclude that within 2 months of implantation, the saphenous vein in the aortocoronary position becomes a "stiff, fibrous-tissue conduit" [15].

II. BIOLOGY OF VEIN GRAFT DISEASE

A. Vein Graft Thrombosis

Immediately after implantation, the engrafted vein segment becomes largely denuded of endothelium, even with meticulous surgical technique, and the graft surface is covered by a layer of fibrin and adherent platelets. Early thrombotic occlusion may occur when these events are combined with poor flow through the graft due to surgical factors (such as proximal or distal anastomotic stenosis), distal native vessel disease, or a large mismatch between the size of the graft and the native coronary artery. Regeneration of the vein graft endothelium confers some protection against mural thrombus formation. However, it is probable that the newly regenerated endothelium does not provide the resistance to thrombosis of the original endothelium for several weeks. Previous studies [16] have suggested, for example, that recovery of vasomotor function after arterial injury is delayed well beyond the period required for complete endothelial regeneration. Although not well studied in an experimental vein graft model, the synthesis by regenerated endothelium of glycosaminoglycans, including heparin sulfate, has been studied in the balloon denuded rabbit aorta model. In the study of Alavi and colleagues [17], when compared with control vessels, synthesis of glycosaminoglycans by aortic segments with a re-endothelialized neointima was increased threefold. However, glycosaminoglycan release into the medium was markedly reduced when compared to controls, suggesting that the regenerated endothelium may function as a "reverse barrier," preventing release of anticoagulant glycosaminoglycans at the luminal surface of the vessel [17]. Similar studies have not been reported for the synthesis of plasminogen activators. However, it is possible that the release of these antithrombotic proteins from the neoendothelium is also compromised for several months after endothelial denudation and repair, not only in injured arteries, but also in surgically manipulated, denuded vein graft segments.

In addition to changes in propensity for thrombosis related to surgical injury, veins may be inherently more susceptible to thrombus formation than arteries, particularly when placed in the arterial circulation. Yang and colleagues [18], while studying the effects of saphenous vein nitric oxide on the vessel wall–platelet interaction, noted that basal nitric oxide release in the saphenous vein is less than that in the internal mammary artery. They postulated that saphenous vein endothelium is less capable than arterial endothelium of inhibiting platelet binding to the vessel wall. To test this hypothesis, they studied in vitro a series of 5-mm rings of internal mammary artery and saphenous vein [19]. Internal mammary artery rings, precontracted with noradrenaline, relaxed when exposed to aggregating platelets, and this platelet-induced relaxation of the artery was inhibited by L-*N*-monomethylarginine

(L-NMMA), an inhibitor of nitric oxide formation. In contrast, similarly prepared saphenous vein rings contracted further when exposed to platelet aggregates. These studies support the postulate that platelet-mediated ADP release causes release of nitric oxide from the internal mammary artery but not from the saphenous vein endothelium. Because endogenous nitric oxide also inhibits platelet adhesion to vascular endothelium [20], this implies that the saphenous vein may be more susceptible to platelet adhesion and aggregation than the internal mammary artery [19]. Thus, the native vein, which is well suited to inhibiting the fibrin-dependent mechanisms that predominate in the low-pressure, venous circulation [21], is less well suited to inhibiting the platelet-mediated thrombotic events that predominate in the arterial circulation.

B. Neointimal Thickening

Histopathology

After the initial phase of platelet adhesion and fibrin formation at the surface of the engrafted vein, a second phase follows in which the vessel wall thickens over a period of 6–12 months. Within several days of engraftment, the denuded subendothelial tissue and inner media of the vein segment become infiltrated with inflammatory cells. Smooth muscle cell proliferation follows, with connective tissue matrix production and replication of the internal elastic lamina and elastic fibers in the media. Using a pig model of vein grafting in the carotid artery, Angelini and coworkers [22] performed sequential histologic and DNA concentration and density studies over a 39-week period. Whereas intimal thickness remained unchanged 1 week after grafting, medial expansion occurred in association with prominent medial smooth muscle cell proliferation. Between 1 and 4 weeks, this rapid medial hyperplasia continued, in conjunction with neointimal thickening, which developed without an increase in overall cell number. In fact, cell density declined over this time, implying that medial and intimal thickening resulted from events other than cell proliferation, such as cell migration, hypertrophy, and extracellular matrix deposition. A similar experiment, using thymidine incorporation to detect cell turnover [23], showed progressive intimal and medial thickening, with declining rates of cell proliferation up to 12 weeks after grafting, highlighting the importance of cell migration, hypertrophy, and matrix deposition in the later stages of development of the neointima (Figure 1).

Stimuli for Neointimal Thickening

   Surgical Manipulation.   The events just outlined are stimulated by a variety of factors, including the autocrine and paracrine release of mitogens and chemoattractant factors, and infiltration of the vessel wall by circulating

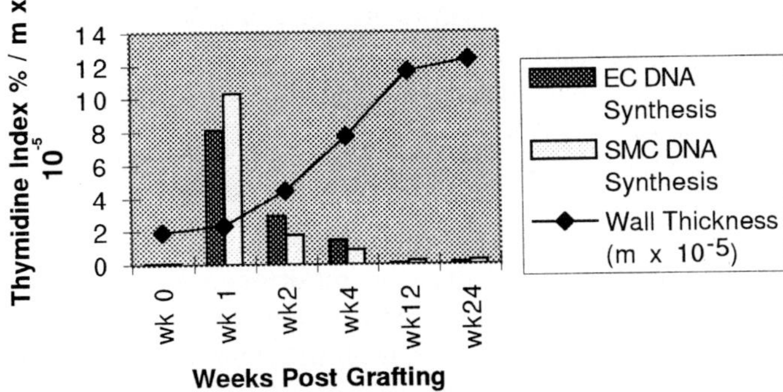

Figure 1 Vein graft DNA synthesis and hypertrophy: Although DNA synthesis of endothelial cells (EC) and smooth muscle cells (SMC) in the transplanted vein starts to decline after week 1, progression of wall thickness continues through week 12. This demonstrates the importance of cell migration and protein synthesis in vessel wall hypertrophy. EC = endothelial cells; SMC = smooth muscle cells. (Adapted from Ref. 23.)

inflammatory cells. These events are promoted both by the injury of surgical manipulation and by the hemodynamic changes associated with arterialization of the thin-walled vein. The trauma associated with surgical manipulation alone may be sufficient to promote neointimal thickening. Moggio and colleagues [24], for example, demonstrated expression of the immediate-early genes, c-*fos* and c-*myc*, within 1 hour of vein graft harvesting, even with very minimal tissue manipulation. c-*fos* and c-*myc* typically increase transiently after growth factor stimulation and are believed to encode transcription factors that regulate subsequent gene activation and entry into the cell cycle. Expression of these immediate-early genes also occurs after endothelial denudation [25] and after vascular injury [26,27].

Endothelial injury.   The second major stimulus to intimal thickening is the endothelial denudation that results from perioperative vein injury. Like the arterial endothelium, the intact venous endothelial layer controls vasomotor tone, platelet adhesion, thrombus formation, and the level of cellular proliferation. Disruption of the endothelial layer, whether through surgical handling or changes in wall stress, has clear implications for vessel wall neointimal formation and vessel patency [23,28]. Soyombo and colleagues [28] examined the influence of the endothelium on smooth muscle cell proliferation and showed a preferential, intimally directed vascular smooth muscle cell proliferative response. They speculated that intimal regulation is mediated by the subendothelial environment through concentration gradients of a variety of cytokines. These include the endothelium-derived vasodilators, nitric oxide (NO) and prostacyclin, which suppress medial smooth muscle cell proliferation, and a variety of mitogens that promote proliferation, including platelet-derived growth factor (PDGF) and basic fibroblast growth factor (FGF). Disruption or disease of the endothelium results in an altered balance of these regulatory factors and loss of normal inhibition of cell proliferation.

Nitric oxide, in particular, appears to have an important role in the regulation of vascular cell proliferation. Early in vitro studies showed that nitric oxide inhibits mitogenesis and proliferation of rat vascular smooth muscle cells [29]. Neointimal formation in balloon-injured rat aortas was also found to be inhibited by the nitric oxide precursor L-arginine [30]. Similarly, in a carotid vein graft model, Davies and colleagues [31] reported a 47% reduction in intimal area after treatment with L-arginine, with evidence of preserved endothelial integrity and function as demonstrated by a vasodilator response to acetylcholine and serotonin. Another study, intriguing because it highlights the complex interaction between vessel wall cells and their products, was performed by Fukuo and colleagues [32]. These investigators showed that while induction of nitric oxide synthase in vascular smooth muscle cells cocultured with endothelial cells inhibited the proliferation of smooth muscle cells, it also caused the release of basic fibroblast growth factor and stimulated migration and proliferation of endothelial cells. Thus, high concentrations of nitric oxide, which are cytotoxic to vascular smooth muscle cells, may lead to the release of basic fibroblast growth factor, which facilitates endothelial cell proliferation. This mechanism may be important in vascular repair after injury, including the repair associated with arterialization of saphenous vein grafts.

It is of interest to note that there may be important differences between saphenous veins and mammary arteries in their response to cytokines. Nguyen and colleagues [33], for example, demonstrated that the number of basic FGF receptors (high affinity and low affinity) in nondistended vein segments was significantly higher in saphenous veins than in internal mammary arteries, and that high-pressure distension to 200 mm Hg resulted in a significantly greater rise in FGF receptor density in the veins than in the mammary artery segments. The potency for smooth muscle cells of PDGF also appears to be far greater for human saphenous veins than for internal mammary arteries.

Mononuclear Cell Infiltration.   Neointimal thickening after vein grafting is also mediated by mononuclear cell infiltration and activation. Mononuclear cells possess several unique properties. Unlike hypoxic endothelial cells, which do not proliferate when cultured alone [34], macrophages do express and secrete mitogenic substances under hypoxic stress [35]. To explore further the macrophage–endothelial cell interaction and the mechanism behind vessel wall repair with hypoxia, Kuwabara and colleagues [36] studied endothelial cells, macrophages, and growth factor levels at various levels of hypoxic stress. Northern blot analysis of hypoxic capillary endothelial cells revealed a dramatic downregulation of FGF mRNA and upregulation of FGF receptor transcripts (flg), a finding consistent with previous studies showing greater high-affinity cell surface binding sites for [^{125}I]FGF on hypoxic endothelial cells [34]. When medium from hypoxic macrophage cultures was added to hypoxic capillary and aortic endothelial cells, a dose-dependent stimulation of growth was observed. In contrast, conditioned medium from macrophages at normal oxygenation, from hypoxic smooth muscle cells, and from fibroblasts caused no increase in incorporation of tritiated thymidine by cultured endothelial cells.

These findings suggest that macrophage cell death and the release of intracellular contents did not account for the observed endothelial cell growth. Cell cycle inhibitors, but not metabolic inhibitors, blocked the increased expression of FGF and PDGF, signifying de novo synthesis of these growth factors. When these same macrophages were returned to normoxic conditions, they no longer stimulated endothelial cell proliferation. Polyclonal antibodies directed against various growth factors mixed with the hypoxic macrophage medium identified acid FGF, basic FGF, and PDGF as mitogens, with basic FGF having the greatest endothelial cell mitogenic effect. When antibodies to the three growth factors were added to hypoxic macrophage medium, endothelial cell proliferation was blocked by 80%. In a hypoxic milieu therefore, macrophages present early in the reparative process and express growth factors that act to stimulate endothelial growth. It is highly likely, therefore, that mononuclear cell infiltration is a major stimulus to neointimal thickening after vein grafting.

Influence of Hemodynamic Changes. In addition to direct vessel wall trauma, hemodynamic stresses are likely to play an important role in promoting neointimal thickening in arterialized vein grafts. The increased wall tension to which the initially thin-walled, large-lumen vein is exposed when placed in the arterial circulation appears to stimulate a specific adaptive response that results in normalization of the wall stress according to the law of LaPlace. With a constant luminal pressure, tangential wall stress is proportional to the ratio of radius-to-wall thickness [23]. Over time, the radius-to-wall thickness ratio of the transplanted vein decreases until it approaches that of the native artery, and then it remains constant. A similar phenomenon has been described in both the coronary arteries, which dilate in response to luminal narrowing [37], and arterio-venous fistulas, which increase in diameter in response to increased flow and increased mean shear stress [38]. These observations argue for an endothelium-dependent mechanism, since an intact endothelial layer must be established before the vessel adapts to achieve a wall shear stress suitable for the new circulatory environment. Consistent with the concept of preserved wall stress is the observation that there is conservation of radius-to-thickness ratio throughout a variety of artery types and animal species. Comparison of luminal diameter-to-wall thickness in 10 different mammalian species of different size, when perfused at a fixed pressure, revealed a constant ratio [39]. This finding, along with that of transposed vein graft thickening and dilatation, suggest a wall tension–dependent conservation of the wall thickness-to-diameter relationship.

Of the hemodynamic changes to which the transplanted vein is subjected, pulsatile stretch may be the most important stimulus to smooth muscle cell proliferation [40]. High pressure alone may not be sufficient to promote the adaptive response, since pressures within the lower extremity veins often approximate arterial pressures (70–80 mm Hg) during prolonged standing, and yet these vessels do not undergo a pathological degree of intimal thickening. The relationship between pulsatile stretch and tritiated thymidine incorporation, a marker for DNA synthesis and cell proliferation, was tested in one study in an in vitro model using internal mammary artery and saphenous vein smooth muscle cells cultured on deformable membranes [40]. After 24 hours of pulsatile stretch that mimicked the frequency and extent of stretch found in the proximal arterial circulation, tritiated thymidine incorporation doubled in the cultured saphenous vein smooth muscle cells while thymidine incorporation in the internal mammary cells was unchanged. Cell number at 24 hours was the same for both smooth muscle cell types, but at 6 days saphenous vein cell number had increased while the cell number from internal mammary artery segments remained constant. These observations support the concept that arterial smooth muscle cells are already adapted to pulsatile flow, whereas smooth muscle cells from veins, when transplanted from a linear to a pulsatile flow environment, respond by proliferating, a finding consistent with the preceding human histologic studies and with light microscopy data showing the lack of intimal thickening in internal mammary grafts [41,42].

Blood flow velocity waveforms and shear rates have also been studied in saphenous vein and internal mammary artery grafts to help elucidate the effects of hemodynamics on vessel wall change. While having a similar peak diastolic velocity, the saphenous vein graft, because of its larger diameter, has a lower shear rate than does the internal mammary artery [43]. Kraiss and coworkers [44] studied the effect of shear stress on neointimal thickening in a porous polytetrafluoroethylene graft model, a model that is free of confounding vasomotor changes. They noted that, in this model, elevated shear stress inhibits smooth muscle cell proliferation and neointimal thickening. These two observations suggest that high shear stress is protective, whereas lower shear stress, as occurs after saphenous vein grafting, stimulates intimal hyperplasia.

In related studies, Malek and colleagues [45] examined the influence of shear stress on basic FGF and PDGF B chain gene expression. Whereas endothelial gene expression of basic FGF was found to increase with high shear stress, downregulation of PDGF was observed with physiologic levels and with markedly elevated levels of fluid shear stress [45]. Thus, the proclivity for intimal hyperplasia of arterialized saphenous vein grafts may stem, in part, from shear stress-related changes in cytokine expression. Lower shear stress in the vein graft would lead to lower basic FGF expression, potentially leading to a loss of integrity of the endothelial cell layer, and to higher PDGF gene expression, resulting in smooth muscle cell proliferation and vasoconstriction. In contrast, the internal mammary artery graft is exposed to normal shear stresses, and thus to normal FGF and PDGF gene expression.

C. Changes in Vasoreactivity

In addition to developing the structural changes associated with neointimal thickening, arterialized vein grafts undergo a series of changes that render them more responsive to circulating vasoconstrictor hormones. These changes include an increased vasoconstrictor response to norepinephrine and the development of a constrictor response to serotonin [46–48]. Experimental studies suggest that these changes may be secondary to the induction of expression of novel G proteins involved in transmembrane signal transduction [49]. An increase in vasoreactivity may be important in normalizing shear stresses in vein grafts, and thus may contribute to the overall narrowing of the graft and eventually to a reduction of flow in the conduit.

III. VEIN GRAFT ATHEROSCLEROSIS

The early intimal hyperplastic changes that occur in vein grafts are followed by lipid uptake and the formation of more typical atherosclerotic vascular occlusions [50]. Histologic analyses have documented atherosclerotic changes, including fatty streaks, lipid-laden foam cells, and lipid inclusions in smooth muscle cells, in vein grafts in place for as little as 1 year [51,52]. The late atherosclerotic changes of aortocoronary vein grafts, seen after the first year, are histologically similar to those seen in native coronary arteries, but with one important difference: The lipid deposits observed in aging vein grafts are not typically encapsulated by a fibrous cap, but rather have a thin intimal endothelial layer and are thus more susceptible to thrombus formation and to distal atheroembolism. Clinical factors thought to influence the extent of atherosclerosis in vein grafts include hyperlipidemia, cigarette smoking, diabetes, the coronary vascular bed supplied, and graft age [2,53].

Dysfunction of the venous endothelium, like that of arterial endothelium, has been demonstrated in animals with vein grafts subjected to a high-cholesterol diet. These animals show changes in cell adhesion to the endothelial surface, particularly monocyte cell adhesion [54]. One of the mechanisms of atherosclerosis and endothelial dysfunction involves LDL oxidation by endothelial cells, which results in expression of vascular cell adhesion molecule (VCAM), a mononuclear leukocyte adhesion molecule [55]. Activated monocytes expressing the VLA_4 ligand then adhere to the endothelial surface and migrate to the subintima, where they ingest modified LDL, further oxidize LDL, and become foam cells. This leads to cytokine release and further macrophage proliferation and the formation of a typical fatty streak. These changes promote smooth muscle cell proliferation and migration. Progression of the lesion is marked by accumulation of necrotic debris, by cholesterol deposition, and by mural thrombosis, thrombus organization, matrix deposition, and cell proliferation. Plaque rupture and hemorrhage, which is made more likely by the absence of a well-defined fibrous cap, is thought to be the final event in the development of vessel occlusion.

It is probable that the accelerated vein graft atherosclerosis observed in clinical practice is augmented by the presence of a neointima. Clinical studies have suggested that the extent of lipid accumulation is proportional to the extent of neointimal thickening [56]. Furthermore, experimental studies have suggested that inhibition of intimal thickening may be associated with relative resistance to lipid deposition in the vein graft wall [57]. Other factors may also contribute to the vein graft's propensity for atherosclerotic change. Recent studies [58] have suggested, for example, that there may be differences in expression of matrix metalloproteinases (MMPs) between veins and arterial grafts. Metalloproteinases have been implicated in the pathogenesis of a number of vascular disease processes, including plaque rupture, and restenosis after PTCA. In the study of Guarda and colleagues [58], MMP-2 expression in vein grafts was much higher than in arterial grafts, but MMP-9 was expressed at lower levels. Both MMP-2 and MMP-9 were inhibited significantly by doxycycline [58]. Other inhibitors of metalloproteins, such as tissue inhibitor of metalloproteinase (TIMP), have been identified and offer potential novel therapies to stabilize vein graft plaque [59,60].

Whether arteries and veins do indeed differ in their propensity to lipid accumulation and atherosclerotic occlusion remains to be determined. Sophisticated molecular biology techniques, such as subtraction cloning of differentially expressed genes, is currently under way to determine whether or not the apparent resistance to atherosclerosis of the internal mammary artery is related to the expression of protective genes that are not expressed in vein graft segments [61].

IV. MOLECULAR/GENETIC APPROACHES TO THERAPY

Advances in surgical technique and medical therapies have undoubtedly had a salutary impact on vein graft patency [62,63]. In spite of these improvements, however, the event-free survival of patients with established saphenous vein graft disease remains very poor (see Chapters 9–11). For this reason, several novel approaches to inhibition of vein graft attrition have been explored. These include gene transfer using DNA encoding a variety of proteins that inhibit thrombus formation, monocyte binding, and cellular proliferation, and antisense oligonucleotide-mediated inhibition of cell cycle regulatory proteins.

A. Gene Transfer

In 1989, Wilson and colleagues [64] established the feasibility of implanting genetically modified synthetic vascular grafts. Endothelial cells cultured from canine jugular veins were infected with a replication-defective retrovirus containing a reporter gene expressing β-galactosidase. Dacron grafts seeded with these modified endothelial cells were implanted as carotid interposition grafts. After 5 weeks, the grafts were harvested, scanned by electron microscopy, and analyzed for the β-galactosidase enzyme product of the *lacZ* reporter gene. Scanning electron microscopy revealed a monolayer of cells with endothelial-like morphology in 10 of the 12 grafts studied. Of the populated grafts, all had β-galactosidase-positive cells. Although only 25–50% of the genetically modified cells seeded were detected after explantation, this study showed that seeding the surface of grafts with genetically modified endothelial cells is feasible, and that transfecting the endothelial cells with genes that confer protection against thrombosis or intimal hyperplasia could favorably impact graft patency.

Ex vivo gene transfer to harvested saphenous veins is also technically feasible and is a potential means of conferring resistance to vein graft atherosclerosis [65]. Because mononuclear cell infiltration has been identified as an early event in the process of neointima formation, blocking the binding of circulating monocytes to venous endothelium was explored in a model of saphenous vein grafting by Chen and colleagues by overexpressing a soluble form of vascular cell adhesion molecule (VCAM-1) [65]. VCAM-1 is a protein that is not constitutively expressed by uninjured endothelial cells. When induced by various cytokines, VCAM-1 is expressed by endothelial cells as well as by smooth muscle cells and macrophages in human atherosclerotic plaques [66,67]. When expressed, the molecule normally remains bound to the cell surface and mediates binding to activated mononuclear cells via its interaction with the VLA$_4$ ligand on the monocyte cell surface. In the study of Chen and colleagues [65], a soluble form of VCAM-1 (sVCAM) that competitively

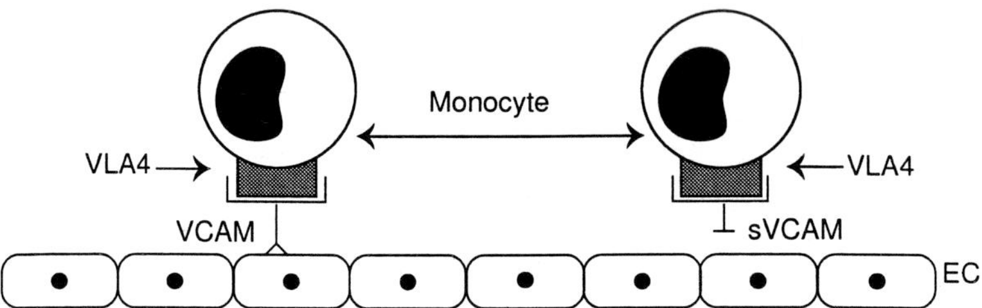

Figure 2 Vascular cell adhesion molecule (VCAM-1) mediates the binding of activated monocytes to the endothelial cell (EC) layer through a monocyte ligand (VLA$_4$). A soluble form of vascular cell adhesion molecule (sVCAM) inhibits monocyte binding by competitively binding the VLA$_4$ ligand. VLA$_4$ = monocyte receptor; VCAM = vascular cell adhesion molecule; sVCAM = soluble vascular cell adhesion molecule; EC = endothelial cell layer.

inhibits mononuclear cell binding to endothelial cells was used. The soluble VCAM was generated by site-directed mutagenesis to exclude the transmembrane domain of the VCAM molecule, thereby causing the sVCAM to be secreted into the extracellular space, where it competitively blocks binding of the mononuclear cell VLA$_4$ ligand to cell-bound VCAM (Figure 2). Recombinant adenoviruses containing the cDNA for sVCAM-1 were used to infect segments of human saphenous vein ex vivo, by exposing the luminal surface to the adenoviral solution for 90–120 minutes. The vein graft segments were excised 3 days after being interposed in the carotid artery position. Immunohistochemical staining and in situ hybridization studies demonstrated that gene transfer and expression (ex vivo and in vivo) were achieved with short incubation periods and high levels of gene transfer (Figure 3). These findings suggest that local in vivo gene expression is possible and may inhibit mural lipid accumulation by blocking macrophage infiltration. Long-term graft patency rates could therefore be improved by blocking one of the early "table-setting" events leading the saphenous vein graft atherosclerosis.

B. Antisense Technology

Before undergoing the dramatic process of cell division, the cell must undergo a growth phase during which time it prepares for division. This part of the cell cycle, known as interphase, starts with the G1 phase, when biosynthetic activity is prominent [68]. The S phase follows and represents DNA synthesis. G2 marks the time between DNA replication and nuclear and cytoplasmic division, which occurs during the M phase. Activation of cell cycle regulatory genes

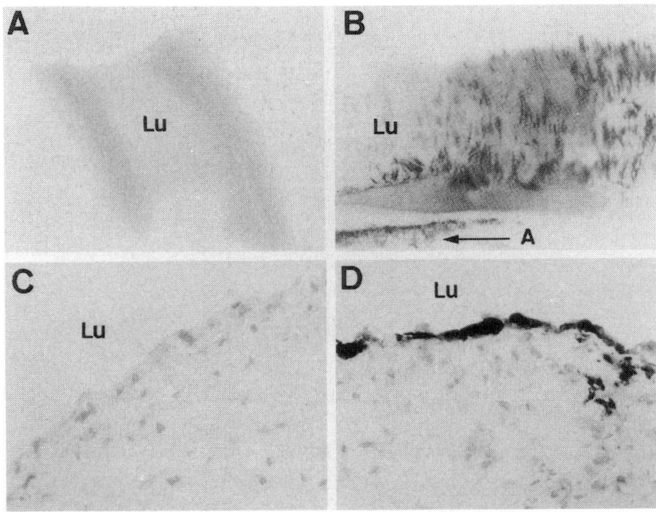

Figure 3　β-Galactosidase expression detected by en face section (A and B) and frozen section (C and D). X-Gal staining of vein grafts explanted on day 3. *LacZ* gene expression was not apparent in veins infected with AD.CB*sVCAM* (A and C) but was apparent in veins infected with Ad.CMV*lacZ* (B and D), particularly at the luminal surface (Lu) and in the adventitia (A). (From Ref. 65.)

controls the process of cell growth and division through cell division cycle (cdc) kinases [69,70].

Antisense oligonucleotide technology, a relatively new strategy used to inhibit the expression of specific genes, represents one strategy potentially useful in blocking the effects of genes that encode unwanted proteins. Antisense oligonucleotides hybridize with their target mRNAs, preventing them from being translated. When translation of the mRNA transcript is blocked, the protein encoded by the target gene cannot be synthesized. Targeting the *c-myb* gene, an important cell cycle regulatory gene, Simons and colleagues [71] were the first to demonstrate that mRNA translation and arterial neointima formation could be reduced by periadventitially delivering antisense oligonucleotides.

Morishita and colleagues [72] employed a similar strategy (Figure 4) to target cdk 2 kinase with oligonucleotides delivered intraluminally using hemagglutinating virus of Japan (HVJ)-liposome-mediated transfer. This method enhances uptake of oligonucleotides packaged in liposomes coated with inactivated HVJ by promoting fusion of the liposome with vascular cells,

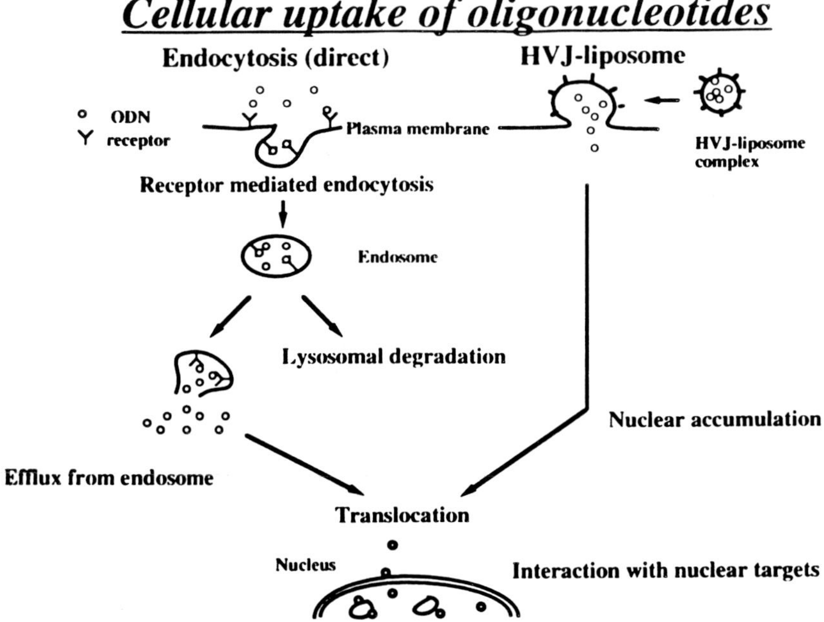

Figure 4   Postulated mechanisms of cellular uptake of oligos with HVJ-liposome method versus passive uptake. Oligos are taken up by endocytostic pathway and released from endosome. In contrast, oligos with HVJ-liposome method are transfected directly into cytoplasm and move rapidly into the nuclei. (From Ref. 72.)

thereby delivering the oligonucleotide intracellularly [73–75]. Using the balloon-injured rat carotid artery model, Morishita and colleagues [75] abolished the expected increase in cdk 2 kinase mRNA after balloon injury with a single intraluminal administration of antisense cdk 2 kinase oligonucleotide. Successful yet incomplete inhibition of neointima formation was observed at 2 weeks. Neointima formation was completely inhibited with the addition of antisense blockade of cdc 2 kinase (a second regulatory enzyme important in the G2/M phase).

Mann and colleagues [57] applied this technology to the vein graft. They argued that as an adaptive response, the vein graft undergoes remodeling through vascular hyperplasia and hypertrophy in order to normalize its diameter-to-wall-thickness ratio, thereby reducing wall tension and increasing wall shear stress to arterial levels. In the vein graft, hyperplasia leads to neointimal formation, a potentially maladaptive response that lends itself to accelerated atherosclerosis. The investigators set out to prove that by blocking vascular smooth muscle cell progression through the cell cycle by G0/1 phase arrest, they could engineer vein grafts that would arterialize by hypertrophy rather than by hyperplasia, without neointima formation and with a reduced susceptibility to atherosclerosis.

Using the previously described in vivo HVJ-liposome-mediated transfer method, Mann and colleagues [57] administered antisense oligonucleotides directed against both cdc 2 kinase and proliferating cell nuclear antigen (PCNA) to New Zealand white rabbit jugular veins. This combination of antisense oligonucleotide blockade was previously shown to be effective in preventing neointimal hyperplasia in an arterial balloon injury model by Morishita and colleagues [76]. Transfection entailed perfusing the dissected vein segment with the HVJ-liposome complex preparation for 20 minutes before anastomosing it into the ipsilateral carotid position. Untreated and sense- and missense-oligonucleotide-treated vein grafts served as controls.

Fluorescence studies revealed nuclear localization of the oligonucleotides in medial cells. The fivefold to tenfold increase in cdc 2 kinase and PCNA protein levels seen in controls was diminished by 90% in treated vein segments [57]. The antisense-treated veins also had markedly fewer cells undergoing DNA replication. Morphometric analysis showed that antisense-oligonucleotide-treated grafts underwent overall vessel wall thickening to the same degree as controls, but predominantly in the form of medial hypertrophy, with a medial thickness of treated grafts approximating the overall thickness of control grafts. In contrast, the increase in wall thickness of the control grafts occurred predominantly by extensive neointimal hyperplasia.

The authors also showed that with high-cholesterol feeding, large numbers of foam cells were found in the intima and in areas of macroscopic plaque of untreated and control transfected grafts. No plaque formation was seen in the antisense-treated vein segments, and only rare macrophages were noted [57]. These observations suggest that by blocking the proliferative, hyperplastic response that occurs in vein segments interposed in an arterial circuit, mechanical stability and wall stress adjustments can still occur without predisposing the grafted vein to accelerated atherosclerosis and ultimate graft failure.

C. Alternative Molecular Therapies

Under conditions of normal homeostasis, cell proliferation is balanced by programmed cell death or apoptosis. Early population dynamics and cell kinetic studies by Thomas and colleagues [77,78] examined the occurrence of apoptosis in atherosclerotic lesions. Using the hypercholesterolemic balloon-injured swine model, these investigators showed a link between cell proliferation in atherosclerotic plaques and nonrandom cell death. Medial cells in nonlesion areas showed low levels of random cell death and necrosis, whereas cells in atherosclerotic lesions showed a prominence of nonrandom cell death. There is now evidence that this cell death is not secondary to local toxins but instead is a regulated phenomenon [79]. This process, unlike necrosis or nonprogrammed cell death, occurs by cell shrinkage with maintenance of membrane integrity. The resultant apoptotic bodies are then phagocytosed by neighboring cells without inciting an inflammatory response [79]. Unlike cell necrosis, apoptosis also requires de novo gene expression and protein synthesis. Apoptotic pathways have been established in various organisms. In the mammal, the interleukin-1 beta converting (ICE) gene encodes proteases that are believed to be responsible for executing the process of cell death [80]. The gene that protects against apoptosis is the proto-oncogene *bcl-2*. Using morphologic, immuno-histochemical, and in situ terminal deoxynucleotidyl transferase–mediated dUTP nick end labeling (TUNEL) analysis as markers for apoptosis, Geng and colleagues [81] and Isner and colleagues [82] identified apoptotic vascular smooth muscle cells and macrophages in primary and restenotic atherosclerotic coronary and peripheral arteries. The highest degrees of apoptosis were seen in areas of ongoing cellular proliferation. The mammalian cell death gene ICE has been shown to localize to areas of TUNEL-positive smooth muscle cells and macrophages [83]. These more recent data strongly argue for the role of programmed cell death in modulating cell proliferation and atheroma development.

Whether dysfunction of the apoptotic pathways is also important in the genesis of vein graft degeneration remains to be determined. Conceivably, local overexpression of the proteases that cause apoptosis may also minimize the extent of intimal thickening and lipid uptake that occur in arterialized vein grafts.

V. CONCLUSION

The very early experimental observations that vein grafts undergo structural wall changes that may be maladaptive forewarned of the great potential for graft failure after saphenous vein coronary artery bypass surgery. Endothelial cell damage, through surgical handling, loss of vasa vasorum, and increased wall stress, initiates a process that involves the complex interplay between mononuclear leukocytes, platelets, vascular smooth muscle cells, growth factors, and cell cycle regulatory elements, leading to an adaptive increase in wall thickness through neointimal hyperplasia and medial hypertrophy.

Neointimal formation increases the graft susceptibility to accelerated atherosclerosis, a process that is accentuated by established risk factors, especially elevated LDL cholesterol. Ultimately, plaque progression and thrombotic closure results in attrition of more than 75% of grafts in place for 10 years. New advances in endothelial cell modification through gene therapy and blockade of intimal hyperplasia through antisense therapy, together with appropriate risk factor modification, offer the potential for substantial improvements in the longevity of arterialized vein grafts, with a corresponding improvement in the clinical efficacy of surgical revascularization.

REFERENCES

1. Carrel A. Results of the transplantation of blood vessels, organs and limbs. JAMA 1908; 20:1662–1667.
2. Campeau L, Enjalbert M, Lesperance J, Bourassa MG, Kwiterovich P, Jr, Wacholder S, Sniderman A. The relation of risk factors to the development of atherosclerosis in saphenous-vein bypass grafts and the progression of disease in the native circulation. A study 10 years after aortocoronary bypass surgery. N Engl J Med 1984; 311:1329–1332.
3. FitzGibbon GM, Leach AJ, Keon WJ, Burton JR, Kafka HP. Coronary bypass graft fate. Angiographic study of 1,179 vein grafts early, one year, and five years after operation. J Thorac Cardiovasc Surg 1986; 91:773–778.
4. Grondin CM, Campeau L, Lesperance J, Enjalbert M, Bourassa MG. Comparison of late changes in internal mammary artery and saphenous vein grafts in two consecutive series of patients 10 years after operation. Circulation 1984; 70(3 Pt 2): I208–I212.
5. Assad-Morell JL, Frye RL, Connolly DC, Davis GD, Pluth JR, Wallace RB, Barnhorst DA, Elveback LR, Danielson GK. Aorta-coronary artery saphenous vein bypass surgery: clinical and angiographic results. Mayo Clin Proc 1975; 50:379–386.
6. Borboriak JJ, Batayias GE, Korns ME. Scanning electron microscope study of human veins and aorta-coronary artery vein grafts. J Thorac Cardiovasc Surg 1976; 71:673–679.
7. Solymoss BC, Leung TK, Pelletier LC, Campeau L. Pathologic changes in coronary artery saphenous vein grafts and related etiologic factors. Cardiovasc Clin 1991; 21:45–65.
8. Waller BF, Roberts WC. Remnant saphenous veins after aortocoronary bypass grafting: analysis of 3,394 centimeters of unused vein from 402 patients. Am J Cardiol 1985; 55:65–71.
9. Amano J, Suzuki A, Sunamori M, Tsukada T, Numano F. Cytokinetic study of aortocoronary bypass vein grafts in place for less than six months. Am J Cardiol 1991; 67:1234–1236.
10. Unni KK, Kottke BA, Titus JL, Frye RL, Wallace RB, Brown AL. Pathologic changes in aortocoronary saphenous vein grafts. Am J Cardiol 1974; 34:526–532.
11. Grondin CM, Meere C, Castonguay Y, Lepage G, Grondin P. Progressive and late obstruction of an aorto-coronary venous bypass graft. Circulation 1971; 43:698–702.

12. Vlodaver Z, Edwards JE. Pathologic changes in aortic-coronary arterial saphenous vein grafts. Circulation 1971; 44:719–728.

13. Marti MC, Bouchardy B, Cox JN. Aortocoronary bypass with autogenous saphenous vein grafts: histopathological aspects. Virchows Arch Pathol Anat Physiol Klin Med 1971; 352:255–266.

14. Kern WH, Dermer GB, Lindesmith GG. The intimal proliferation in aortic-coronary saphenous vein grafts. Light and electron microscopic studies. Am Heart J 1972; 84:771–777.

15. Spray TL, Roberts WC. Changes in saphenous veins used as aortocoronary bypass grafts. Am Heart J 1977; 94:500–516.

16. La Veau PJ, Sarembock IJ, Sigal SL, Yang TL, Ezekowitz MD. Vascular reactivity after balloon angioplasty in an atherosclerotic rabbit. Circulation 1990; 82:1790–1801.

17. Alavi M, Moore S. Glycosaminoglycan composition and biosynthesis in the endothelium-covered neointima of de-endothelialized rabbit aorta. Exp Mol Pathol 1985; 42:389–400.

18. Yang ZH, von Segesser L, Bauer E, Stulz P, Turina M, Luscher TF. Different activation of the endothelial L-arginine and cyclooxygenase pathway in the human internal mammary artery and saphenous vein. Circ Res 1991; 68:52–60.

19. Yang ZH, Stulz P, von Segesser L, Bauer E, Turina M, Luscher TF. Different interactions of platelets with arterial and venous coronary bypass vessels. Lancet 1991; 337:939–943.

20. Radomski MW, Palmer RM, Moncada S. Endogenous nitric oxide inhibits human platelet adhesion to vascular endothelium. Lancet 1987; 2(8567):1057–1058.

21. Arnman V, Nilsson A, Stemme S, Risberg B, Rymo L. Expression of plasminogen activator inhibitor-1 mRNA in healthy, atherosclerotic and thrombotic human arteries and veins. Thromb Res 1994; 76:487–499.

22. Angelini GD, Bryan AJ, Williams HM, Soyombo AA, Williams A, Torey J, Newby AC. Time-course of medial and intimal thickening in pig venous arterial grafts: relationship to endothelial injury and cholesterol accumulation. J Thorac Cardiovasc Surg 1992; 103:1093–1103.

23. Zwolak RM, Adams MC, Clowes AW. Kinetics of vein graft hyperplasia: association with tangential stress. J Vasc Surg 1987; 5:126–136.

24. Moggio RA, Ding JZ, Smith CJ, Tota RR, Stemerman MB, Reed GE. Immediate-early gene expression in human saphenous veins harvested during coronary artery bypass graft operations. J Thorac Cardiovasc Surg 1995; 110:209–213.

25. Miano J, Tota R, Vlasic N, Danishefsky K, Stemerman M. Early proto-oncogene expression in rat aortic smooth muscle cells following endothelial removal. Am J Pathol 1990; 137:761–765.

26. Miano JM, Vlasic N, Tota RR, Stemmerman MB. Smooth muscle immediate early gene and growth factor activation follows vascular injury: a putative in vivo mechanism for autocrine growth. Arteriosclero Thromb 1993; 13:211–219.

27. Bauters C, de Groote P, Adamantidis M, Delcayre C, Hamon, Lablanche JM, Bertrand ME, Dupois B, Swynghedauw B. Proto-oncogene expression in rabbit aorta after wall injury. First marker of the cellular process leading to restenosis after angioplasty? Eur Heart J 1992; 13:556–559.

28. Soyombo AA, Angelini GD, Bryan AJ, Newby AC. Surgical preparation induces injury and promotes smooth muscle cell proliferation in a culture of human saphenous vein. Cardiovasc Res 1993; 27:1961–1967.
29. Garg UC, Hassid A. Nitric oxide–generating vasodilators and 8-bromo-cyclic guanosine monophosphate inhibit mitogenesis and proliferation of cultured rat vascular smooth muscle cells. J Clin Invest 1989; 83:1774–1777.
30. Taguchi J, Abe J, Okazaki H, Takuwa Y, Kurokawa K. L-arginine inhibits neointima formation following balloon injury. Life Sci 1993; 53:PL387–PL392.
31. Davies MG, Kim JH, Dalen H, Makhoul RG, Svendsen E, Hagen PO. Reduction of experimental vein graft intimal hyperplasia and preservation of nitric oxide–mediated relaxation by the nitric oxide precusor L-arginine. Surgery 1994; 116:557–568.
32. Fukuo K, Inoue T, Morimoto S, Nakahashi T, Yasuda O, Kitano S, Sasada R, Ogihara T. NO mediates cytotoxicity and basic fibroblast growth factor release in cultured vascular smooth muscle cells. J Clin Invest 1995; 95:669–676.
33. Nguyen HC, Grossi EA, LeBoutillier M, 3rd, Steinberg BM, Rifkin DB, Baumann FG, Colvin SB, Galloway AC. Mammary artery versus saphenous vein grafts: assessment of basic fibroblast growth factor receptors. Ann Thorac Surg 1994; 58: 308–310; discussion 310–311.
34. Shrceniwas R, Ogawa S, Cozzolino F, Torcia G, Brainstein N, Butura C, Brett J, Lieberman HB, Furie MB, Joseph-Silverstein J, et al. Macrovascular and microvascular endothelium during long-term hypoxia: alterations in cell growth, monolayer permeability, and cell surface coagulant properties. J Cell Physiol 1991; 146: 8–17.
35. Knighton DR, Hunt TK, Scheuenstuhl H, Halliday BJ, Werb Z, Banda MJ. Oxygen tension regulates the expression of angiogenesis factor by macrophages. Science 1983; 221:1283–1285.
36. Kuwabara K, Ogawa S, Matsumoto M, Koga S, Clauss M, Pinsky DJ, Lyn P, Leavy J, Witte L, Joseph-Silverstein J, et al. Hypoxia-mediated induction of acidic/basic fibroblast growth factor and platelet-derived growth factor in mononuclear phagocytes stimulates growth of hypoxic endothelial cells. Proc Natl Acad Sci USA 1995; 92:4606–4610.
37. Glagov S, Weisenberg E, Zarins CK, Stankunavicius R, Koletsis GJ. Compensatory enlargement of human atherosclerotic coronary arteries prevents narrowing of lumen. N Engl J Med 1987; 316:1371–1375.
38. Kamiya A, Togawa T. Adaptive regulation of wall shear stress to flow change in the canine carotid artery. Am J Physiol 1980; 239:H14–H21.
39. Wolinsky H, Glagov S. A lamellar unit of aortic medial structure and function in mammals. Circ Res 1967; 20:99–111.
40. Predel HG, Yang Z, von Segesser L, Turina M, Buhler FR, Luscher TF. Implications of pulsatile stretch on growth of saphenous vein and mammary artery smooth muscle. Lancet 1992; 340:878–879.
41. Sims FH. A comparison of coronary and internal mammary arteries and implications of the results in the etiology of arteriosclerosis. Am Heart J 1983; 105:560–566.
42. Ferro M, Conti M, Novero D, Micca FB, Palestro G. The thin intima of the internal mammary artery as the possible reason for freedom from atherosclerosis and success in coronary bypass [editorial]. Am Heart J 1991; 122(4 Pt 1):1192–1195.

43. Fujiwara T, Kajiya F, Kanazawa S, Matsuoka S, Woda Y, Hiramtsu O, Kagiyawa M, Ogasawura Y, Tsujioka K, Katsumura T. Comparison of blood-flow velocity waveforms in different coronary artery bypass grafts. Sequential saphenous vein grafts and internal mammary artery grafts. Circulation 1988; 78(5 Pt 1):1210–1217.

44. Kraiss LW, Kirkman TR, Kohler TR, Zierler B, Clowes AW. Shear stress regulates smooth muscle proliferation and neointimal thickening in porous polytetrafluoroethylene grafts. Arterioscler Thromb 1991; 11:1844–1852.

45. Malek AM, Gibbons GH, Dzau VJ, Izumo S. Fluid shear stress differentially modulates expression of genes encoding basic fibroblast growth factor and platelet-derived growth factor B chain in vascular endothelium. J Clin Invest 1993; 92: 2013–2021.

46. Steen S, Willen R, Sjoberg T, Carlen B. Contractile and morphologic properties of saphenous vein after 12 years as an aortocoronary bypass graft. Blood Vessels 1991; 28:349–353.

47. Makhoul RG, Davis WS, Mikat EM, McCann RL, Hagen PO. Responsiveness of vein bypass grafts to stimulation with norepinephrine and 5-hydroxytryptamine. J Vasc Surg 1987; 6:32–38.

48. Ku DD, Caufield JB, Kirklin JK. Endothelium-dependent responses in long-term human coronary artery bypass grafts. Circulation 1991; 83:402–411.

49. Davies MG, Ramkumar V, Gettys TW, Hagen P-O. The expression and function of G-proteins in experimental intimal hyperplasia. J Clin Invest 1994; 94:1680–1689.

50. Mautner SL, Mautner GC, Hunsberger SA, Roberts WC. Comparison of composition of atherosclerotic plaques in saphenous veins used as aortocoronary bypass conduits with plaques in native coronary arteries in the same men. Am J Cardiol 1992; 70:1380–1387.

51. Kennedy JH, Wieting DW, Hwang NH, Anderson MS, Bayardo RJ, Howell JF, DeBakey ME. Hydraulic and morphologic study of fibrous intimal hyperplasia in autogenous saphenous vein bypass grafts. J Thorac Cardiovasc Surg 1974; 67:805–813.

52. Barboriak JJ, Pintar K, Korns ME. Atherosclerosis in aortocoronary vein grafts. Lancet 1974; 2:621–624.

53. Chesebro JH, Clements IP, Fuster V, Elveback LR, Smith HC, Bardsley WT, Frye RL, Holmes Dr, Jr, Vliestra RE, Pluth JR, Wallace RB, Puga FJ, Orszulak TA, Piehlei JM, Schoff HV, Danielson GK. A platelet-inhibitor-drug trial in coronary-artery bypass operations: benefit of perioperative dipyridamole and aspirin therapy on early postoperative vein-graft patency. N Engl J Med 1982; 307:73–78.

54. Cybulsky MI, Gimbrone MA, Jr. Endothelial expression of a mononuclear leukocyte adhesion molecule during atherogenesis. Science 1991; 251:788–791.

55. Dzau VJ. Pathobiology of atherosclerosis and plaque complications. Am Heart J 1994; 128:1300–1304.

56. Solymoss BC, Nadeau P, Millette D, Campeau L. Late thrombosis of saphenous vein coronary bypass grafts related to risk factors. Circulation 1988; 78(3 Pt 2): I140–I143.

57. Mann MJ, Gibbons GH, Kernoff RS, Diet FP, Tsao PS, Cooke JP, Kaneday, Dzau VJ. Genetic engineering of vein grafts resistant to atherosclerosis. Proc Natl Acad Sci USA 1995; 92:4502–4506.

58. Guarda E, Grez R, Irarrazabal MJ, Acevedo C. Effects of doxycycline on metalloproteinase activity of mammary arteries and saphenous veins. Eur Heart J 1996; 17:103 (abst).

59. Baker AH, Wilkinson GWG, Hembry RM, Murphy G, Newby AC. Characterization of recombinant adenoviruses engineered to express high levels of metalloproteinase-9 or tissue inhibitor of metalloproteinase-1, -2, or -3 genes. Eur Heart J 1996; 17:329 (abst).

60. Kranzhofer A, Bajer AH, Newby AC. Neointimal expression of tissue inhibitors of metalloproteinases in human saphenous vein (abstr). Eur Heart J 1996; 17:530.

61. Hishikawa K, Oemar BS, Schrami P, Luscher TF. Subtraction cloning of differentially expressed gene from internal mammary arteries: implications for atherosclerosis (abstr). Eur Heart J 1996; 17:97.

62. Fuster V, Chesebro JJ. Aortocoronary artery vein-graft disease: experimental and clinical approach for the understanding of the role of platelets and platelet inhibitors. Circulation 1985; 72(6 Pt 2):V65–V70.

63. Fuster V, Chesebro JH. Role of platelets and platelet inhibitors in aortocoronary artery vein-graft disease. Circulation 1986; 73:227–232.

64. Wilson JM, Birinyi LK, Salomon RN, Libby P, Callow AD, Mulligan RC. Implantation of vascular grafts lined with genetically modified endothelial cells. Science 1989; 244:1344–1346.

65. Chen S-J, Wilson JM, Muller DWM. Adenovirus-mediated gene transfer of soluble vascular cell adhesion molecule to porcine interposition vein grafts. Circulation 1994; 89:1922–1928.

66. O'Brien KD, Allen MD, McDonald TO, Chait A, Harlan JM, Fishbein D, McCarty J, Ferguson M, Hudkins K, Benjamin CD, et al. Vascular cell adhesion molecule-1 is expressed in human coronary atherosclerotic plaques: implications for the mode of progression of advanced coronary atherosclerosis. J Clin Invest 1993; 92:945–951.

67. Carlos TM, Schwartz BR, Kovach NL, Yee E, Rosa M, Osborn L, Chi-Rosso G, Newman B, Lobb R, Rosso M, Harlan JM. Vascular cell adhesion molecule-1 (VCAM-1) mediated lymphocyte adherence to cytokine-activated cultured human endothelial cells. Blood 1990; 76:965–970.

68. Pardee A. G1 events and regulation of cell proliferation. Science 1989; 246:603–608.

69. Freeman R, Donoghue D. Protein kinases and protooncogenes: biochemical regulators of the eukaryotic cell cycle. Biochemistry 1991; 30:2293–2302.

70. Hartwell L, Kastan M. Cell cycle control and cancer. Science 1994; 266:1821–1828.

71. Simons M, Edelman ER, Dekeyser J-L, Langer R, Rosenberg RD. Antisense c-myb oligonucleotides inhibit intimal arterial smooth muscle cell accumulation in vivo. Nature 1992; 359:67–70.

72. Morishita R, Gibbons GH, Ellison KE, Nakajima M, von der Leyen H, Zhang L, Kaneda Y, Ogihara T, Dzau VJ. Intimal hyperplasia after vascular injury is inhibited by antisense cdk2 kinase oligonucleotides. J Clin Invest 1994; 93:1458–1464.

73. Okada Y, Koseki I, Kim J, Maeda Y, Hashimoto T. Modification of cell membranes with viral envelopes during fusion of cells with HVJ (Sendai virus). Exp Cell Res 1975; 93:368–378.

74. Tomita N, Higaki J, Morishita R, Kato K, Mikami H, Kaneda Y, Ogihara T, Dzau VJ. Direct in vivo gene introduction into rat kidney.Biochem Biophys Res Commun 1992; 186:129–134.

75. Morishita R, Gibbons GH, Kaneda Y, Ogihara T, Dzau VJ. Pharmacokinetics of antisense oligodeoxyribonucleotides (cyclin B1 and CDC 2 kinase) in the vessel wall in vivo: enhanced therapeutic utility for restenosis by HVJ-liposome delivery. Gene 1994; 149:13–19.

76. Morishita R, Gibbons GH, Ellison KE, Nakajima M, Zhang L, Kaneda Y, Ogihara T, Dzau VVJ. Single intraluminal delivery of antisense cdc2 kinase and proliferating-cell nuclear antigen oligonucleotides results in chronic inhibition of neointimal hyperplasia. Proc Natl Acad Sci USA 1993; 90:8474–8478.

77. Thomas WA, Reiner JM, Florentin FA, Lee KT, Lee WM. Population dynamics of arterial smooth muscle cells. V. Cell proliferation and cell death during initial 3 months in atherosclerotic lesions induced in swine by hypercholesterolemic diet and intimal trauma. Exp Mol Pathol 1976; 24:360–374.

78. Thomas WA, Scott RF, Florentin RA, Reiner JM, Lee KT. Population dynamics of arterial cells during atherogenesis. XI. Slowdown in multiplication and death rates of lesion smooth muscle cells in swine during the period 105–165 days after balloon endothelial cell denudation followed by a hyperlipidemic diet. Exp Mol Pathol 1981; 35:153–162.

79. Steller H. Mechanisms and genes of cellular suicide. Science 1995; 267:1445–1449.

80. Xia Z, Dickens M, Raingeaud J, Davis RJ, Greenberg ME. Opposing effects of ERK and JNK-p38 MAP kinases on apoptosis. Science 1995; 270:1326–1331.

81. Geng Y, Wu Q, Muszynsjki M, Hansson G, Libby P. Apoptosis of vascular smooth muscle cells induced by in vitro stimulation with interferon-gamma, tumor necrosis factor-alpha, and interleukin-1 beta. Arterioscler Thromb Vasc Biol 1996; 16:19–27.

82. Isner J, Kearney M, Bortman S, Passeri J. Apoptosis in human atherosclerosis and restenosis. Circulation 1995; 91:2703–2711.

83. Geng YJ, Libby P. Evidence for apoptosis in advanced human atheroma. A J Pathol 1995; 147:251–266.

6
Noninvasive Diagnosis of Saphenous Vein Bypass Graft Disease

Liwa T. Younis and Bernard Raymond Chaitman
St. Louis University Health Sciences Center, St. Louis, Missouri

I. INTRODUCTION

Coronary artery bypass surgery was introduced in the late 1960s, and the procedure results have been improved by the development of new methods of cardioplegia, the use of the internal mammary artery (IMA) conduit, the increased experience of surgeons and anesthesiologists, and the use of antiplatelet therapy. The indications to perform coronary bypass surgery have been expanded to include patients who were previously rejected for the operation because of an unacceptably high operative mortality rate [1–10]. One-month survival is reported at 95–98%, 1-year survival at 94–98%, and 5-year survival at 80–95%. The favorable outcome after surgery is extended to 10–15 years, where survival is reported at 60–80% [11–14]. In addition to its beneficial role in survival, coronary artery bypass surgery has a favorable outcome on other endpoints, including angina pectoris, quality of life, and return to work [15]. Important factors for the short- and long-term success of this procedure are related to the completeness of coronary revascularization and to the type of conduit used, since the 10-year patency rate of coronary bypass grafts is 95% when the IMA is anastomosed to the left anterior descending artery [16]. Patency rates are lower when the arterial conduit is anastomosed to other arteries, and are not significantly different than those for vein grafts.

Table 1 Noninvasive Testing Used to Evaluate Coronary Artery Bypass Graft Patency

- Exercise testing
- Stress myocardial perfusion imaging (exercise, dipyridamole, dobutamine)
- Stress echocardiography (exercise, dobutamine)
- Positron emission tomography
- Radionuclide ventriculography (resting, exercise)
- Ambulatory 24-hour Holter monitoring (ST-segment) analysis
- Magnetic resonance imaging
- Ultrafast computed tomography

Saphenous vein grafts demonstrate intimal hyperplasia after being in place for more than 1 year, with a 10% incidence of early postoperative closure of the graft and a 50% incidence of vein graft closure at 10 years [17–19]. Several factors influence graft patency, including arterial diameter, regional myocardial wall motion, and location of the native artery [20]. Coronary angiography is the standard method to diagnose graft atherosclerosis and to determine both the extent and the morphology of graft disease [21,22]. However, the procedure is expensive and inconvenient and is associated with limited mortality and morbidity and with significant interobserver and intraobserver variation when visual interpretation is used [23]. In this review, we will attempt to identify the role and the value of several modalities of noninvasive testing (Table 1) in identifying coronary artery bypass graft disease and the prognostic value of these tests in predicting short- and long-term outcome after coronary artery bypass grafting.

II. EXERCISE TESTING IN THE DIAGNOSIS OF SAPHENOUS VEIN GRAFT DISEASE

Exercise testing has been widely used for the last 20 years as a diagnostic tool in evaluating suspected coronary artery disease, with evolving diagnostic and prognostic implications to assess patients with chronic ischemic coronary artery disease. Despite the fact that the exercise electrocardiogram has limitations, it remains an important, relatively inexpensive, and widely available technique to assess patients with documented coronary artery disease [24].

A. Diagnostic Value of Exercise Testing

The use of Bayesian theory to estimate the pretest likelihood of coronary artery disease has substantially increased the predictive accuracy of the test [25,26]. The use of multiple-lead analysis, maximal and symptom-limited exercise, and computerized electrocardiogram results has enhanced the sensitivity and specificity of exercise parameters. The overall sensitivity of ST-segment depression in the diagnosis of obstructive coronary artery disease ranges from 56% to 81%, and specificity ranges from 72% to 96%. The sensitivity of ST-segment criteria for 1-, 2-, and 3-coronary artery disease (>70% luminal stenosis) is 40–84%, 63–91%, and 79–100%, respectively [27–29]. The use of exercise testing for diagnostic purposes following coronary artery bypass surgery has an inherent limitation, in that the abnormal response of ST-segment depression can be related to either progression of native coronary artery disease or disease of the coronary artery bypass grafts. Another limiting factor is the effect of drugs following coronary artery bypass surgery, such as beta blockers or nitrates, specifically in cases of incomplete revascularization. The influence of drug therapy can prolong the time to onset of ischemic ST-segment depression, and in a small minority of patients can normalize an initial ischemic response.

Although extensive data are available regarding the effect of exercise testing performed following coronary artery bypass surgery on symptoms, exercise performance, and survival, relatively few data are available regarding the diagnostic accuracy of the test in predicting postoperative occlusion of coronary artery bypass grafts [30,31]. Gohlke et al. [32] reported on 435 patients who had serial exercise tests following coronary artery bypass surgery 1–6 years after the procedure. All patients had postoperative angiography within 12 months·of surgery to determine the degree of revascularization achieved. The percentage of patients with significant ST-segment depression ($\geq$1 mm of ST-segment depression during exercise) correlated with the degree of revascularization and time from surgery (Table 2). All patients in this study had improvement in angina symptoms and degree of ST-segment depression after coronary artery bypass surgery, with the highest benefit reported when revascularization was complete or near complete. There was progressive loss in the improvement in all groups over 6 years of follow-up. Hultgren et al. [30] reported results from the Veteran Administrative Cooperative Study, which evaluated the effect of CABG on angina pectoris and exercise performance. At entry, 27% of the patients had <1 mm of ST-segment depression at peak exercise vs. 73% who showed >1 mm of ST-segment depression. Postoperatively the percentage of patients who had <1 mm of ST-segment depression at peak exercise increased to 59% at 1 year and to 62% at 5 years, and the percentage of patients with abnormal ST-segment depression decreased to 40% and 48% at 1 and 5 years, respectively.

Table 2 Preoperative and Post-CABG Exercise ST-Segment Depression

	Pre-CABG	Post-CABG	
		1 year	5 years
Degree of revascularization:			
Complete ($n = 182$)	76%	20%	34%
Incomplete ($n = 233$)	78%	34%	43%
Occluded grafts ($n = 20$)	85%	35%	33%

Adapted from Ref. 32 with permission.

B. Prognostic Value of Exercise Testing Following CABG

In the CASS study, Ryan et al. [33] reported the results of exercise testing performed in 81% of 780 randomized patients. The cumulative survival at the end of 7-year follow-up was 90% for patients assigned to the surgical intervention vs. 88% for patients who received medical therapy. When the patients were stratified using the degree of ST-segment depression and the workload performed, there were no significant differences in 7-year survival rates between the medically and surgically assigned groups; however, the presence of preoperative-exercise-induced angina identified patients who had a survival advantage when surgery was the therapy, with a 7-year survival rate of 94% vs. 87% for medically treated patients ($P = 0.007$). In an analysis of 1,005 patients [34], post-CABG exercise testing demonstrated an average increase of 41% in exercise capacity, and the maximal heart rate increased from 123 to 134. Although only 17% of patients had exercise-induced angina compared with 67% preoperatively, ST-segment depression persisted in 34% of patients. These results and others suggest that postoperative exercise tests, when performed in a selected population, provide significant prognostic information in surgically treated patients. However, the diagnostic value of the postoperative exercise test specifically to identify graft stenosis, occlusion, or progression in the native coronary circulation using variable exercise parameters remains limited [31,35,36].

III. AMBULATORY 24-HOUR ELECTROCARDIOGRAPHIC ST SEGMENT MONITORING

The improvement in angina after coronary artery bypass is reported by the majority of patients, independent of graft patency. Therefore detection of myocardial ischemia objectively during daily activity can theoretically enhance detection of incomplete revascularization [37–40].

Crea et al. [41] reported on 45 patients with incomplete myocardial revascularization by coronary angiography who had Holter monitoring to evaluate the diagnostic value of this modality in the detection of ischemic episodes in patients with stable angina pectoris. Twenty-six patients had both episodes of ST-segment depression during Holter monitoring and ischemia during exercise testing. Ten patients had normal Holter results but abnormal exercise ST-segment depression. The remaining patients had negative exercise tests and Holter monitoring. The sensitivity was 38% for the exercise test vs. 23% for Holter monitoring, both suboptimal. The specificity was 64% and 66% for exercise testing and Holter monitoring, respectively. The results suggest that both techniques have limited utility in the diagnosis of coronary artery bypass graft patency in patients with stable angina.

In a prospective study of 278 patients examined within 12 months after coronary artery bypass surgery by 24-hour ambulatory electrocardiography, Kennedy et al. [42] reported that silent myocardial ischemia was not associated with the presence of graft occlusion, low graft flow rates, grafted arteries with significant distal residual stenosis, or a nongrafted stenotic coronary artery, whether the test was performed early (within 3 months after coronary artery bypass surgery) or at 12 months. In addition, silent myocardial ischemia was not associated with an adverse clinical outcome within the 5 years following the procedure. Thus, the use of ambulatory electrocardiography ST-segment analysis provides limited diagnostic and prognostic information in the assessment of degree of revascularization and graft patency in patients following coronary artery bypass surgery (Table 3).

IV. MYOCARDIAL PERFUSION IMAGING AND IDENTIFICATION OF CORONARY ARTERY BYPASS GRAFT DISEASE

A. Diagnostic Role of Myocardial Perfusion Imaging

Coronary artery bypass surgery is associated with significant improvement in myocardial perfusion when preoperative studies are compared with postop-

Table 3 Diagnostic Accuracy of Noninvasive Cardiac Stress Testing after CABG

	Sensitivity	Specificity	Accuracy
Exercise ST-segment depression (n = 560 patients) [32,54]	42%	77%	71%
Ambulatory Holter monitoring (n = 161 patients) [42]	48%	71%	68%
Serial exercise thallium-201 (n = 55 patients) [45]	80%	88%	86%
Exercise echocardiography (n = 315 patients) [54,55]	92%	82%	90%

erative images. The postoperative myocardial perfusion study can be used to document improvement in myocardial perfusion as well as serving as a baseline for subsequent studies when symptoms recur or when new indications exist for these studies. The stress perfusion images are useful in patients who demonstrate resting ST-T changes due to conduction abnormalities, use of digitalis, or other electrocardiographic abnormalities. Gibson et al. [43] reported 47 patients undergoing coronary artery bypass surgery who had 4-week preoperative and 8-week postoperative thallium-201 quantitative images. Ninety-three percent of totally redistributing ischemic segments became normal postoperatively; however, only 73% of myocardial segments with partial redistribution consistent with severe ischemia and/or infarction normalized postoperatively. There was significant improvement in regional wall motion, which correlated with the improvement in the perfusion pattern in these patients. The presence of a fixed thallium-201 defect postoperatively was associated with only 45% normalization of wall motion following bypass surgery. However, fixed defects that showed improved perfusion postoperatively were associated with improvement in wall motion following revascularization.

Although successful and complete revascularization by coronary bypass surgery is associated with significant improvement in myocardial perfusion and graft patency (Figure 1), an abnormal perfusion pattern may persist in patients with baseline abnormal left ventricular function. Iskandrian et al. [44] reported that 95 patients with normal ejection fraction and no history of previous myocardial infarction preoperatively after uncomplicated coronary artery bypass surgery had a significantly higher incidence of normal SPECT images postoperatively when compared with those who had abnormal baseline left ventricular function (65% vs. 16%; $p < 0.0001$). There was a significant correlation between the ejection fraction and the extent of the perfusion abnormality ($R = 0.44$; $p < 0.0001$). Therefore, it appears that the specificity of postoperative myocardial perfusion images (SPECT) can vary with baseline left ventricular function and segmental wall motion [43,44].

The importance of serial testing over time was assessed in 55 patients undergoing preoperative, 2-week, and 1-year postoperative exercise thallium-201 imaging [45]. A sensitivity of 80%, a specificity of 88%, and a diagnostic accuracy of 86% was reported for detecting or excluding graft occlusion. At 1-year postoperatively, new occlusions were successfully localized in 11 of 18 patients. The mislocalizations were found in the posterior circulation (right coronary artery, obtuse marginal, and circumflex arteries). Eighty-three percent of left anterior descending coronary artery system lesions were successfully identified using exercise thallium-201 imaging [45] (Table 3). The serial evaluation of patients following coronary artery bypass surgery showed a progressive decrease in bypass graft patency, with a 15–30% stenosis-occlusion rate within the first 2 years after surgery followed by a subsequent patency loss

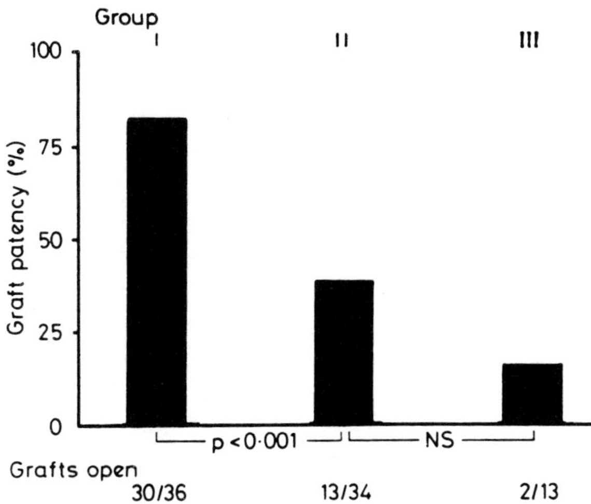

Figure 1 Saphenous graft patency rate relative to post-CABG thallium-201 scan finding. Group I = normal scan; group II = unchanged perfusion scan compared with preoperative scan; and group III = worsened scan. (From Hirzel HO, et al. Br Heart J 1980; 43:426–435, with permission.)

of 1–2% annually. It is estimated that 10 years postoperatively, 60% of grafts remain patent, but only 40% of all grafts are entirely free of angiographic-determined disease.

The problem of persistent or fixed defects without reversibility is frequently encountered in assessing patients following revascularization. The myocardial perfusion defects can represent areas of severe ischemia perfused by high-grade stenoses. The addition of 24-hour delayed imaging or reinjection can enhance the identification of these areas by demonstrating the presence of a reversible defect. The appearance of a new fixed defect without reversibility is probably due to an intraoperative myocardial infarction.

If the exercise myocardial perfusion study is normal following surgery, the majority of patients will have patent grafts. However, an abnormal postoperative scan, specifically one with redistribution, cannot suggest with reasonable accuracy graft occlusion or stenosis, incomplete revascularization, or progression of native disease.

B. Timing of Performance of Stress Myocardial Perfusion Study

Although serial testing probably increases the accuracy of detecting graft disease or occlusion, it is difficult to justify the cost and the inconvenience of performing serial testing in all patients following coronary revascularization. The reliance on recurrence of angina can be used as a reasonable guideline to repeat these studies. The recurrence of presurgery angina pattern is associated with a 70–80% incidence of graft disease or occlusion, whereas atypical chest pain is associated with about a 30% incidence of graft occlusion at 1 year postoperatively (Figure 2). The presence of any type of chest pain is probably a sufficient indication to perform a myocardial perfusion study, since 83% of patients in one series had new thallium-201 defects associated with occluded grafts on angiography. The absence of chest pain or nonspecific chest pain without a new thallium defect was associated with only a 9% incidence of graft occlusion. It is of extreme importance to evaluate the symptoms carefully and possibly to enhance the diagnostic accuracy of the myocardial perfusion studies by assessment of regional wall motion as well. The absence of new perfusion defects is 90% predictive that all grafts will be patent and is the usual finding in asymptomatic patients [45] (Table 3). In a recent study, Palmas et al. [46]

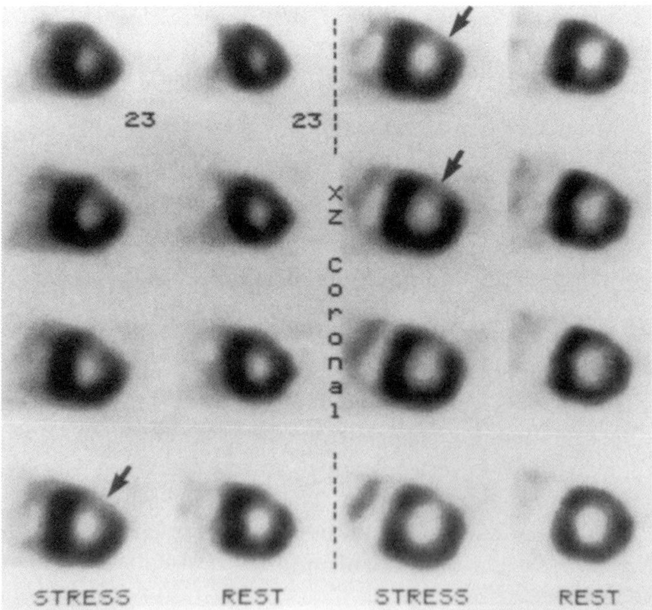

Figure 2   Rest and postoperative exercise and resting short-axis Tc-99m sestamibi tomogram in a post-CABG patient who developed angina. The images demonstrate partially reversible transmural anterior defect. (From Beller GA, Clinical nuclear cardiology. 1994, p. 343, with permission.)

reported the prognostic value of exercise thallium-201 SPECT in 294 patients 5 or more years after CABG. After 2.5 years of follow-up, 14% had died or had myocardial infarction. The summed reversibility score and stress-induced measured lung uptake were the most significant predictors of these events, with odds ratios of 1.13 and 1.77 ($p < 0.001$ and $p = 0.016$, respectively), and added incremental information to peak exercise heart rate.

Therefore, in post-CABG patients an early myocardial perfusion study is not recommended unless the patient is symptomatic. However, the test can provide significant prognostic information, even in mildly symptomatic patients when done 5 or more years after CABG and is predictive of cardiac events.

C. Positron Emission Tomography

In a head-to-head comparison, Marwick et al. [47] reported on 50 patients who underwent coronary artery bypass surgery and had myocardial perfusion assessment using rubidium-82 positron imaging tomography and thallium-201 SPECT following dipyridamole handgrip stress. The mean interval of the non-invasive evaluation was 6.5 years after surgery. All patients underwent coronary arteriography. Forty-six patients had recurrent or residual stenoses on angiography. Ninety-three percent of the patients had a perfusion defect that was identified by positron emission tomography, whereas SPECT imaging identified only 76% of these patients ($p = 0.04$). Stress-induced perfusion defects were demonstrated by PET in 19 patients, only 11 of these 19 patients had reversible defects identified with thallium SPECT. Graft disease (more than 70% stenosis) was present in 33 patients with quantitative angiography, and positron emission tomography identified 30 patients (91%) compared to 24 patients (73%) identified by SPECT thallium ($p = $ NS). Therefore, PET imaging may be superior to thallium SPECT in assessing patients following coronary artery bypass surgery (Figure 3); however, PET is expensive and limited to a few medical centers around the country, which renders the use of myocardial perfusion tomography, specifically in combination with new technetium-based isotopes, more available and practical.

The degree of improvement in myocardial perfusion images obtained after coronary artery bypass surgery correlates with the completeness of coronary revascularization. The use of quantitative analyses provides a tool to identify incomplete or minimal redistribution on thallium images, which can be associated with viable or ischemic myocardium and can be useful in assessing patients presenting with symptoms following coronary artery bypass surgery [48].

The assessment of changes in left ventricular ejection fraction during exercise provides significant prognostic information following coronary artery

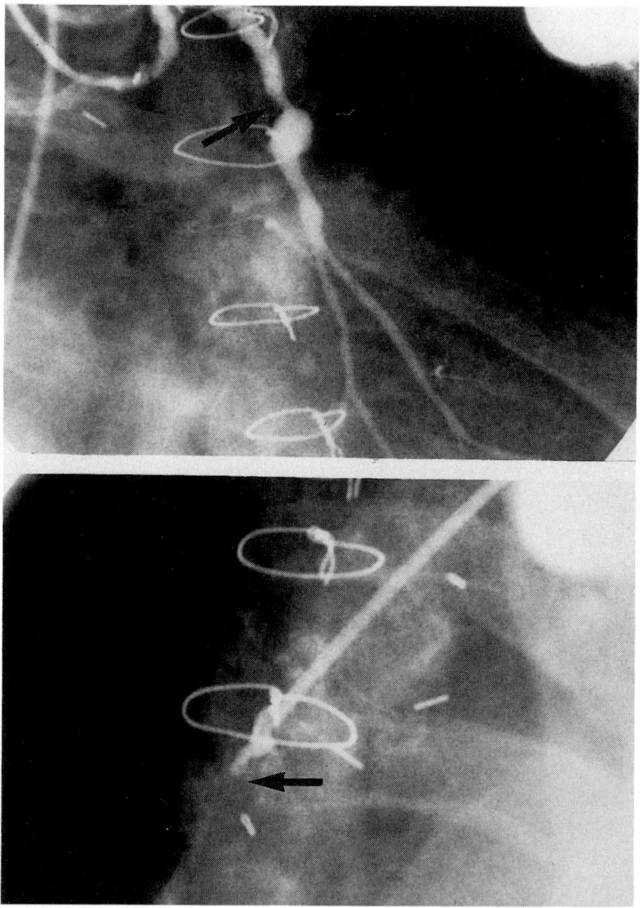

(A)

Figure 3 Angiographic (A) images obtained from a 71-year-old patient who had previous CABG. The SVG to circumflex-obtuse marginal branch showed 80% stenosis (↑) and the SVG to RCA is totally occluded (↑). (B) Scintigraphic 99mTc sestamibi tomogram shows a partially reversible inferior posterolateral defect. (C) Positron emission tomography showed a mismatch defect in the inferior wall with a perfusion defect (NH₃) and normal FDG uptake (↑), suggesting viability in this segment.

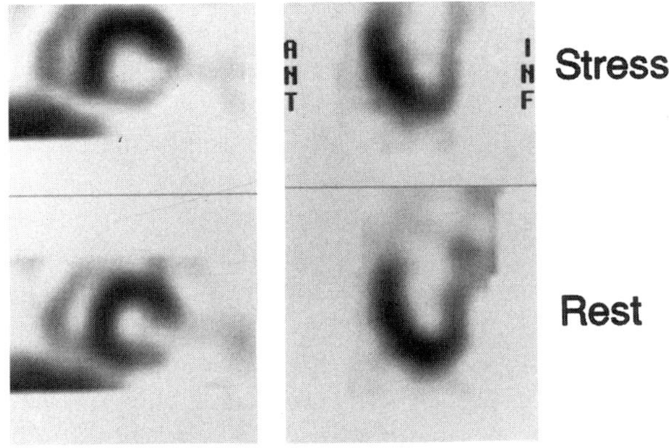

(B)

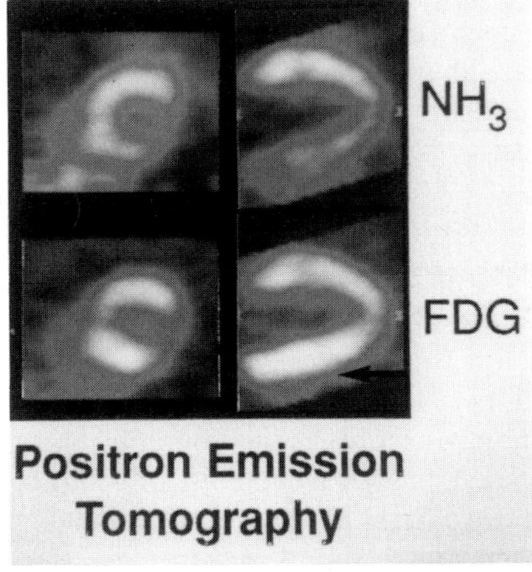

(C)

Figure 3 Continued.

bypass surgery. There is an incremental increase in the risk of cardiac death associated with failure to increase left ventricular ejection fraction during exercise by 10%. Patients who respond normally by increasing their ejection fraction during exercise have an excellent outcome [49]. However, the diagnostic information obtained from exercise radionuclide ventriculography in this patient population appears limited.

In summary, postoperative myocardial perfusion imaging is useful to assess the functional status of bypass grafts. There is significant improvement in both perfusion and function associated with complete revascularization in areas with preserved wall motion. The presence of reversible myocardial perfusion images during stress may be the early indication of incomplete revascularization or graft disease and can precede the recurrence of angina. However, a preoperative scan or a baseline postoperative scan is needed to evaluate the significance of these abnormalities.

Patients with patent bypass grafts usually have no or minimal chest pain, and those who do not suffer an intraoperative myocardial infarction should theoretically normalize their regional myocardial perfusion following surgery, provided that the revascularization is complete. The timing of this noninvasive evaluation should be decided based on the symptoms of the patient. The choice of the stress test in this population will depend on the ability of these patients to perform adequate exercise; otherwise, pharmacologic stress testing with dipyridamole or with dobutamine can be used to assess perfusion improvements following coronary artery bypass surgery.

V. STRESS ECHOCARDIOGRAPHY ASSESSMENT OF SAPHENOUS VEIN GRAFT DISEASE

Stress echocardiography has established its role in the diagnosis of coronary artery disease, with an excellent correlation with coronary angiography, using exercise or pharmacological stress [50–52]. The wide availability of echocardiography, the relative ease in incorporating stress modalities with imaging, the excellent diagnostic accuracy of this imaging technique in coronary artery disease, and increased experience have resulted in increased indications for this noninvasive test. Several reports have demonstrated the usefulness of exercise echocardiography or pharmacologic echocardiography in detecting coronary artery stenoses following successful angioplasty [53]. However, the diagnostic accuracy of this technique following CABG is not well established. Crouse et al. [54] evaluated the diagnostic accuracy of exercise echocardiography after coronary artery bypass surgery in 125 patients who were seen because of recurrence of symptoms or as a postoperative evaluation. The sensitivity, specificity, and positive and negative predictive accuracy of the test were

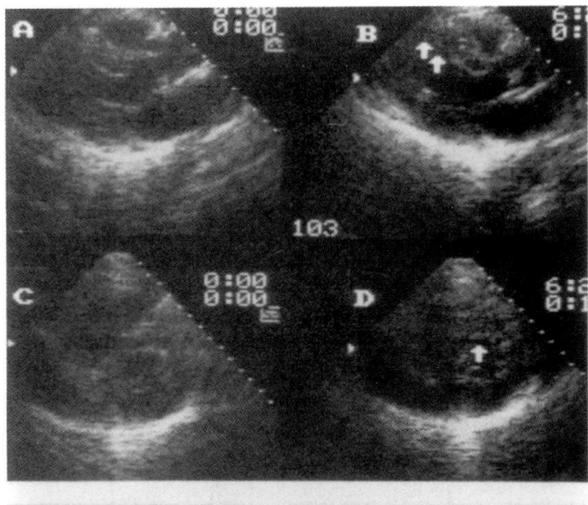

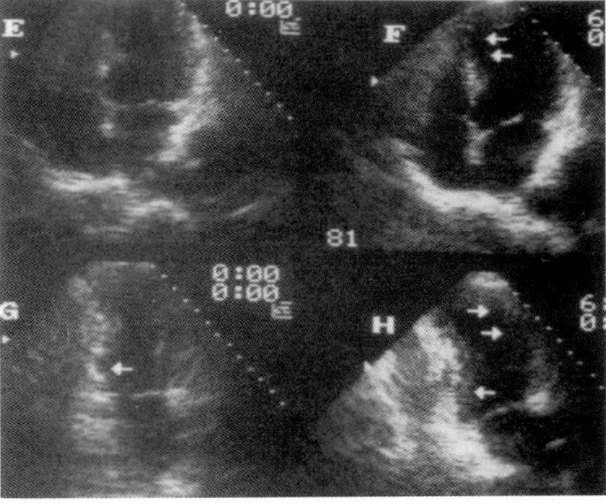

Figure 4 Rest and postexercise echocardiography of a CABG patient who developed interscapular pain. The resting images show severe anteroapical hypokinesis. Postexercise there is anteroseptal apical akinesis and inferior akinesis. The exercise electrocardiogram is normal. Coronary angiography demonstrated patent SVG to the diagonal branch; however, the LAD graft was occluded. Seventy percent mid-RCA stenosis was present. (From Ref. 54, with permission.)

98%, 92%, 99%, and 86%, respectively. The sensitivity of exercise echocardiography in detection of a single region with abnormal vascular supply was 88%, but there were no detailed angiographic results regarding the accuracy of exercise echocardiography in identifying the patency of the coronary artery bypass graft (Figure 4).

In a recent study, Kafka et al. [55] reported on 182 patients who underwent exercise echocardiography 2 weeks to 21 years after CABG. All patients had coronary angiography within 6 weeks of the test. Twenty-eight percent and 9% of exercise treadmill and echocardiography tests, respectively, were inconclusive. The positive predictive values of the exercise echocardiogram and exercise ECG were 85% and 62%, respectively; the negative predictive values were 81% and 52%, respectively. The overall sensitivity of exercise echocardiography in one vascular territory was 77%, compared to 96% when two or more vascular territories were involved (Table 2). The preliminary observations are indicative of the usefulness of exercise echocardiography in evaluating graft patency. The combination of dobutamine with echocardiography can potentially expand the patients who can be evaluated using stress echocardiography to those who are unable to exercise, specifically early after coronary artery bypass surgery. However, data are still lacking regarding dobutamine echocardiography after CABG. There are a few limitations that might influence the results of stress echocardiography, including the presence of septal wall motion abnormality and the difficulty in obtaining appropriate echocardiographic windows using the transthoracic echocardiogram, which can render image acquisition suboptimal.

VI. RADIOLOGY TECHNIQUES IN THE DETECTION OF CORONARY ARTERY BYPASS GRAFT DISEASE

A. Magnetic Resonance Imaging

Magnetic resonance imaging (MRI) is an excellent imaging technology for evaluating the heart based on identification of soft tissue contrast without the actual need for contrast agent administration. This technique has an excellent correlation with coronary angiography in identifying native proximal coronary artery disease, with a sensitivity and specificity approaching 100% for left main coronary artery disease, 90% for left anterior descending artery and right coronary artery, and 80% for left circumflex coronary artery [56].

Cine MRI is based on the analysis of blood flow dynamics through the coronary artery, with laminar blood flow represented as a bright signal and high-velocity turbulent flow showing no evidence of signal. Aurigemma et al. [57] assessed the diagnostic accuracy of cine MRI and the determination of coronary artery bypass graft patency in 20 patients with 45 proximal CABG anastomoses. There were 21 left anterior descending grafts, 12 left circumflex grafts, and 12 right coronary grafts. All patients underwent coronary angiography. The overall sensitivity of identification of patent grafts was 88%; the specificity was 100%, for the cine MRI identified all of the occluded grafts. The diagnostic accuracy was similar whatever the type of graft used

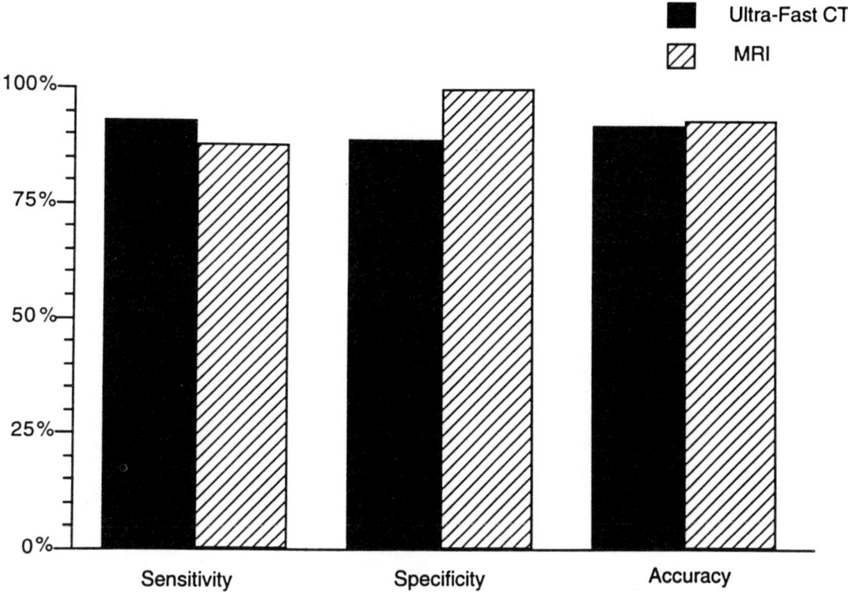

Figure 5 Assessment of coronary bypass graft patency by magnetic resonance imaging and ultrafast computed tomography. (Adapted from Refs. 57 and 60, with permission.)

(saphenous vein vs. left internal mammary artery graft) and the site of anastomosis (Figure 5). Therefore these preliminary data demonstrate a potential role for cine MRI in the routine postoperative evaluation of graft patency. Larger series are required to confirm the excellent diagnostic accuracy of this technology [56–58].

B. Ultrafast Computed Tomography

Ultrafast computed tomographic imaging has excellent temporal and spatial resolution that permits the acquisition of sequential images during bolus injections of contrast agent in a peripheral vein. The use of this technology has been tested in the diagnosis of coronary artery disease and found to be relatively accurate [59]. Stanford et al. [60] reported that in 74 patients who had coronary artery bypass surgery performed with the use of 179 grafts, ultrafast CT tomography is technically feasible in 84% of the patients. The sensitivity of detecting angiographically patent grafts was 93%; the specificity of detecting angiographically occluded grafts was 89%, with a predictive accuracy of

Table 4 Comparative Analysis of Noninvasive Cardiac Testing in Assessment of Post-CABG Graft Patency

Method	Diagnostic accuracy	Prognostic information	Availability	Cost ($)
ETT	+ +	+ + +	+ + + +	250
Stress nuclear imaging	+ + +	+ + + +	+ + +	1,000–1,500
Stress echocardiography	+ + +	+ + +	+ + +	750–1,000
Positron emission tomography	+ +	N/A	+	3,000
Cardiac MRI	+ +	N/A	+	2,000
Cardiac ultrafast CT	+ +	N/A	+	1,000

+ + = fair; + + + = good; + + + + = excellent.

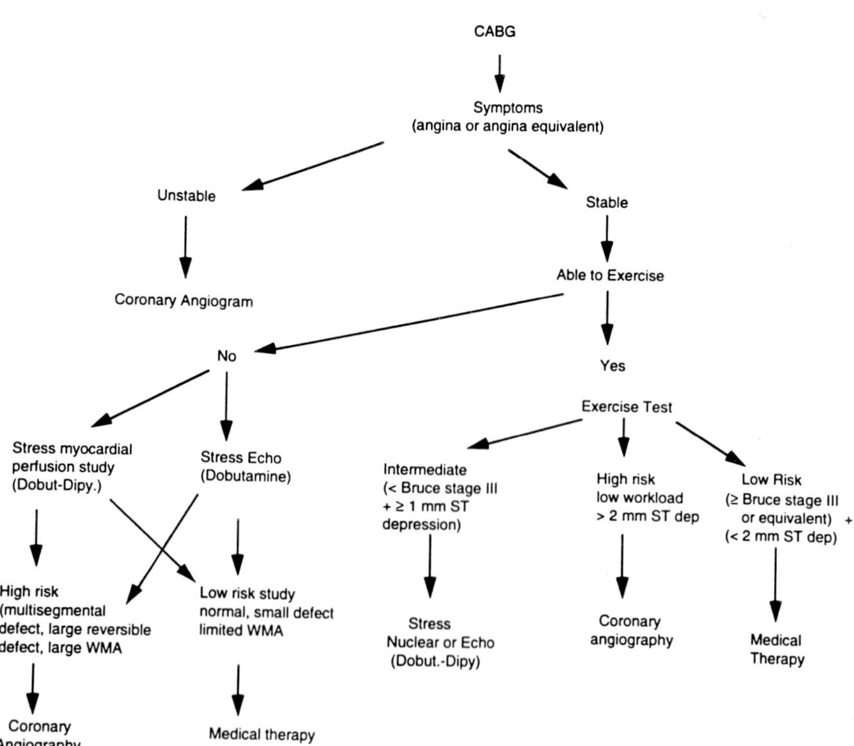

Figure 6 Managment strategy for the use of cardiac testing after CABG.

92%. The predictive accuracy of assessing left anterior descending grafts was 96%, that for left circumflex and the right coronary artery grafts were 92% and 86%, respectively. There was no difference between the diagnostic accuracy of the test when left internal mammary artery vs. saphenous vein grafts were assessed (92% vs. 91%) (Figure 5). The potential limitation of this technology when compared with other noninvasive modalities for assessing coronary bypass grafts is the need to inject intravenous contrast medium and exposure to a moderate amount of radiation, in addition to the technical difficulty in obtaining satisfactory studies in about 20–30% of patients.

VII. CONCLUSION

The noninvasive diagnosis of coronary artery bypass graft atherosclerosis remains the center of debate due to significant limitations associated with noninvasive cardiac imaging in this patient subset, the need for a control (preoperative or early postoperative) study, and the cost versus convenience of the noninvasive test (Table 4). It appears that chest pain should be the main determinant for pursuing noninvasive stress imaging with radionuclide myocardial perfusion or echocardiography. If the results of these tests are markedly abnormal, coronary angiography should follow (Figure 6).

REFERENCES

1. Garrett HE, Dennis EW, DeBakey ME. Aortocoronary bypass with saphenous vein graft: seven-year follow-up. JAMA 1973; 223:792–794.
2. Vigilante GJ, Weintraub WS, Klein LW, Schneider RM, Seelaus PA, Parr GVS, Lemole G, Agarwal JB, Helfant RH. Improved survival with coronary bypass surgery in patients with three-vessel coronary disease and abnormal left ventricular function. Matched case-control study in patient with potentially operable disease. Am J Med 1987; 82:697–702.
3. Loop FD, Golding LR, Macmillan JP, Cosgrove DM, Lytle BW, Sheldon WC. Coronary artery surgery in women compared with men: analyses of risks and long-term results. J Am Coll Cardiol 1983; 1:383–389.
4. Gersh BJ, Kronmal RA, Schaff HV, Frye RL, Ryan TJ, Mock MB, Myers WO, Athearn MW, Gosselin AJ, Kaiser GC, Bourassa MG, Killip T, and the participants in the Coronary Artery Surgery Study. Comparison of coronary artery bypass surgery and medical therapy in patients 65 years of age or older: a nonrandomized study from the Coronary Artery Surgery Study (CASS) Registry. N Engl J Med 1985; 313:217–224.
5. Chesebro JH, Fuster V, Elveback LR, Clements IP, Smith GC, Holmes DR, Bardsley WT, Pluth JR, Wallace RB, Puga FJ, Orszulak TA, Piehler JM, Danielson GK,

Schaff HV, Frye RL. Effect of dipyridamole and aspirin on late vein-graft patency after coronary bypass operations. N Engl J Med 1984; 310:209–215.

6. Killip T, Passamani E, Davis K, and the CASS Principal Investigators and their Associates. Coronary Artery Surgery Study (CASS): a randomized trial of coronary bypass surgery. Eight-year follow-up and survival in patients with reduced ejection fraction. Circulation 1985; 72(suppl V):102–108.

7. Caracciolo EA, Davis KB, Kaiser GC, Schaff H, Taylor HA, Corley S, Sopko G, Chaitman BR, for the CASS investigators. Comparison of surgical and medical group survival in patients with left main coronary artery disease. Long-term CASS experience. Circulation 1995; 91:2325–2334.

8. Varnauskas E, and The European Coronary Surgery Study Group. Twelve-year follow-up of survival in the randomized European Coronary Surgery Study. N Engl J Med 1988; 319:332–338.

9. CASS Principal Investigators and their Associates. Coronary Artery Surgery Study (CASS): a randomized trial of coronary artery bypass surgery. Survival data. Circulation 1983; 68:939–944.

10. European Coronary Surgery Study Group. Long-term results of prospective randomized study of coronary artery bypass surgery in stable angina pectoris. Lancet 1982; 2:1173–1179.

11. Alderman EL, Bourassa MG, Cohen LS, Davis KB, Kaiser GG, Killip T, Mock MB, Pettinger M, Robertson TL, for the CASS Investigators. Ten-year follow-up of survival and myocardial infarction in the randomized Coronary Artery Surgery Study. Circulation 1990; 82:1629–1635.

12. Caracciolo EA, Davis KB, Sopko G, Kaiser GC, Corley SD, Schoff H, Taylor HA, Chaitman BR. Comparison of surgical and medical group survival in patients with left main equivalent coronary artery disease. Long-term CASS experience. Circulation 1995; 91:2335–2344.

13. Kirklin JW, Naftel DC, Blackstone EH, Pohost GM. Summary of a consensus concerning death and ischemic events after coronary artery bypass grafting. Circulation 1989; 79(suppl I):81–86.

14. The VA Coronary Artery Bypass Surgery Cooperative Study Group. Eighteen-year follow-up in the Veterans Affairs Cooperative Study of Coronary Artery Bypass Surgery for Stable Angina. Circulation 1992; 86:121–130.

15. Kirklin JW, Akins CW, Blackstone EH, Booth DC, Califf RM, Cohen LS, Hall RJ, Harrell FE, Kouchoukos NT, McCallister BD, Naftel DC, Parker JO, Sheldon WC, Smith HC, Wechsler AS, Williams JF Jr. ACC/AHA guidelines and indications for coronary artery bypass graft surgery. A report of the American College of Cardiology/American Heart Association Task Force on assessment of diagnostic and therapeutic cardiovascular procedures. Circulation 1991; 83:1125–1131.

16. Loop FD, Lytle BW, Cosgrove DM, Steward RW, Goormastic M, Williams GW, Golding LAR, Gill CC, Taylor PC, Sheldon WC, Proudfit WL. Influence of the internal mammary artery graft on 10-year survival and other cardiac events. N Engl J Med 1986; 314:1–7.

17. Bourassa MG, Fisher LD, Campeau L, Gillespie MJ, McConney M, Lesperance J. Long-term fate of bypass grafts: the Coronary Artery Surgery Study (CASS) and Montreal Heart Institute experiences. Circulation 1985; 72(suppl V):V-71–V-78.

18. Grondin CM, Campeau L, Lesperance J, Enjalbert M, Bourassa MG. Comparison of late changes in internal mammary artery and saphenous vein grafts in two consecutive series of patients 10 years after operation. Circulation 1984; 70(suppl I): I-208–I-212.

19. Campeau L, Enjalbert M, Lesperance J, Vaislic C, Grondin CM, Bourassa MG. Atherosclerosis and late closure of aortocoronary saphenous vein grafts: sequential angiographic studies at 2 weeks, 1 year, 5 to 7 years, and 10 to 12 years after surgery. Circulation 1983; 68(suppl II):II-1–II-7.

20. Cataldo G, Braga M, Pirotta N, Lavezzari M, Rovelli F, Marubini E, on behalf of Studio Indobufene nel Bypass Aortocoronarico (SINBA). Factors influencing 1-year patency of coronary artery saphenous vein grafts. Circulation 1993; 88(part II):II-93–II-98.

21. Lytle BW, Loop FD, Cosgrove DM, Ratliff NB, Easly K, Taylor PC. Long-term (5–12 years) serial studies of internal mammary artery and saphenous vein coronary bypass grafts. J Thorac Cardiovasc Surg 1985; 89:248–258.

22. Fuster V, Chesebro JJ. Aortocoronary artery vein-graft disease: experimental and clinical approach for the understanding of the role of platelets and platelet inhibitors. Circulation 1985; 72(suppl V):V-65–V-70.

23. Shub C, Vlietstra RD, Smith HC, Fulton RE, Elveback L. The unpredictable progression of symptomatic coronary artery disease: a serial clinical-angiographic analysis. Mayo Clin Proc 1981; 56:155–160.

24. Chaitman BR. The changing role of the exercise electrocardiogram as a diagnostic and prognostic test for chronic ischemic heart disease. J Am Coll Cardiol 1986; 8: 1195–1210.

25. Detrano R, Yiannikas J, Salcedo EE, Rincon G, Go RT, Williams G, Leatherman J. Bayesian probability analysis: a prospective demonstration of its clinical utility in diagnosing coronary disease. Circulation 1984; 69:541–547.

26. Detry JMR, Kapita BM, Cosyns J, Sottiaux B, Brasseur LA, Rousseau MF. Diagnostic value of history and maximal exercise electrocardiography in men and women with suspected coronary heart disease. Circulation 1977; 56: 756–761.

27. Froelicher VF, Yanowitz FG, Major AJT, Lancaster MC. The correlation of coronary angiography and the electrocardiographic response to maximal treadmill testing in 76 asymptomatic men. Circulation 1973; 48:597–604.

28. Borer JS, Brensike JF, Redwood DR, Itscoitz SB, Passamani ER, Stone NJ, Richardson JM, Levy RI, Epstein SE. Limitations of the electrocardiographic response to exercise in predicting coronary artery disease. N Engl J Med 1975; 293: 267–371.

29. Chaitman BR, Bourassa MG, Wagniart P, Corbara F, Ferguson RJ. Improved efficiency of treadmill exercise testing using a multiple-lead ECG system and basic hemodynamic exercise response. 1978; 57:71–79.

30. Hultgren HN, Peduzzi P, Detre K, Takaro T, and the Study Participants. The 5-year effect of bypass surgery on relief of angina and exercise performance. Circulation 1985; 72(suppl V):V-79–V-83.

31. Weiner DA, Ryan TJ, Parsons L, Fisher LD, Chaitman BR, Sheffield LT, Tristani FE. Prevalence and prognostic significance of silent and symptomatic ischemia

after coronary bypass surgery: a report from the Coronary Artery Surgery Study (CASS) randomized population. J Am Coll Cardiol 1991; 18:343–348.

32. Gohlke H, Gholke-Barwolf C, Samek L, Sturzenofecker P, Schmuziger M, Roskamm H. Serial exercise testing up to 6 years after coronary bypass surgery: behavior of exercise parameters in groups with different degrees of revascularization determined by postoperative angiography. Am J Cardiol 1983; 51:1301–1306.

33. Ryan TJ, Weiner DA, McCabe CH, Davis KB, Sheffield LT, Chaitman BR, Tristani FE, Fisher LD. Exercise testing in the Coronary Artery Surgery Study randomized population. Circulation 1985; 72:V31–V38.

34. Dubach P, Froelicher V, Atwood JE, Myers J, Sandhu SS, Lehmann K. A comparison of the exercise test responses pre/post revascularization: does coronary artery bypass surgery produce better results than percutaneous transluminal coronary angioplasty? J Cardiovasc Rehab 1990; 10:120–125.

35. Dubach P, Froelicher V, Klein J, Detrano R. Use of the exercise test to predict prognosis after coronary artery bypass grafting. Am J Cardiol 1989; 63:530–533.

36. Yli-Mayry S, Huikuri HV, Airaksinen J, Ikaheimo MJ, Linnaluoto MK, Takkunen JT. Usefulness of a postoperative exercise test for predicting cardiac events after coronary artery bypass grafting. Am J Cardiol 1992; 70:56–59.

37. Benchimol A, dos Santos A, Desser KB. Relief of angina pectoris in patients with occluded coronary bypass grafts. Am J Med 1976; 60:339–343.

38. Block TA, Murray JA, English MT. Improvement in exercise performance after unsuccessful myocardial revascularization. Am J Cardiol 1977; 40:673–680.

39. Slegel W, Lim JS, Proudfit WL, Sheldon WC, Loop FD. The spectrum of exercise test and angiographic correlations in myocardial revascularization surgery. Circulation 1975; 52(suppl I):I-156–I-162.

40. Hartman CW, Kong Y, Margolis JR, Warren SG, Peter RH, Behar VS, Oldham HN. Aortocoronary bypass surgery. Correlation of angiographic, symptomatic, and functional improvement at 1 year. Am J Cardiol 1976; 37:352–357.

41. Crea F, Kaski JC, Fragasso G, Hackett D, Stanbridge R, Taylor KM, Maseri A. Usefulness of Holter monitoring to improve the sensitivity of exercise testing in determining the degree of myocardial revascularization after coronary artery bypass grafting for stable angina pectoris. Am J Cardiol 1987; 60:40–43.

42. Kennedy HL, Seiler SM, Sprague MK, Homan SM, Whitlock JA, Kern MJ, Vandormael MG, Barner HB, Codd JE, Willman VL. Relation of silent myocardial ischemia after coronary artery bypass grafting to angiographic completeness of revascularization and long-term prognosis. Am J Cardiol 1990; 65:14–22.

43. Gibson RS, Watson DD, Taylor GJ, Crosby IK, Wellons HL, Holt ND, Beller GA. Prospective assessment of regional myocardial perfusion before and after coronary revascularization surgery by quantitative thallium-201 scintigraphy. J Am Coll Cardiol 1983; 1:804–815.

44. Iskandrian AE, Kegel JG, Tecce MA, Wasserleben V, Cave V, Heo J. Simultaneous assessment of left ventricular perfusion and function with technetium-99m sestamibi after coronary artery bypass grafting. Am Heart J 1993; 126:1199–1203.

45. Pfisterer M, Emmenegger H, Schmitt HE, Muller-Brand J, Hasse J, Gradel E, Laver MB, Burckhardt D, Burkart F. Accuracy of serial myocardial perfusion scin-

tigraphy with thallium-201 for predictiion of graft patency early and late after coronary artery bypass surgery. Circulation 1982; 66:1017–1024.

46. Palmas W, Bingham S, Diamond GA, Denton TA, Kiat H, Friedman JD, Scarlata D, Maddahi J, Cohen I, Berman DS. Incremental prognostic value of exercise thallium-201 myocardial single-photon emission computed tomography late after coronary artery bypass surgery. J Am Coll Cardiol 1995; 25:403–409.

47. Marwick TH, Lafont A, Go RT, Underwood DA, Saha GB, MacIntyre WJ. Identification of recurrent ischemia after coronary artery bypass surgery: a comparison of positron emission tomography and single photon emission computer tomography. Int J Cardiol 1992; 35:33–41.

48. Ohtani H, Tamaki N, Mohiuddin IH, Yonekura Y, Konishi J, Hirata K, Ban T. Minimal redistribution of thallium-201 representing reversible ischemia after coronary artery bypass surgery: value of quantitative analysis of exercise thallium-201 SPECT. J Cardiol 1991; 21:835–846.

49. Wallis JB, Supino PG, Borer JS. Prognostic value of left ventricular ejection fraction response to exercise during long-term follow-up after coronary artery bypass graft surgery. Circulation 1993; 88:99–109.

50. Beleslin BD, Ostojic M, Stepanovic J, Djordjevic-Dikic A, Stojkovic S, Nedeljkovic M, Stankovic G, Petrasinovic Z, Gojkovic, Vasiljevic-Pokrajcic, Nedeljkovic S. Stress echocardiography in the detection of myocardial ischemia. Head-to-head comparison of exercise, dobutamine, and dipyridamole tests. Circulation 1994; 90:1168–1176.

51. Quinones MA, Verani MS, Haichin RM, Mahmarian JJ, Suarez J, Zoghbi WA. Exercise echocardiography versus 201 Tl single-photon emission computer tomography in evaluation of coronary artery disease. Analysis of 292 patients. Circulation 1992; 85:1026–1031.

52. Segar DS, Brown SE, Sawada SG, Ryan T, Feigenbaum H. Dobutamine stress echocardiography: correlation with coronary lesion severity as determined by quantitative angiography. J Am Coll Cardiol 1992; 19:1197–1202.

53. Heinle SK, Lieberman EB, Ancukiewicz M, Waugh RA, Bashore TM, Kisslo J. Usefulness of dobutamine echocardiography for detecting restenosis after percutaneous transluminal coronary angioplasty. Am J Cardiol 1993; 72:1220–1225.

54. Crouse LJ, Vacek JL, Beauchamp GD, Porter CB, Rosamond TL, Kramer PH. Exercise echocardiography after coronary artery bypass grafting. Am J Cardiol 1992; 70:572–576.

55. Kafka H, Leach AJ, Fitzgibbon GM. Exercise echocardiography after coronary artery bypass surgery: correlation with coronary angiography. J Am Coll Cardiol 1995; 25:1019–1023.

56. Manning WJ, Li W, Edelman RR. A preliminary report comparing magnetic resonance coronary angiography with conventional angiography. N Engl J Med 1993; 328:828–832.

57. Aurigemma GP, Reichek N, Axel L, Schiebler M, Harris C, Kressel HY. Noninvasive determination of coronary artery bypass graft patency by cine magnetic resonance imaging. Circulation 1989; 80:1595–1602.

58. Pennell DJ, Keegan J, Firmin DN, Gatehouse PD, Underwood SR, Longmore DB. Magnetic resonance imaging of coronary arteries: technique and preliminary results. Br Heart J 1993; 70:315–326.

59. Bateman TM, Gray RJ, Whiting JS, Sethna DH, Berman DS, Matloff JM, Swan HJC, Forrester JS. Prospective evaluation of ultrafast cardiac computed tomography for determination of coronary bypass graft patency. Circulation 1987; 75:1018–1024.
60. Stanford W, Brundage BH, MacMillan R, Chomka EV, Bateman TM, Eldredge WJ, Lipton MJ, White CW, Wilson RF, Johnson MR, Marcus ML. Sensitivity and specificity of assessing coronary bypass graft patency with ultrafast computed tomography: results of a multicenter study. J Am Coll Cardiol 1988; 12:1–7.

7

Invasive Diagnosis of Saphenous Vein Bypass Graft Disease

William L. Mecca* and John McB. Hodgson[†]
University Hospitals of Cleveland, Cleveland, Ohio

The most widely available imaging technique for the evaluation of saphenous vein bypass grafts (SVBGs) is contrast angiography. Although useful in many ways, no other imaging modality has been able to provide enough detail to be used as a stand-alone technique for the evaluation and treatment of SVBG disease (Table 1). In this chapter we review invasive techniques for the evaluation of SVBG pathology. The relative strengths and weaknesses of each modality will be discussed and contrasted with those of selective angiography.

I. CONVENTIONAL SELECTIVE ANGIOGRAPHY

Antiography remains the gold standard for the diagnosis of SVBG disease as well as for the diagnosis of atherosclerotic disease of the native coronary and internal mammary arteries. As expected, angiographic variables such as lesion location and morphology play a significant role in guiding catheter-based treatment strategies such as balloon angioplasty, atherectomy, laser angioplasty, and balloon-expandable endoluminal stenting.

Selective cannulation of the graft ostium and injection of 5–10 cc of a radiopaque contrast using standard diagnostic coronary catheters is required

---

Current affiliations:
*Hammot Medical Center, Erie, Pennsylvania.
[†]MetroHealth Medical Center, Cleveland, Ohio.

Table 1 Invasive Evaluation of SVBG
Patency and Function

Conventional contrast angiography
Digital subtraction angiography
Intracoronary ultrasound (ICUS)
Doppler flow studies
Coronary angioscopy

for adequate imaging. Frequently, all SVBGs can be cannulated using a Judkins right coronary 4.0 (JR4) catheter. Occasionally, a saphenous vein graft to the right coronary artery will point at a steep downward angle so that a JR4 cannot be positioned coaxial to the graft ostium, resulting in poor filling of the graft and producing streaming artifacts and inadequate visualization of the graft ostium. Under these circumstances, a multipurpose catheter is usually the best choice, for it points inferiorly when positioned at the level of the graft. If the aortic root size is large, an Amplatz left coronary 2.0 (AL2) catheter or a left bypass catheter is a good choice for saphenous vein grafts that anastomose with left coronary artery targets.

The total number of grafts to be injected and the position of the grafts must be known prior to attempting angiography. This information is not always available, particularly when cardiac catheterization is performed for emergent indications. Incomplete imaging leading to inappropriate assumptions regarding the overall status of the patient's revascularization is a significant concern during these conditions. An aortic root injection can be used to identify the origins of vein grafts that have been difficult to find and may assist in determining if all vein grafts had been selectively injected. If an aortic root injection is to be used to exclude the possibility of unidentified vein grafts, two views should be performed, preferably with digital enhancement (see later), and with adequate contrast to opacify the aorta. During attempts to cannulate vein grafts selectively, large amounts of contrast may be administered if the proximal anastomosis is difficult to locate or if an ostial occlusion is not recognized. This increased contrast load must be considered when imaging patients with underlying renal insufficiency in order to maintain an acceptable risk of renal failure.

Contrast flow patterns can provide a crude indication of the hemodynamic significance of borderline lesions. Slow flow, swirling, or hang-up of contrast at the lesion suggests unfavorable lesion geometry. Although contrast "staining" can be seen with intimal disruption or complex plaque dissections, extravasation of contrast is diagnostic of perforation. Venous valves and bends may be difficult to distinguish from atherosclerotic plaque and frequently produce irregular flow patterns. The plaque composition in vein grafts tends to

Table 2 Angiographic Variables Associated with Unfavorable Outcome of PTCA in SVBG Disease

Extent of disease: length >10 mm or diffuse disease
Lesion location: proximal anastomosis or body
Presence of thrombus
Vein graft age >4–6 years
Single vs. sequential SVBG
Total occlusion

be softer and more friable than atherosclerotic disease of the native coronary arteries; however, contrast angiography does not convey this information.

In a retrospective review of balloon angioplasty for the treatment of saphenous vein bypass graft disease, de Feyter et al. [1] were able to stratify patients according to outcome on the basis of angiographic variables, vein graft age, and the risk of cardiogenic shock in the event of total graft closure. Factors influencing outcome of PTCA in SVBG disease are shown in Table 2. Initial success and restenosis rates vary in proportion to the total extent of disease in the vein graft. Restenosis rates are influenced by lesion location, with restenosis as high as 58% for lesions in the proximal segments and body of SVBG, down to 28% for lesions at the distal anastomosis. Vein graft age also has an impact on both initial success and restenosis, with a restenosis rate of 83% for grafts 36 or more months old vs. 42% for younger grafts. Although the presence of thrombus markedly reduces initial success rates, total occlusion of the vein graft is associated with almost 100% restenosis rates.

II. INTRACORONARY ULTRASOUND

Intracoronary ultrasound (ICUS) is a catheter-based imaging modality that provides a unique cross-sectional view of the SVBG. Several ICUS systems are currently in use. Mechanical catheters utilize a rotating transducer element at the catheter tip. A second type of ultrasound catheter employs a multielement synthetic aperture array consisting of multiple transducer elements that are electronically switched to produce the sweeping ultrasound beam. ICUS catheters display a continuous tomographic image of the vessel wall, which is viewed in gray scale and recorded in real time onto videotape.

The electronic array ICUS catheter (Endosonics, Pleasanton, CA), used in our laboratory, is available as a 3.5F monorail catheter that accommodates a 0.014-inch angioplasty guide wire. The ICUS catheter is advanced over the angioplasty guide wire through a minimum 6F angioplasty guiding catheter to the region of interest. As with angioplasty, a "road map" of the vessel to be imaged must be obtained, via contrast angiography, prior to the introduction of the guide wire and ICUS catheter. The operator must be skilled in the manipulation of intracoronary wires, angioplasty balloon, and guiding catheters. The patient must be heparinized to prevent thrombotic complications.

In a comprehensive review of early validation studies, Liebson and Klein [2] noted excellent reproducibility and accuracy of dimensional measurements obtained by ICUS. When lumen area and lumen diameter measurements obtained by ICUS were compared to histologic measurements, an excellent correlation ($r = 0.85$–0.99) was found for normal and atherosclerotic arteries in animal and human studies [3–5]. The correlation between ICUS dimensional measurements and angiography was excellent in animal studies [6] ($r = 0.96$–0.98). But the correlation was often lower in human studies [7–9] of angiographically normal arteries, and loses statistical significance in the presence of atherosclerotic disease ($r = 0.26$–0.92). The inadequate correlation between ICUS and angiography is in part explained by necropsy studies [10,11], which demonstrate that angiography consistently underestimates the extent of atherosclerosis. In minimally diseased vessels, discordance between ICUS and angiography results from the detection of significant atherosclerosis by ICUS in vessels that may appear normal by angiography. In more diseased vessels, the discordance becomes more significant, because lesion geometry becomes more complex.

Nase-Hueppmeier et al. [12] used ICUS during the evaluation of saphenous vein bypass grafts (4 months to 11 years of age) in patients undergoing repeat catheterization for recurrent angina. In saphenous vein grafts appearing normal by both angiography and intracoronary ultrasound, the vessel walls were homogeneous, and separate layers such as the intima, media, and adventitia could not be distinguished (Figure 1a). This homogeneous appearance of the vein graft by ultrasound is the result of an incomplete internal elastic lamina and absent external elastic lamina. The wall thickness in normal grafts (0.54–0.63 mm, median 0.59 mm) was significantly different from the wall thickness of normal-appearing segments (0.99–1.07 mm, median 1.02 mm; $p < 0.001$) in vein grafts that demonstrated focal lesions. Concentric thickening of the entire vein graft wall is detected by ICUS simultaneous with the development of angiographically focal lesions (Figure 1a and 1b). This increased wall thickness corresponds to the diffuse intimal hyperplasia seen on histopathologic studies. Similar to findings in native coronary arteries, ICUS was more sensitive than angiography, which identified only 51% of the lesions demonstrated by ICUS.

III. CORONARY FLOW RESERVE

Percent diameter stenosis is only one of several factors that contribute to the hemodynamic effects of a particular lesion. The influence of other factors,

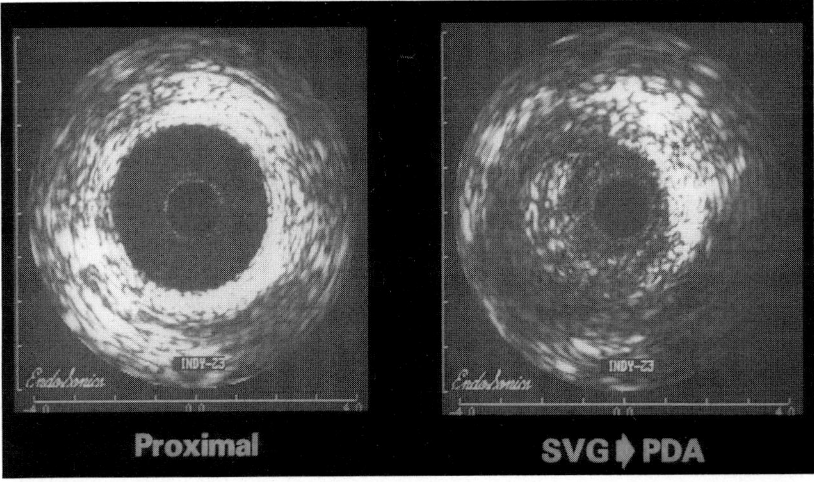

(a)

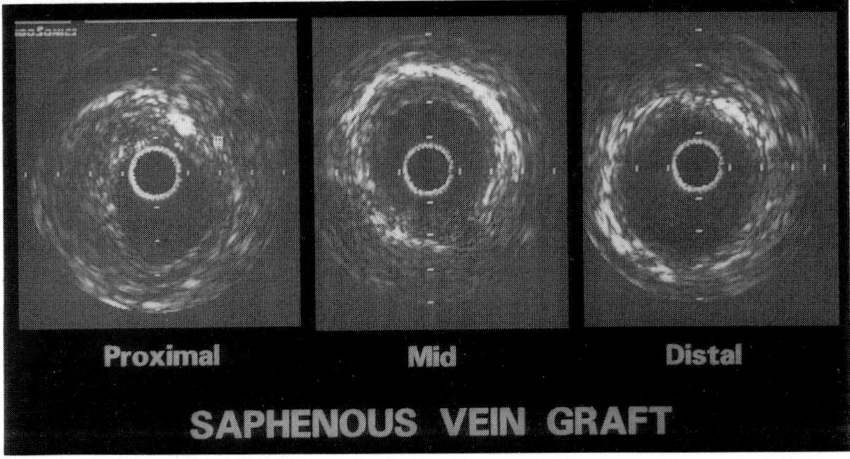

(b)

Figure 1 Intracoronary ultrasound (ICUS) imaging in SVBG. (a) Saphenous vein graft (SVG) to the posterior descending artery (PDA): In the proximal graft, the wall appears normal. At the junction with the PDA (right) there is significant eccentric atheroma occluding the lumen. (b) Example of the variability of disease within a single SVBG: Proximally there is an eccentric atheroma between 6:00 and 12:00. In the mid-graft, there is mild concentric atheroma. Distally, the graft appears normal. Since the lumen remains nearly constant, angiography in this case was unremarkable and did not demonstrate significant disease.

such as lesion length and laminar flow characteristics, are more difficult to predict. Lesion geometry significantly affects the accuracy of angiographically determined percent diameter stenosis. As a result of the important limitations of angiography, alternative criteria have been sought.

Coronary flow reserve (CFR), the ratio of maximal to resting coronary blood flow, has been recognized as an important physiologic parameter that is indicative of the ability of the vascular bed to meet its metabolic demands. Under conditions of maximal stress, the normal functioning coronary vasculature can augment blood flow five to six times over the basal flow rates [13]. Near-maximal coronary blood flow can be induced pharmacologically using intravenous dipyridamole and intracoronary adenosine or papaverine. Although resting coronary blood flow remains normal until coronary diameter stenosis is greater than 90%, maximal coronary blood flow begins to decrease when coronary diameter stenosis exceeds 50% [14]. Several factors can influence coronary blood flow measurements (Table 3), and these factors need to be considered when results are interpreted.

Various methods of measuring coronary blood flow or coronary flow reserve have been applied clinically (Table 4). The most recent of these is the Doppler flow wire (Flowire; Cardiometrics, Inc.), which has the advantage of doubling as an angioplasty guide wire if an intervention must be performed. It can be introduced through standard diagnostic catheters, helping to offset costs.

The Doppler guide wire is available in two sizes; the 0.014-inch Flowire operates at a frequency of 15 MHz, and the 0.018-inch Flowire operates at 12 MHz. The Doppler signal is processed and displayed as a phasic velocity signal along with single-lead electrocardiogram. Unlike the Doppler velocity probe, which is limited to open chest procedures or animal studies, the Doppler guide wire is readily applied to awake patients during diagnostic catheterization or catheter-based interventions. This technique requires that the operator be familiar with the handling of standard angioplasty guides wires. The Flowire does not require angioplasty guiding catheters; however, the patient must be treated with heparin to reduce thrombotic complications. With a cross-sectional area of 0.164 mm^2 for the 0.018-inch Flowire and 0.099 mm^2 for the

Table 3 Factors Influencing Coronary Blood Flow

Noncardiac	Cardiac	Pharmacologic
Body temperature	Tachycardia	Beta-blockers
Hypoxia	Epicardial stenosis	Calcium channel blockers
Anemia	Impaired microvascular circulation	Vasodilators
		Vasoconstrictors

Table 4   Clinical Measurement
of CFR

Digital radiography
Doppler velocity probe
Doppler coronary catheter
Doppler flow wire

0.014-inch Flowire, this system is less likely to alter the flow velocity profile and peak velocities than the Doppler catheters (3F) with a cross-sectional area of 1 mm^2. Studies of flow characteristics across artificial stenosis by Folts et al. [15] determined that maximal flow was not limited until approximately 59% of the cross-sectional area of the vessel was occluded. Based upon these observations, the 0.014-inch Flowire should accurately reflect velocity profiles in vessels as small as 0.5 mm in diameter.

By comparing the average peak velocity (APV) signal proximal and distal to a lesion during resting and hyperemic conditions, coronary flow reserve can be determined. Lesions that are hemodynamically significant will demonstrate a reduced coronary flow reserve. In addition to coronary flow reserve, other characteristics of native coronary and saphenous vein bypass graft blood flow have been described, including peak diastolic velocity (PV_d), peak systolic velocity (PV_s), diastolic systolic peak velocity ratio (DSVR), and proximal/distal flow velocity ratio.

In vitro and in vivo studies by Doucette et al. [16] compared Doppler guide wire flow (Q_D) rates and the time-average spectral peak velocity (APV) with electromagnetic flow (Q_{EMF}) rates. These investigators found a high correlation between APV and Q_{EMF} ($r^2 = 0.98–0.99$) in straight plastic tubes ranging from 0.76 mm to 4.76 mm in diameter. This correlation was less accurate in the largest tube (7.94 mm in diameter) and was especially poor at flow rates above 922 mL/min, with Q_D consistently underestimating Q_{EMF} by over 20%. When comparing Q_D to Q_{EMF} in the left circumflex artery (LCx) of dogs, a good linear correlation was found ($r^2 = 0.85$). Comparison of the time-average spectral peak velocity (APV) to Q_{EMF} demonstrated a higher correlation in the proximal segments of the LCx ($r^2 = 0.93–0.99$) than in the distal segments of the LCx ($r^2 = 0.86–0.99$).

Ofili et al. [17] compared coronary flow characteristics in angiographically appearing normal and abnormal arteries. As expected, these investigators found that normal arteries had a significantly higher coronary flow reserve ($p < 0.02$) as compared to angiographically diseased arteries. They discovered that a predominantly diastolic flow pattern was characteristic of normal arteries,

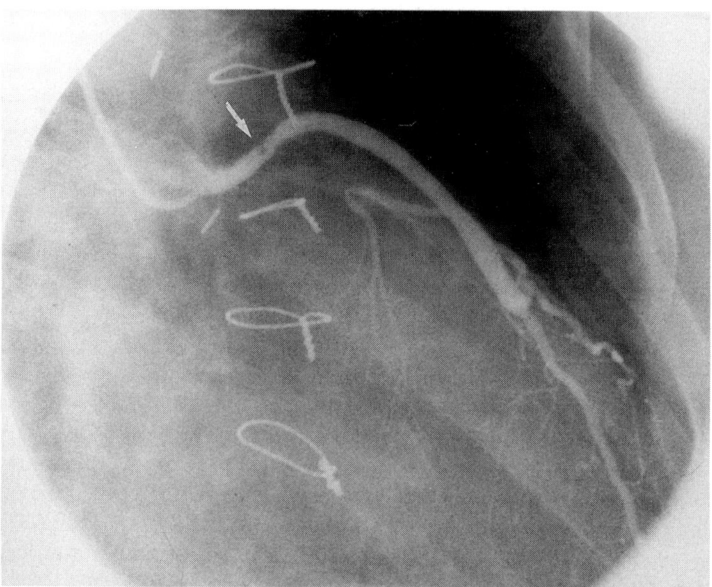

(a)

Figure 2 Evaluation of a questionable stenosis. (a) Right anterior oblique selective angiogram showing a filling defect (arrow) in the proximal SVBG to the left anterior descending artery. (b) Left anterior oblique projection of the same SVBG. (c) Coronary flow reserve (CFR) measured distal to the filling defect using a 0.014-inch Doppler wire. *Lower left*: baseline flow pattern with diastolic predominance [diastolic/systolic velocity ratio (DSVR) of 1.7] and average peak velocity (APV) of 21. *Lower right*: hyperemic flow pattern after 12 μg adenosine. The APV increased to 50, yielding a CFR of 2.4 Based on these results, intervention was not performed.

with a shift towards a predominantly systolic flow pattern in abnormal arteries. This is measured as the diastolic systolic velocity ratio (DSVR), which is the ratio of peak diastolic velocity to peak systolic velocity. In angiographically diseased arteries, all flow velocities were lower distal to the lesion as compared to flow in the proximal vessel. This is called the proximal/distal flow velocity ratio.

Bach et al. [18] described the phasic blood flow characteristics of angiographically normal appearing saphenous vein bypass grafts and internal mammary artery bypass grafts. Similar to the native coronary circulation, they found a predominantly diastolic flow pattern in the SVBG (proximal DSVR,

(b)

ARDIOMETRICS
09:37:24
17 APR 95
APV:43
DSVR:1.5
BASELINE
APV:21
DSVR:1.7
PEAK
APV:50
DSVR:1.5
CFR:2.4
THR:21 P#:2
BASE 09:36:38
PEAK 09:37:15

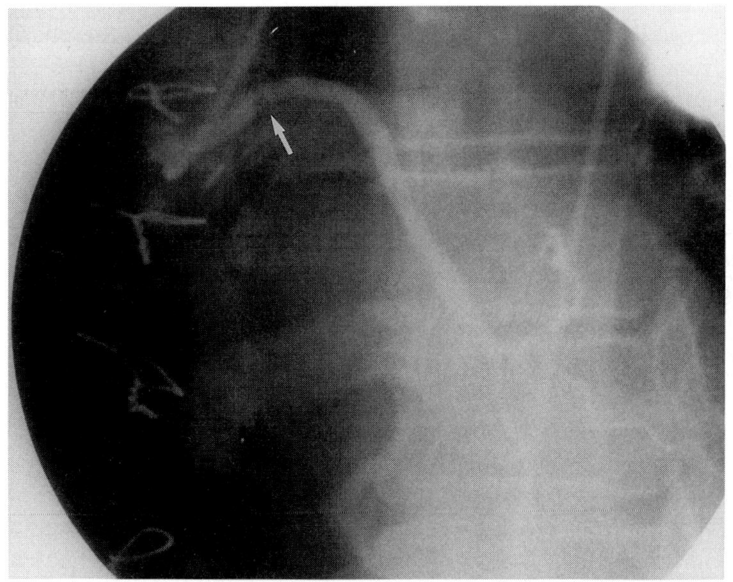

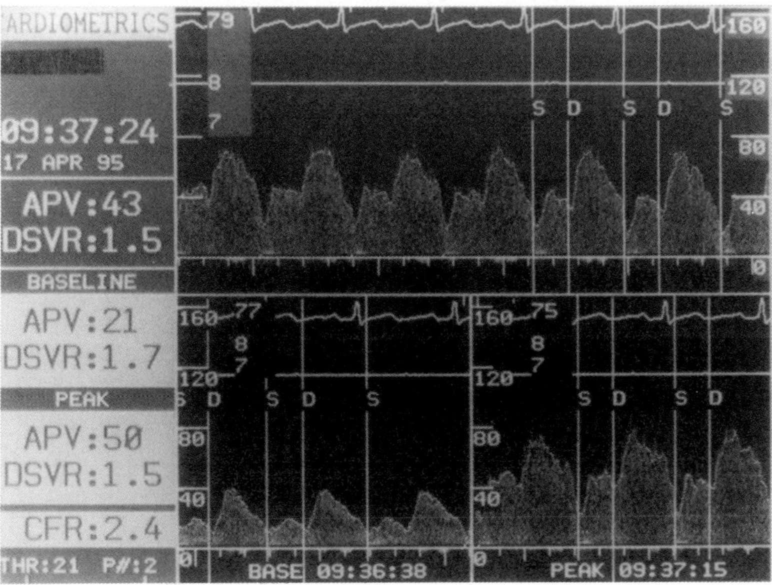

(c)

1.4 ± 0.6; distal DSVR, 1.5 ± 0.7; p = NS). The internal mammary artery bypass grafts, however, demonstrated a longitudinal transition in the phasic flow pattern from a predominantly systolic flow pattern proximally (DSVR, 0.6 ± 0.2) to a predominantly diastolic flow pattern distally (DSVR, 1.4 ± 0.3) (p < 0.001).

The Doppler flow wire is useful in the evaluation of borderline stenosis (Figure 2). It provides physiologic data indicative of the hemodynamic impact that a particular stenosis has on the vasculature. This is particularly true if exercise testing combined with nuclear or echo imaging has not been performed prior to angiography. The use of Doppler flow wire data to determine the efficacy of catheter-based interventions in SVBG remains to be studied.

IV. DIGITAL ANGIOGRAPHY

Digital angiography may be utilized to evaluate graft patency and function. The major use of digital angiography is to perform simple mask subtraction and provide enhanced images for immediate review while in the catheterization laboratory. Use of mask subtraction is important when reviewing aortography, because vein graft filling may be slow or limited in the setting of disease. By subtracting the background structures, we avoid mistakenly thinking that these faintly filling grafts are occluded. Several studies have documented the accuracy of this approach [19–28]. Although effective for establishing the patency of grafts, the distal anastomosis, distal coronary bed, and even vein graft body stenosis may not be well seen via this technique. Therefore, in symptomatic patients, selective cannulation and standard angiography are needed to evaluate graft pathology fully.

Two other forms of digital subtraction angiography have been described for the evaluation of vein grafts. Intravenous injection of contrast with subsequent subtraction imaging of the aortic root has been used to assess vein graft patency [23,27–29]. Sievert et al. [29] showed a sensitivity of 92.5% and specificity of 70% for the diagnosis of an occluded graft using intravenous injection of 40 cc contrast. Guthaner et al. [23] compared intravenous and intraaortic injection in the same population. They found that only 41% of the patent grafts seen by intraaortic injection were seen by intravenous injection. While an intravenous approach was initially felt to be a potential tool for outpatient screening of graft patency, studies such as these have shown the technique to be too limited in accuracy for widespread application.

Digital subtraction angiography has also been used to evaluate the function of vein grafts. By obtaining a series of EKG-gated images after a carefully gated contrast injection, it is possible to evaluate the wash-in and wash-out of contrast in the vascular bed supplied by the graft. Generally these studies employ a second injection after administration of a vasodilator such as papaverine or adenosine. By comparing the basal to the hyperemic images, a measure of coronary flow reserve can be calculated [30].

This technique has been used to assess the acute and chronic flow responses in various coronary graft conduits [31–33]. Bates et al. [32,33] found the coronary flow reserve after bypass to be improved compared to nonbypassed vessels and similar to that in vessels after balloon angioplasty. Flow reserve remains less than in normal vessels, however, probably due to chronic microvascular disease. Hodgson et al. [31] compared vein grafts to internal mammary artery grafts and found the flow reserve provided by both types of conduit to be similar 4 weeks following surgery.

Digital subtraction angiography is most useful when aortic injections are performed to assess graft patency. Neither intravenous nor functional imaging is widely used, in large part due to technical complexity and limited diagnostic application.

V. ANGIOSCOPY

Coronary angioscopy has been shown to be more sensitive than conventional angiography for the diagnosis of intravascular thrombi and complex lesion morphology [34]. The coronary angioscope is a 4.3F catheter. A balloon capable of occluding blood flow in the vessel to be imaged is required. A third channel carries a 2,000-element fiberoptic imaging bundle that is connected to a color video monitor. The fourth channel accommodates a specially designed 0.014-inch guide wire and allows for infusion of crystalloid used to clear blood from the field of view.

Angioscopy is performed by advancing the guide wire through an 8F PTCA guiding catheter into the distal vessel, past the stenosis or segment to be visualized. The angioscope is then advanced to within a few millimeters of the target. The balloon is inflated, occluding flow to the vessel being imaged while crystalloid is injected down the guide wire lumen to clear blood from the field of view. The distal end of the catheter is positioned by rotating and withdrawing the specially designed guide wire, which has preformed sinusoidal bends that allow the catheter to be steered into coaxial alignment.

Imaging time is limited by ischemia induced by the occlusion balloon. Angioscopy is not able to evaluate ostial disease or to be used in vein grafts larger than the effective diameter of the occlusion balloon (2.5–4.0 mm) since the field of view cannot be kept free of blood. Intramural thrombi appear red and may be either firmly adherent to the vessel wall or mobile globular masses projecting into the lumen. The usual appearance of the vessel wall is a pale yellow, which contrasts well with thrombi. Dissections may appear as mobile white flaps of tissue projecting into the lumen of the vein or as deep fissures in the vessel wall.

A comparison of angioscopy and conventional angiography for the evaluation of saphenous vein bypass grafts by White et al. [34] found that thrombi were identified by angioscopy in 71% of the vein grafts they evaluated but was recognized by conventional angiography in only 19% ($p < 0.001$). These investigators also noted intimal tears in 33% of the vein grafts they evaluated prior to angioplasty, all of which were unrecognized by conventional angiography. Following angioplasty, conventional angiography identified only 2 of 11 dissections noted by angioscopy ($p < 0.01$). Although angioscopy appears superior to conventional angiography for the detection of thrombi and dissections in saphenous vein bypass grafts, the impact that angioscopy will have on catheter-based interventions remains unclear. It will be difficult to demonstrate the cost effectiveness of angioscopy unless angioscopic criteria can be developed that affect interventional outcomes. In the study by White et al. [34], distal embolization of plaque did not occur in any of the saphenous vein bypass grafts undergoing balloon angioplasty, including 11 SVBGs identified by angioscopy to have friable plaque. Larger studies are needed to address these questions.

Table 5 Equipment Requirements of Techniques for Invasive Diagnosis of SVBG Disease

Contrast angiography	Standard cardiac catheterization laboratory
	Diagnostic catheters
	Contrast
Digital subtraction angiography	Subtraction angiography laboratory
	Contrast
Intracoronary ultrasound	Catheterization laboratory
	PTCA guiding catheters and guide wires
	ICUS catheter and image processor
	Contrast
Doppler flow studies	Catheterization laboratory
	Diagnostic catheters
	Doppler flow wire and image processor
	Contrast
	Hyperemic agent
Angioscopy	Catheterization laboratory
	PTCA guiding catheters
	Special angioscopy guide wire
	Balloon inflation device
	Angioscopy catheters and image processor
	Contrast

VI. CONCLUSION

While newer technologies have been developed to provide information that is difficult to obtain from angiography, none of them can be used as a stand-alone imaging modality (Table 5). One must consider additional costs as well as additional risks when evaluating the need for these devices (Table 6).

Intracoronary ultrasound, Doppler flow wire, and angioscopy all require heparinization to reduce the risk of developing intracoronary thrombi, and they are associated with the risks of guide wires and catheter-induced vessel

Table 6 Comparison of Various Techniques for Invasive Diagnosis of SVBG Disease

Technique	Pros	Cons
Conventional contrast angiography	Adequate detail of the vein graft anatomy to allow for intervention. Does not require interventional (PTCA) skills. Gives overview of entire graft.	Requires knowledge of the number and location of bypass grafts. Unable to determine plaque morphology. Unable to provide functional data.
Digital subtraction i.v. angiography	Can be performed by technician. Does not require knowledge of the number or location of grafts. No risk of arterial puncture.	Inadequate detail of vein graft anatomy to allow for intervention. Contrast load is the same as for selective angiography.
Intracoronary ultrasound	Provides information regarding vessel wall and plaque morphology. Useful evaluating ostial lesions. Useful in ambiguous lesions.	Requires interventional (PTCA) skills and heparinization. Contrast angiography must still be performed. Limited to single tomographic image at one time.
Doppler flow studies	Useful for determining the functional significance of borderline lesions.	Requires interventional (PTCA) skills and heparinization. Contrast angiography must still be performed.
Angioscopy	Useful for distinguishing plaque from thrombus.	Requires interventional (PTCA) skills and heparinization. Contrast angiography must still be performed. Can not evaluate ostial lesions. Controlled ieschemia will occur.

wall trauma and plaque disruption. Intracoronary ultrasound and angioscopy must be performed through guiding catheters, which are capable of inflicting increased vascular injury during insertion and may traumatize graft ostia. Angioscopy carries the risks associated with controlled ischemia produced during inflation of the occluding balloon. Although intravenous digital subtraction angiography would be an attractive alternative to selective angiography, the current technology is incapable of providing adequate detail and exposes the patient to the same contrast-related risks.

When complex lesion geometry produces ambiguous angiographic results or when plaque morphology characteristics must be determined, intracoronary ultrasound is the imaging modality of choice. The tomographic orientation of the ICUS image combined with longitudinal assessment of the vein graft during "pull-back" allows the operator to construct a three-dimensional representation of the region of interest. Although crude assessment of the function capacity of vascular territories can be obtained from digital subtraction functional studies, Doppler velocity studies provide the most accurate means of establishing saphenous vein graft function. If thrombus detection is imperative, angioscopy is the procedure of choice.

Despite the advantages of these newer technologies, contrast angiography is likely to remain the dominant invasive imaging modality for SVBGs for years to come.

REFERENCES

1. de Feyter PJ, van Suylen RJ, de Jaegere, Topol EJ, Serruys PW. Balloon angioplasty for the treatment of lesions in saphenous vein bypass grafts. J Am Coll Cardiol 1993; 21:1539–1549.
2. Liebson PR, Klein LW. Intravascular ultrasound in coronary atherosclerosis: a new approach to clinical assessment. Am Heart J 1992; 123:1643–1660.
3. Hodgson JM, Graham SP, Savakus AD, Dame SG, Stephens DN, Dhillon PS, Brands D, Sheehan H, Eberle MJ. Clinical percutaneous imaging of coronary anatomy using an over-the-wire ultrasound catheter system. Int J Card Imaging 1989; 4:187–193.
4. Pandian NG, Kreis A, Brockway B, Isner JM, Sacharoff A, Boleza E, Caro R, Muller D. Ultrasound angioscopy: real-time, two-dimensional, intraluminal ultrasound imaging of blood vessels. Am J Cardiol 1988; 62:493–494.
5. Potkin BN, Bartorelli AL, Bessert JM, Neville RF, Almagor Y, Roberts WC, Leon MB. Coronary artery imaging with intravascular high-frequency ultrasound. Circulation 1990; 81:1575–1585.
6. Nissen SE, Grines CL, Gurley JC, Sublett K, Haynie D, Diaz C, Booth DC, DeMaria AN. Application of a new phased-array ultrasound imaging catheter in the assessment of vascular dimensions. Circulation 1990; 81:660–666.

7. Hodgson JM, Graham SP, Sheehan H, Savakus AD. Percutaneous intracoronary ultrasound imaging: initial applications in patients. Echocardiography 1990; 7: 403–413.

8. Tobis JM, Mallery J, Mahon D, Lehman K, Zalesby P, Griffith J, Gessert O, Moriuchi M, Dwyer ML, McRae M, et al. Intravascular ultrasound imaging of human coronary arteries in vivo analysis of tissue characterizations with comparison to in vitro histological specimens. Circulation 1991; 83:913–926.

9. Nissen SE, Gurley JC, Grines CL, Booth DC, McLure R, Berk M, Fischer C, DeMaria AN. Intravascular ultrasound assessment of lumen size and wall morphology, in normal subjects and patients with coronary artery disease. Circulation 1991; 84:1087–1099.

10. Vlodaver Z, Frech R, van Tassel RA, Edwards JE. Correlation of the antemortem coronary angiogram and the postmortem specimen. Circulation 1973; 47:162–168.

11. Roberts WC, Jones AA. Quantitation of coronary arterial narrowing at necropsy in sudden coronary death. Am J Cardiol 1979; 44:39–44.

12. Nase-Hueppmeier S, Uebis R, Doerr R, Hanrath P. Intravascular ultrasound to assess aortocoronary venous bypass grafts in vivo. Am J Cardiol 1992; 70: 455–458.

13. Katz LN, Linder E. Quantitative relation between reactive hyperemia and the myocardial ischemia which it follows. Am J Physiol 1939; 126:283.

14. Gould KL, Lipscomb K, Hamilton GW. Physiologic basis for assessing critical coronary stenosis. Am J Cardiol 1974; 33:87.

15. Folts JD, Gallagher K, Rowe GG. Hemodynamic effects of controlled degrees of coronary artery stenosis in short-term and long-term studies in dogs. J Thorac Cardiovasc Surg 1977; 73:722–727.

16. Doucette JW, Corl PD, Payne HM, Flynn AE, Goto M, Nassi M, Segal J. Validation of a doppler guide wire for intravascular measurement of coronary artery flow velocity. Circulation 1992; 85:1899–1911.

17. Ofili EO, Morton KJ, Labotiz AJ, St Vrain JA, Segal J, Aguirre FV, Castello R. Analysis of coronary blood flow velocity dynamics in angiographically normal and stenosed arteries before and after endolumen enlargement by angioplasty. J Am Coll Cardiol 1993; 21:308–316.

18. Bach RG, Kern MJ, Donohue TJ, Aguirre FV, Caracciolo EA. Comparison of phasic blood flow velocity characteristics of arterial and venous coronary artery bypass conduits. Circulation 1993; 88 (part 2):133–140.

19. Myerowitz PD, Turnipseed WD, Swanson DK, Van Lysel M, Peppler W, Mistretta C, Chopra PS, Berkoff H, Kroncke G, Hasegawa B, Steighorst M, Turski P, Crummy AB. Digital subtraction angiography as a method of screening for coronary artery disease during peripheral vascular angiography. Surgery 1982; 92(6): 1042–1048.

20. Vandenbosch G, Delcour C, Delatte P, Struyven J. Evaluation de permeabilité des pontages aort-coronariens par angiographie numerisée. Journal de Radiologie 1988; 69:25–28.

21. Grigg LE, Chan W, Hunt D, Thomson K. Assessment of aortocoronary bypass graft patency by intra-arterial digital subtraction angiography compared to selective graft angiography. Aust NZ J Med 1988; 18:651–655.

22. Hayward R, Hunter GJS. Digital subtraction angiography in coronary artery bypass graft assessment: clinical applicability. Br Heart J 1985; 54:357–361.
23. Guthaner DF, Wexler L, Bradley B. Digital subtraction angiography of coronary grafts: optimization of technique. Am J Radiol 1985; 145:1185–1190.
24. Luska VG, Hendrickx Ph, Kuhl A, Lichtlen P. Peripher venose digitale Subtraktionsangiographie (DSA) zur Kontrolle von aortokoronaren Venenbypassgrafts (ACVB). Fortschr Rontgenstr 1985; 142(1):35–40.
25. Heuser L, Krestin GP, Hannekum H, Wimmer G. Dsrstellung aortokoronarer Venenbruken mit der digitalen Subtraktionsangiographie. Dtsch Med Wschr 1985; 110:243–247.
26. Witte VG, Jacobs G, Grabbe E, Rodiger W, Kalmar P, Bucheler E. ARterielle DSA zur Darstellung des aortokoronaren Venenbypass (ACVB). Fortschr Rontgenstr 1984; 140(3):251–253.
27. Mancini GBJ, Higgins CB. Digital subtraction angiography: a review of cardiac applications. Prog Cardiovasc Dis 1985; 18(2):111–141.
28. Wholey MH. Cardiovascular applications of digital subtraction angiography. Radiol Clin North Am 1985; 23(4):627–639.
29. Sievert H, Rauber K, Kunkel B. Schork A, Satter A, Riemann H, Kaltenbach M, Kober G. Darstellung aortokoronarer Bypasses mit der intravenosen digitalen Subtraktionsangiographie. Z Kardiol 1987; 76:733–736.
30. Hodgson JMcB, LeGrand V, Bates ER, Mancini GBJ, Aueron FM, O'Neill WW, Simon SB, Beauman GJ, LeFree MT, Vogel RA. Validation in dogs of a rapid angiographic technique to measure relative coronary blood flow during routine cardiac catheterization. Am J Cardiol 1985; 55:188–193.
31. Hodgson JMcB, Singh AK, Drew TM, Riley RS, Williams DO. Coronary flow reserve provided by sequential internal mammary artery grafts. J Am Coll Cardiol 1986; 7:32–37.
32. Bates ER, Vogel RA, LeFree MT, Kirlin PC, O'Neill WW, Pitt B. The chronic coronary flow reserve provided by saphenous vein bypass grafts as determined by digital coronary radiography. Am Heart J 1984; 108:462–468.
33. Bates ER, Aueron FM, LeGrand V, LeFree MT, Mancini GBJ, Hodgson JM, Vogel RH. Comparative long-term effects of coronary artery bypass graft surgery and percutaneous transluminal coronary angioplasty on regional coronary flow reserve. Circulation 1985; 72:833–839.
34. White CJ, Ramee SR, Collins TJ, Mesa JE, Jain A. Percutaneous angioscopy of saphenous vein bypass grafts. J Am Coll Cardiol 1993; 21:1181–1185.

8
Medical Interventions for Saphenous Vein Bypass Graft Disease

Eric R. Bates, Robert J. Lederman, and Jorge Saucedo
University of Michigan Medical Center, Ann Arbor, Michigan

I. INTRODUCTION

Coronary artery bypass graft (CABG) surgery acutely relieves symptoms in the large majority of patients and prolongs survival in certain subsets. However, the long-term benefits are eroded by late deterioration of the saphenous vein bypass graft (SVBG) [1] conduits (Figure 1). SVBG attrition results from thrombosis and accelerated atherosclerosis. Acute SVBG occlusion producing myocardial infarction is associated with twice the mortality risk of native artery occlusion, presumably because CABG patients are more likely to have multivessel disease and left ventricular dysfunction [2]. Chronic SVBG attrition and native disease progression after surgery lead to recurrent angina and the risk of myocardial infarction, congestive heart failure, and sudden death. Repeat revascularization constitutes the indication for 10–20% of CABG procedures and an unknown number of PTCA procedures performed in the United States. Therefore, preventing SVBG attrition is an important treatment goal for reducing long-term morbidity, mortality, and health care costs.

There have been dramatic advances in understanding the role of risk factor control in patients with atherosclerotic vascular disease. Application of these principles in patients after CABG is of paramount importance. Whereas native coronary artery disease atherosclerosis develops over decades, SVBG disease becomes clinically evident within years. This chapter reviews

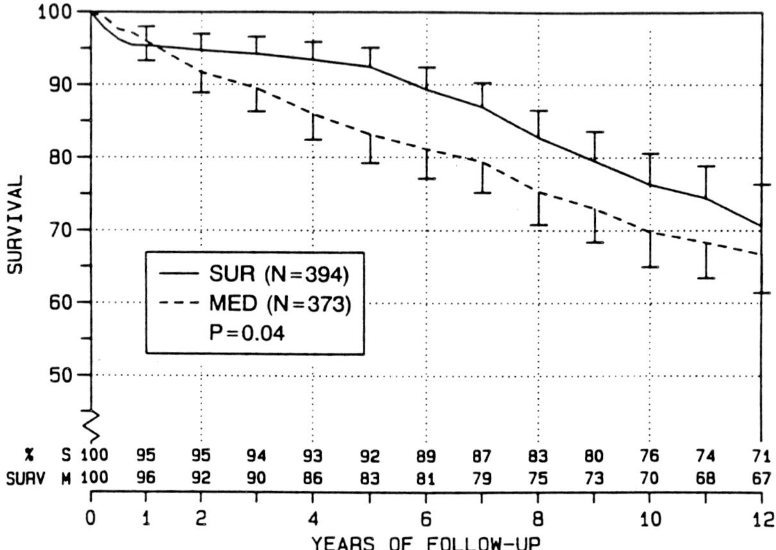

Figure 1 Cumulative survival curves for patients in the European Coronary Surgery Study randomized to surgical (SUR) or medical (MED) treatment. A smaller difference in survival rates is present at 10 and 12 years as compared with 5 years.

the clinical data regarding risk factor control after surgical revascularization and makes treatment recommendations.

II. RISK FACTOR CONTROL AND SVBG DISEASE

A. Hyperlipidemia

Hyperlipidemia appears to be the main risk factor for SVBG atherosclerosis and is the only risk factor implicated in every nature history study. The association between hyperlipidemia and coronary SVBG disease was first reported by Barboriak et al. [3] in 1974. Campeau et al. [4] performed an angiographic study 10 years after surgery and found atherosclerotic lesions in patients with higher levels of total cholesterol, LDL cholesterol, LDL apoprotein B, and triglycerides and in patients with lower levels of HDL cholesterol. Neitzel et al. [5] made the observation that patients requiring a second bypass graft operation had higher total cholesterol and triglyceride levels and lower HDL cholesterol levels than those not requiring reoperation. Hoff et al. [6] found serum lipoprotein LP(a) levels doubled in patients with SVBG stenoses, compared than those with no stenoses. Recently, Daida and colleagues [7] demonstrated significant SVBG stenoses 7 years after surgery in 12% of patients with total cholesterol <200 mg/dL, in 39% of patients with levels between 200 and 239 mg/dL, and in 43% of patients with cholesterol levels >240 mg/dL.

B. Cigarette Smoking

Campeau et al. [4] did not find smoking to be a risk factor for developing SVBG disease, but had only 15 patients without new lesions to compare with 67 patients with new lesions in the grafts or native arteries. In contrast, Neitzel et al. [5] studied grafts from 42 patients 6–12 years after surgery and compared the incidence of risk factors with that of 535 patients without repeat CABG. The frequency of SVBG disease was increased in smokers. An association between graft thrombosis and smoking was documented in a histologic study of 173 resected grafts by Solymoss et al. [8].

C. Hypertension

There are no studies suggesting that poor hypertension control is an independent risk factor for SVBG disease. This is not surprising, given that no consistent cardiovascular benefit has been shown in individual randomized trials of medical therapy for hypertension. However, a meta-analysis of 14 randomized trials has demonstrated that a decrease of 5–6 mm Hg in diastolic blood pressure over 5 years was associated with a 42% reduction in the risk of stroke and a 14% reduction in the incidence of nonfatal myocardial infarction in 37,000 patients [9].

D. Diabetes Mellitus

Similarly, there are no consistent data relating hyperglycemia to SVBG disease, although the subject has been inadequately investigated. The underlying mechanisms for accelerated atherogenesis in diabetes are poorly understood and confounded by the association of hyperglycemia with hyperlipidemia, hypertension, and obesity. Only recently have two Finnish studies in 362 newly diagnosed patients with noninsulin diabetes supported the linear association of glycemic control with the risk for coronary heart disease [10]. In the Diabetes Control and Complications Trial [11], the risks for retinopathy, nephropathy, and neuropathy were substantially reduced in the intensively treated patients with insulin-independent diabetes mellitus. Cardiovascular events were reduced by 41%, but this decrease was not statistically significant.

Diabetes does have an adverse effect on survival after CABG, but is not a risk factor for repeat angiography or repeat CABG. Some, but not all, of this risk is due to older age, more extensive coronary disease, and worse left ventricular function at the time of surgery. Lawrie et al. [12] observed preoperative blood glucose level to be a significant independent predictor of 15-year survival after surgery in over 1,400 patients operated on between 1968 and 1973. Morris et al. [13] reported on 5,654 consecutive patients operated on between January 1980 and December 1989 at Duke University. Five-year survival was 91% in nondiabetics and 80% in diabetic patients. More recently, the Bypass Angioplasty Revascularization Investigation (BARI) trial [14] reported a five-year survival of 81% in diabetic patients after CABG, compared with 65% after angioplasty.

III. CLINICAL TRIALS

A. The Cholesterol-Lowering Atherosclerosis Study (CLAS)

The CLAS study [15] randomized 188 normotensive, nonsmoking men a mean of 3.3 years after CABG. During 2 years of treatment, patients received either colestipol (30 g/day) and niacin (4 g/day) plus diet or placebo plus diet. Baseline and follow-up angiography was completed in 162 men. Lipid levels at baseline included total cholesterol 246 mg/dL, triglycerides 151 mg/dL, LDL cholesterol 171 mg/dL, and HDL cholesterol 45 mg/dL. Drug therapy reduced total cholesterol by 26%, triglycerides by 22%, and LDL cholesterol by 43% and increased HDL cholesterol by 37%. The mean LDL cholesterol level was 97 mg/dL during the trial. This was associated with a dramatic reduction in new lesion formation in both native arteries (10% vs. 22%) and grafts (14% vs. 33%). A follow-up report [16] after 4 years of treatment (CLAS-II) documented the results in 103 patients who underwent an additional angiogram. Lipid levels were maintained at the same levels. More drug-treated patients demonstrated nonprogression (52% vs. 15%) and regression (18% vs. 6%) of atherosclerotic lesions in native coronary arteries. Only 16% of drug-treated patients developed new lesions in SVBG grafts versus 38% of placebo-treated patients. The authors suggested that new lesions in grafts were promoted by hyperlipidemia, since lipid lowering markedly reduced their formation. The failure to prevent progression of existing graft lesions in CLAS suggested to the authors that thrombosis might be the mechanism for progression.

B. The Post-Coronary Artery Bypass Graft Trial

The NIH-funded Post-CABG trial [17] enrolled 1,351 stable patients from 1 to 11 years after surgery. Entry criteria included age <75 years, LDL cholesterol 130–175 mg/dL, two patent vein grafts in men, one patent vein graft in women, and an ejection fraction >30%. This was an angiographic trial, not an event trial, with paired angiograms performed a mean of 4.3 years apart. Patients were randomized to either an aggressive lipid-lowering strategy or a moderate lipid-lowering strategy and to treatment with warfarin or placebo. In the aggressive strategy, lovastatin 40–80 mg/dL was prescribed if LDL cholesterol was 80 mg/dL or greater and cholestyramine 8 mg day was added if LDL cholesterol was over 95 mg/dL. This treatment was compared with moderate lipid-lowering therapy of lovastatin 2.5 mg increased to 5 mg/day if LDL cholesterol was over 140 mg/dL and cholestyramine added if LDL cholesterol was over 160 mg/dL.

Baseline values included cholesterol 226 mg/dL, triglycerides 156 mg/dL, HDL cholesterol 39 mg/dL, and LDL cholesterol 156 mg/dL. In the aggressive-treatment group, an average of lovastatin 76 mg with 30% of patients taking cholestyramine reduced mean LDL cholesterol to 93 mg/dL, a 39% reduction. In the moderate-treatment group, an average of lovastatin 4 mg/dL with 5% of patients taking cholestyramine reduced mean LDL cholesterol to 136 mg/dL, a 14% reduction. A total of 66% of patients assigned to aggressive treatment and 5% assigned to moderate treatment had an LDL cholesterol level below 100 mg/dL.

Patients following the aggressive lipid-lowering regimen showed a 31% reduction in progression of atherosclerotic lesions in SVBG conduits (Table 1). Moreover, fewer grafts developed new lesions or total occlusion. The risk for repeat PTCA or CABG surgery was reduced by 29%. Low-dose warfarin (INR 1.4) did not reduce the progression of atherosclerosis. Thus, there are major benefits in patients with SVBGs who can reduce the LDL cholesterol below 100 mg/dL.

C. Smoking Cessation

The Coronary Artery Surgery Study (CASS) randomized 708 patients to medical therapy or CABG surgery. In the entire cohort, 10-year survival was 82%

Table 1 The Post-CABG Trial

	Aggressive treatment	Moderate treatment
Disease progression (%)	27	39
Graft occlusion (%)	10	16
New lesions (%)	10	21
Percent stenosis (Δ)	7.9	13.3
Minimum lumen diameter (Δ)	−0.197	−0.379
Repeat revascularization (%)	6.5	9.2

among patients who reported no smoking during follow-up, compared with 77% among smokers [18]. Survival was 80% among smokers who quit versus 69% among those who continued smoking. For patients randomized to surgery, survival at 10 years was 84% for quitters and 68% for nonquitters. This represents a twofold relative risk of death for nonquitters. At 10 years, more nonsmokers were free of angina (54% vs. 42%) and had no activity limitation (38% vs. 29%). The hospitalization rate for smokers was 3.8 admissions/patient (28.6 days) versus 2.6 admissions/patient (19.6 days) for nonsmokers. Reoperation was performed in 12.8% of smokers and 8.4% of nonsmokers.

Voors et al. [19] followed 446 consecutive patients for 15 years following CABG surgery. There was no difference in outcome between patients who stopped smoking after surgery and nonsmokers. Patients still smoking 1 year after surgery had a relative risk of 2.3 for myocardial infarction and a relative risk of 2.5 for reoperation compared with those who quit. Smokers at 5 years after surgery had relative risks for myocardial infarction, reoperation, angina pectoris, and PTCA of 2.5, 3.3, 2.0, and 1.9, respectively, compared with quitters.

IV. THE POST-CABG REVASCULARIZATION CLINIC

Risk factors are infrequently assessed or treated by the revascularization team that sees the patient in consultation. Furthermore, few primary care providers are organized to provide systematic screening and management in these areas. The American Heart Association has published a special report entitled "Optimal Risk Factor Management in the Patient after Coronary Revascularization" [20]. The recommendations can easily be adapted to establish a comprehensive and coordinated Post-Revascularization Clinic led by cardiovascular specialists and including a multidisciplinary team of nurses, registered dietitians, and exercise physiologists to offer skills in counseling, nutrition, exercise, smoking cessation, and pharmacologic interventions. The goal is aggressive promotion of good health and disease prevention in this highest risk group of patients. Additionally, risk factor assessments are performed in first-degree relatives, who become intimately involved in the process to improve patient compliance. Although it is preferable to initiate appropriate interventions before surgery, practical considerations often delay assessment and investigation until after surgery. One benefit to this strategy is that patients and their families are more receptive to these concepts because of the temporary disruption in normal lifestyle.

A. Evaluation

A comprehensive approach to risk factor assessment is outlined in Table 2. Every patient should have a complete lipid profile, including measurement of

Table 2 Assessment of Risk Factors in the Patient Undergoing Surgical Revascularization

Risk factor	Therapeutic goal
Elevated total cholesterol	<160 mg/dL
Elevated LDL cholesterol	<100 mg/dL
Decreased HDL cholesterol	>35 mg/dL
Elevated triglycerides	<200 mg/dL
Hypertension	<140/90 mm Hg
Physical inactivity	>20 min of physical activity of level walking, 1.5–2 miles/day, 3×/week as a minimum
Smoking	Complete cessation
Obesity	<130% of ideal body weight
Diabetes	<140 mg/dL
Stress	Improved coping skills

LDL: low-density lipoprotein; HDL: high-density lipoprotein.

total cholesterol, HDL cholesterol, LDL cholesterol, and total triglycerides. The National Cholesterol Education Program Adult Treatment Panel II recommendations are that two measurements be performed 1–8 weeks apart [21]. Desirable levels include total cholesterol <160 mg/dL, LDL cholesterol <100 mg/dL, HDL cholesterol >35 mg/dL, and triglycerides <200 mg/dL.

Using an appropriate cuff size, systolic and diastolic blood pressure should be measured in both arms, in the sitting position and with the arm bare, supported, and positioned at the heart level after 5 minutes of quiet rest. Two pressures separated by 2 minutes should be taken and averaged. Elevated levels should be confirmed on at least two subsequent visits or with appropriately calibrated devices at home. A systolic blood pressure less than 140 mm Hg and a diastolic blood pressure less than 90 mm Hg requires no intervention [22].

The level and frequency of physical activity in both occupational and nonoccupational activities should be determined. Physical activity vigorous enough to make the patient breathe hard and/or sweat should be performed at least three times per week unless ischemic symptoms or stress testing suggest limitations. This can often be accomplished by brisk walking for 1.5–2 miles.

A smoking history should include duration and frequency of past and present use of tobacco. The assessment should include inquiring about prior attempts at smoking cessation and the presence of other smokers at work and at home.

Obesity is associated with perioperative morbidity and impaired lung function. Ideal body weight should be calculated from height and weight.

Intensive diet and exercise programs are needed for patients whose body weight is more than 130% of ideal weight.

Diabetes mellitus is an important risk factor for atherosclerosis and late mortality after CABG. A fasting blood glucose >140 mg/dL or a glycosylated hemoglobin >7.5% suggests glucose intolerance.

Finally, assessing the level of perceived psychosocial stress at home and at work is important. Although controversial, some data suggest that stress reduction in type A personalities reduces subsequent cardiac events. It is more certain that poor coping skills decrease the ability to alter risk factors.

B. Nonpharmacologic Interventions

Diet, physical activity, smoking cessation, weight reduction, and stress reduction constitute a comprehensive program of cardiac rehabilitation that can lead to as much as a 25% reduction in future coronary events [23]. All patients should follow the Step II diet recommended by the National Cholesterol Education Program. The Step II diet limits saturated fat to less than 7% of calories, total fat to less than 30% of calories, and dietary cholesterol to less than 200 mg/day. Moreover, to facilitate blood pressure control, dietary sodium should be restricted to 3 g/day and alcohol intake should be limited to 1 oz/day. Appropriate caloric restrictions to achieve a target weight also need to be instituted. A registered dietitian should meet with the patient and key family members to assess current eating patterns and offer advice on shopping, cooking, and dietary changes. A phase II cardiac rehabilitation exercise program has important physical, psychological, occupational, and social consequences. Successful smoking cessation may require the services of a trained counselor or enrollment in a formal program. Likewise, learning to avoid stress or relieve unavoidable stress may require professional counseling.

C. Pharmacologic Interventions

Antiplatelet Drugs

Antiplatelet therapy is essential in reducing early SVBG thrombosis due to endothelial injury and platelet activation. A meta-analysis of antiplatelet therapy after CABG surgery has been published [24], and treatment guidelines have been regularly updated [25]. Chesebro et al. [26–27] initially demonstrated the benefits of antiplatelet therapy on SVBG patency. A regimen of dipyridamole 75 mg/TID started before surgery and aspirin 325 mg/TID started 7 hours after surgery reduced the occlusion rate from 10% to 2% at 1 month and from 23% to 11% at 1 year. Subsequently, Goldman et al. [28] showed that 325 mg of aspirin daily was as effective as 975 mg/day and that dipyridamole offered no additional benefit. In another study, Goldman et al. [29] demonstrated that starting aspirin 6 hours after surgery was as effective in preventing SVBG occlusion 7–10 days after surgery as starting 12 hours before surgery, without the increased bleeding risk associated with preoperative treatment. No reduction in SVBG occlusion rate has been seen when antiplatelet therapy is started more than 48 hours after surgery. For patients sensitive to aspirin, ticlopidine 250 mg twice daily can be substituted. Limet et al. [30] documented a reduction in graft occlusion rate with ticlopidine from 13% to 7% 10 days after surgery, from 24% to 15% after 6 months, and from 26% to 16% after 1 year. Interestingly, a beneficial effect of antiplatelet therapy on maintaining arterial graft patency has not yet been demonstrated, presumably because of high initial patency rates and inadequate sample sizes. Similarly, patency rates have not been improved by aspirin treatment for longer than 1 year, even though aspirin is indicated indefinitely for patients with coronary artery disease.

Lipid-Lowering Drugs

The HMG-CoA reductase inhibitors should be used aggressively to reduce LDL cholesterol levels to less than 100 mg/dL [17,31]. Combination therapy with older agents, such as niacin and resins, may be useful if monotherapy proves inadequate. Patients with SVBG represent the highest risk for progressive atherosclerosis. Therefore, controlling lipids is most likely to reduce subsequent clinical events and be cost effective.

Blood-Pressure-Reducing Drugs

Antihypertensive medications should be started if lifestyle modifications fail to maintain the blood pressure below 140/90 mm Hg. Diuretics and beta-blockers are preferred for initial drug therapy because of cost. Beta-blockers have the added advantage of decreasing myocardial ischemia and reducing nonfatal myocardial infarction and mortality in postinfarction patients [32]. ACE inhibitors also reduce the rates of nonfatal myocardial infarction and death in patients with left ventricular ejection fractions below 40% [33,34].

Other Classes of Drugs

Warfarin is not superior to aspirin for preventing SVBG occlusion. However, warfarin does reduce thromboembolic complications in patients with atrial fibrillation [35] and possibly in those with significant left ventricular dysfunction. Calcium channel blockers have probably been unfairly labeled as dangerous in the treatment of hypertension and advantageous in the treatment of non–Q wave myocardial infarction. They are recommended for approximately

6 months postoperatively in patients with radial artery grafts, to decrease the likelihood of arterial spasm [36]. Postmenopausal hormone replacement therapy and vitamin supplementation are other potential interventions undergoing clinical testing in randomized trials.

V. CONCLUSION

CABG is not a substitute for medical therapy. Rather, it should be an important stimulus to initiate the most intensive medical therapy possible, with the goal of preventing new atherosclerosis and slowing progression of existing atherosclerosis. The best way to avoid SVBG disease is to use arterial grafts whenever possible. Nevertheless, the majority of patients will have at least one SVBG. Graft patency in these patients will best be maintained by early antiplatelet therapy, smoking cessation, and aggressive lipid control.

REFERENCES

1. Varnauskas E and The European Coronary Surgery Study Group. Twelve-year follow-up of survival in the randomized European Coronary Surgery Study. N Engl J Med 1988; 319:332–337.
2. DeFranco AC, Sketch MH, Ellis SG, Abramowitz BM, Stebbins A, Holmes DR, Califf RM, Topol EJ. Outcome of acute myocardial infarction in patients with prior coronary bypass graft surgery receiving thrombolytic therapy. Submitted.
3. Barboriak JJ, Pintar K, Korns ME. Atherosclerosis in aorto-coronary vein grafts. Lancet 1974; 2:621–624.
4. Campeau L, Enjalbert M, Lesperance J, Bourassa MG, Kwiterovich P Jr, Wacholder S, Sniderman A. The relation of risk factors to the development of atherosclerosis in saphenous vein bypass grafts and the progression of disease in the native circulation: a study 10 years after aortocoronary bypass surgery. N Engl J Med 1984; 311:1329–1332.
5. Neitzel GF, Barboriak JJ, Pintar K, Qureshi I. Atherosclerosis in aortocoronary bypass grafts: morphologic study and risk factor analysis 6 to 12 years after surgery. Arteriosclerosis 1986; 6:594–600.
6. Hoff HF, Beck GJ, Skinbinski CI, Jurgens G, O'Neill J, Kramer J, Lytle B. Serum Lp(a) level as a predictor of vein graft stenosis after coronary artery bypass surgery in patients. Circulation 1988; 77:1238–1244.
7. Daida H, Yokoi H, Miyano H, Mokuno H, Satoh H, Kottke TE, Hosoda Y, Yamaguchi H. Relation of saphenous vein graft obstruction to serum cholesterol levels. J Am Coll Cardiol 1995; 25:193–197.

8. Solymoss BC, Nadeau P, Millette D, Campeau L. Late thrombosis of saphenous vein coronary bypass grafts related to risk factors. Circulation 1988; 78(Suppl I): I140–I143.

9. Collins R, Peto R, MacMahon S, Hebert P, Fiebach NH, Eberlein KA, Godwin J, Qizilbach N, Taylor JO, Hennekins CH. Blood pressure, stroke, and coronary heart disease. Part 2, Short-term reductions in blood pressure: overview of randomised drug trials in their epidemiological context. Lancet 1990; 335:827–838.

10. Laakso M. Glycemic control and the risk for coronary heart disease in patients with non-insulin-dependent diabetes mellitus. The Finnish studies. Ann Intern Med 1996; 124:127–130.

11. The Diabetes Control and Complications Trial Research Group. The effect of intensive treatment of diabetes on the development and progression of long-term complications in insulin-dependent diabetes mellitus. N Engl J Med 1993; 329: 977–986.

12. Lawrie GM, Morris GC, Glaeser DH. Influence of diabetes mellitus on the results of coronary bypass surgery. JAMA 1986; 256:2967–2971.

13. Morris JJ, Smith LR, Jones RH, Glower DD, Morris PB, Muhlbaier H, Reves JG, Rankin JS. Influence of diabetes and mammary artery grafting on survival after coronary bypass. Circulation 1991; 84(suppl III):III-275–III-284.

14. The Bypass Angioplasty Revascularization Investigation (BARI) Investigators: Comparison of coronary bypass surgery with angioplasty in patients with multivessel disease. N Engl J Med 1996; 335:217–225.

15. Blankenhorn DN, Nessim SA, Johnson RL, Sammarco ME, Azen SP, Cashin-Hempill L. Beneficial effects of combined colestipol-niacin therapy on coronary athero-sclerosis and coronary venous bypass grafts. JAMA 1987; 257:3233–3240.

16. Cashin-Hemphill L, Mack WJ, Pagoda JM, Sammarco ME, Azen SP, Blankenhorn DH. Beneficial effect of colestipol-niacin on coronary atherosclerosis. A 4-year follow-up. JAMA 1990; 264:3013–3017.

17. The Post Coronary Artery Bypass Graft Trial Investigators. The effect of aggressive lowering of low-density lipoprotein cholesterol levels and low-dose anticoagulation on obstructive changes in saphenous-vein coronary artery bypass grafts. N Engl J Med 1997; 336:153–162.

18. Cavender JB, Rogers WJ, Fisher LD, Gersh BJ, Coggin CJ, Myers WO, CASS Investigators. Effects of smoking on survival and morbidity in patients randomized to medical or surgical therapy in the Coronary Artery Surgery Study (CASS): 10-year follow-up. J Am Coll Cardiol 1992; 20:287–294.

19. Voors AA, Van Brussel BL, Plokker T, Ernst SMP, Ernst N, Koomen E, Tijssen J, Vermeulen EE. Smoking and cardiac events after venous coronary bypass surgery. Circulation 1996; 93:42–47.

20. Pearson T, Rapaport E, Criqui M, Furberg C, Fuster V, Hiratzka L, Little W, Ockene I, Williams G. Optimal risk factor management in the patient after coronary revascularization. Circulation 1994; 90:3125–3133.

21. Summary of the second report of the National Cholesterol Education Program (NCEP) Expert Panel On Detection, Evaluation, And Treatment Of High Blood Cholesterol In Adults (Adult Treatment Panel II). JAMA 1993; 269:3015–3023.

22. National High Blood Pressure Education Program. The Fifth Report of the Joint National Committee on Detection, Evaluation, and Treatment of High Blood Pressure. Bethesda, MD: National Heart, Lung, and Blood Institute, 1993. US Dept of Health, Education, and Welfare publication NIH 93-1088.

23. Oldridge NB, Guyatt GH, Fisher ME, Rimm AA. Cardiac rehabilitation after myocardial infarction: combined experience of randomized clinical trials. JAMA 1988; 260:945–950.

24. Henderson WG, Goldman S, Copeland JG, Moritz TE, Harker LA. Antiplatelet or anticoagulant therapy after coronary artery bypass surgery: a meta-analysis of clinical trials. Ann Intern Med 1989; 111:743–750.

25. Stein PD, Dalen JE, Goldman S, Schwartz L, Théroux P, Turpie AGG. Antithrombotic therapy in patients with saphenous vein and internal mammary artery bypass grafts. Chest 1995; 108:424S–430S.

26. Chesebro JH, Clements IP, Fuster V, Elveback LR, Smith HC, Bardsley WT, Frye RL, Holmes DR Jr, Vlietstra RE, Pluth JR, Wallace RB, Puga FJ, Orszlak TA, Piehler JM, Schaff HV, Danielson GK. A platelet-inhibitor-drug trial in coronary-artery bypass operations: benefit of perioperative dipyridamole and aspirin therapy on early postoperative vein-graft patency. N Engl J Med 1982; 307:73–78.

27. Chesebro JH, Fuster V, Elveback LR, Clements IP, Smith HC, Holmes DR Jr, Bardsley WT, Pluth JR, Wallace RB, Puga FJ, Orszulak TA, Piehler JM, Danielson GK, Schaff HV, Frye RL. Effect of dipyridamole and aspirin on late vein-graft patency after coronary bypass operations. N Engl J Med 1984; 310:209–214.

28. Goldman S, Copeland J, Moritz T, Henderson W, Zadina K, Ovitt T, Doherty J, Read R, Chesler E, Sako Y, Lancaster L, Emery R, Sharma GVRK, Josa M, Pacold I, Montoya A, Parikh D, Sethi G, Holt J, Kirklin J, Shabetai R, Moores W, Aldridge J, Masud Z, DeMors H, Floten S, Haakenson C, Harker LA. Improvement in early saphenous vein graft patency after coronary artery bypass surgery with antiplatelet therapy: results of a Veterans Administration cooperative study. Circulation 1988; 77:1324–1332.

29. Goldman S, Copeland J, Moritz T, Henderson W, Zadina K, Ovitt T, Kern KB, Sethi G, Sharma GVRK, Khuri S, Richards K, Grover F, Morrison D, Whitman G, Chesler E, Sako Y, Pacold I, Montoya A, DeMots H, Floten S, Doherty J, Read R, Scott S, Spooner T, Masud Z, Haakenson C, Harker LA, and the Department of Veterans Affairs Cooperative Study. Starting aspirin therapy after operation: effects on early graft patency. Circulation 1991; 84:520–526.

30. Limet R, David JL, Magotteaux P, Larock MP, Rigo P. Prevention of aorto-coronary bypass graft occlusion: beneficial effect of ticlopidine on early and late patency rates of various coronary bypass grafts: a double blind study. J Thorac Cardiovasc Surg 1987; 94:773–783.

31. 4S Investigators. Randomized trial of cholesterol lowering in 4444 patients with coronary heart disease: the Scandinavian Simvastatin Survival Study (4S). Lancet 1994; 344:1383–1389.

32. Yusuf S, Peto R, Lewis J, Collins R, Sleight P. Beta blockade during and after myocardial infarction: an overview of the randomized trials. Prog Cardiovasc Dis 1985; 27:335–371.

33. SOLVD Investigators. Effect of enalapril on mortality and the development of heart failure in asymptomatic patients with reduced left ventricular ejection fractions. N Engl J Med 1992; 327:685–691.
34. Pfeffer MA, Braunwald E, Moye LA, Basta L, Brown EJ Jr, Cuddy TE, Davis BR, Geltman EM, Goldman S, Flaker GC, Klein M, Lamas GA, Packer M, Rouleau J, Rouleau JL, Rutherford J, Wertheimer JH, Hawkins CM. Effect of captopril on mortality and morbidity in patients with left ventricular dysfunction after myocardial infarction. The SAVE Investigators. N Engl J Med 1992; 327:669–677.
35. Atrial Fibrillation Investigators. Risk factors for stroke and efficacy of antithrombotic therapy in atrial fibrillation. Analysis of pooled data from five randomized controlled trials. Arch Intern Med 1994; 154:1449–1457.
36. Buxton B, Fuller J, Gaer J, Liu JJ, Mee J, Sinclair R, Windsor M. The radial artery as a bypass graft. Curr Opin Cardiol 1996; 11:591–598.

9
Balloon Angioplasty for Saphenous Vein Bypass Grafts

Kirk N. Garratt and David R. Holmes, Jr.
Mayo Clinic, Rochester, Minnesota

I. PREVALENCE AND PATHOLOGY OF SAPHENOUS VEIN GRAFT DISEASE

Coronary artery bypass graft surgery revolutionized the care of chronic ischemic syndromes 30 years ago [1]. The daring use of a reverse saphenous vein graft segment as a conduit from the ascending aorta to a targeted coronary segment replaced entirely the use of the Vineberg procedure [2] and offered the potential for enduring relief of ischemia for patients with ischemic syndromes. However, the technical issues of vein graft thrombosis and accelerated atherosclerosis were quickly recognized as limitations of the procedure. These issues were partially, but not completely, resolved with the introduction of the internal mammary (thoracic) artery selective coronary bypass technique [3]. Other arterial conduits, including the gastroepiploic and free radial arterial grafts, have also proven to be of utility [4], but the limited availability of arterial segments has made the use of reverse saphenous vein segments a standard procedure that persists to this day.

Bypass grafts may fail for several reasons. In the early weeks or months following surgery, graft failure is almost uniformly related to graft thrombosis [5,6]. Graft thrombosis may be induced by poor-quality grafting material, poor distal coronary beds with limited blood flow, coagulation disorders, and surgical technical errors. The incidence of early vein graft failure may be as high as 10% within the first 30 days and 18% within the first year of surgery [6–8].

After the first year or so, graft failure occurs at a rate of 1–2% per year for 5–10 years [6]. During the first few years after placement, graft failure is most commonly related to the development of intimal hyperplasia within the conduit. Although incompletely understood, this intimal hyperplasia is believed related to the deposition of subocclusive thrombus in the graft segment, which becomes organized and replaced with fibromuscular cells. The histopathology of this tissue is similar to that of the coronary restenosis that develops after balloon angioplasty [9]. Characteristically, this process involves most or all of the graft segments.

After 5 years from surgery, most graft failures are related to the development of accelerated atherosclerosis [6]. In vein grafts, the disease process is characterized by excessive foam cell infiltration and the development of a friable cholesterol-laden neointimal layer. Ulceration, local thrombosis, and aneurysmal dilatation are common. Studies conducted at the Montreal Heart Institute suggest that by 10 years after surgery, half of vein grafts are occluded, and there is a high prevalence of advanced disease in the remainder [5,6,10,11]. By comparison, acceleration of disease in the native arteries of patients undergoing bypass surgery occurs at a rate of about 5% per year [11].

These pathologic abnormalities are less common among internal mammary grafts, particularly the late development of atherosclerosis [3]. Nonetheless, graft failure may still occur in about 5% of in situ mammary grafts.

Coronary artery bypass surgery is conducted on thousands of Americans annually. The Healthcare Cost and Utilization Project—3 reported that 300,676 coronary artery bypass surgeries were performed in 1992 at the hospitals participating in the Nationwide Inpatient Survey [12].* Since the median age of bypass surgery in most published series is around 60 years, and since most Americans survive into the eighth decade, it is apparent that a large number of patients with prior bypass surgery are likely to develop recurrent ischemic symptoms related to graft failure. However, a study by Harris et al. [13] from the Mayo Clinic found that the proportion of balloon angioplasty patients with a history of prior bypass surgery rose from 6% to 14% ($p < 0.001$) between 1981 and 1991, while the proportion of such patients undergoing bypass surgical procedures remained stable at about 10% during that interval; in fact, total balloon angioplasty procedures increased dramatically during this period while total bypass surgical procedures remained unchanged (Figure 1). These data

---

*The Healthcare Cost and Utilization Project—3 is operated by the Agency for Health Care Policy and Research. This project records vital statistics drawn from a survey of all inpatient medical records collected from a sampling of 20% of U.S. community hospitals, taken from 11 states. The most recent year for which statistics were available is 1992. During that year, 300,676 coronary artery bypass procedures were done at participating hospitals. The average length of stay was 12.75 days, and the mean charge was $48,591. During the same period, 333, 566 balloon angioplasty procedures were done at these centers. The mean length of stay was 4.99 days, and the average charge was $18,520.

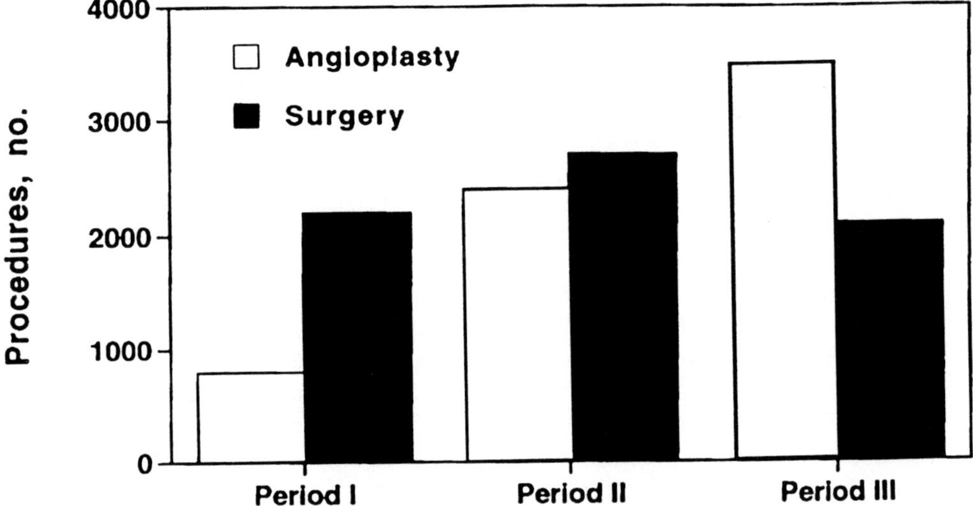

Figure 1 Rates of coronary angioplasty and coronary artery bypass surgery at the Mayo Clinic during three time periods. Period I = January 1, 1982, through April 30, 1985; Period II = May 1, 1985, through August 31, 1988; Period III = September 1, 1988, through December 31, 1991. Although rates of coronary angioplasty rose, rates of coronary artery bypass surgery declined in the last period. The proportion of angioplasty patients with prior coronary artery bypass surgery was 6% in Period I, 12% in Period II, and 14% in Period III ($p = 0.001$). (Data from Ref. 13.)

verify that interventional cardiologists are assuming care responsibilities for an increasing fraction of patients with coronary artery disease, including those with prior thoracic surgical procedures, which underlines the importance of familiarity with the special issues relevant to bypass graft angioplasty.

II. TECHNICAL ISSUES RELATED TO BYPASS GRAFT ANGIOPLASTY

Proximal anastomoses of saphenous vein bypass grafts usually arise from the anterior or right lateral aspect of the ascending aorta. Calcific atherosclerosis of this portion of the aorta will occasionally require that other portions of the aorta be used, and occasionally grafts may originate from a posterior site or from high up on the ascending aorta, near the aortic arch. Rarely, grafts will originate from the right subclavian artery. Originally, Favaloro performed bypasses of right coronary arteries by interposing a graft from the proximal to the distal right coronary segments, but this is now done rarely [1,14]. The variability in location of aortovein graft ostia can make proper guide catheter engagement challenging.

For vein graft ostia originating from the right lateral aspect of the ascending aorta, a Judkins right guide catheter is usually suitable (Figure 2). If the vein graft has a downward angulation in its ostial segment, a multipurpose catheter may provide better engagement. A right bypass graft guide catheter has a distal angulation that is intermediate between the Judkins right and multipurpose tip angulations, and may be the best guide choice for many applications. Uncontrolled slippage of the guide catheter down into the body of the graft can cause disruption of the graft and distal embolization, despite the use of "soft tip" catheters and should be avoided. When the ostial segment of the graft is superiorly or horizontally directed, better engagement and much better guide support may be offered by an Amplatz right guide catheter or a small left Amplatz guide catheter, such as an AL1. In larger roots, an AL2 guide catheter, particularly the short-tip variant, can provide excellent support.

For vein graft ostia rising from the anterior surface of the aorta, Judkins right guide catheters may also be adequate. However, when a Judkins right guide catheter fails to engage properly, a left bypass graft catheter is usually sufficient. This guide catheter has a tip angulation just slightly less than that of a Judkins right guide, but the portion of catheter distal to the primary angulation is longer. This guide may not provide much support, however. When added support is needed, a short-tip AL2 guide catheter is often ideal. If the ostial graft segment is directed sharply inferiorly or laterally, engagement with this catheter can be difficult. In some cases, the Champ guide catheter (USCI, Billerica, Massachusetts) may be easier to engage and can provide nearly equivalent support. In larger aortic roots, an XB (Cordis [division of Johnson & Johnson], Miami, Florida) or Voda (SciMed Life Systems [division of Boston Scientific], Minneapolis, Minnesota) 3.0 or 3.5 guide catheter can be useful.

A significant issue with vein graft angioplasty is balloon size. Since normal saphenous vein segments may be 5 or 6 mm in diameter (or larger), angioplasty aimed at achieving a "zero-percent" residual stenosis is impractical with standard coronary angioplasty balloons, which are typically sized to no more than 4 or 4.5 mm. very compliant balloons capable of significant balloon "overstretch" may help with this problem; but frequently, "off-label" use of peripheral vascular angioplasty balloons may be necessary for an ideal angioplasty result.* Many peripheral angioplasty balloons are now available that are

---

* "Off-label" use of a medical product means that the product is being used by an approved purchaser/operator, usually a physician, for purposes other than those for which the product was given Food and Drug Administration approval for marketing and distribution. Current law permits such action by the purchaser/operator, but restricts manufacturing companies from discussion of such product uses, if these discussions are intended to promote the use of the product for the unapproved application.

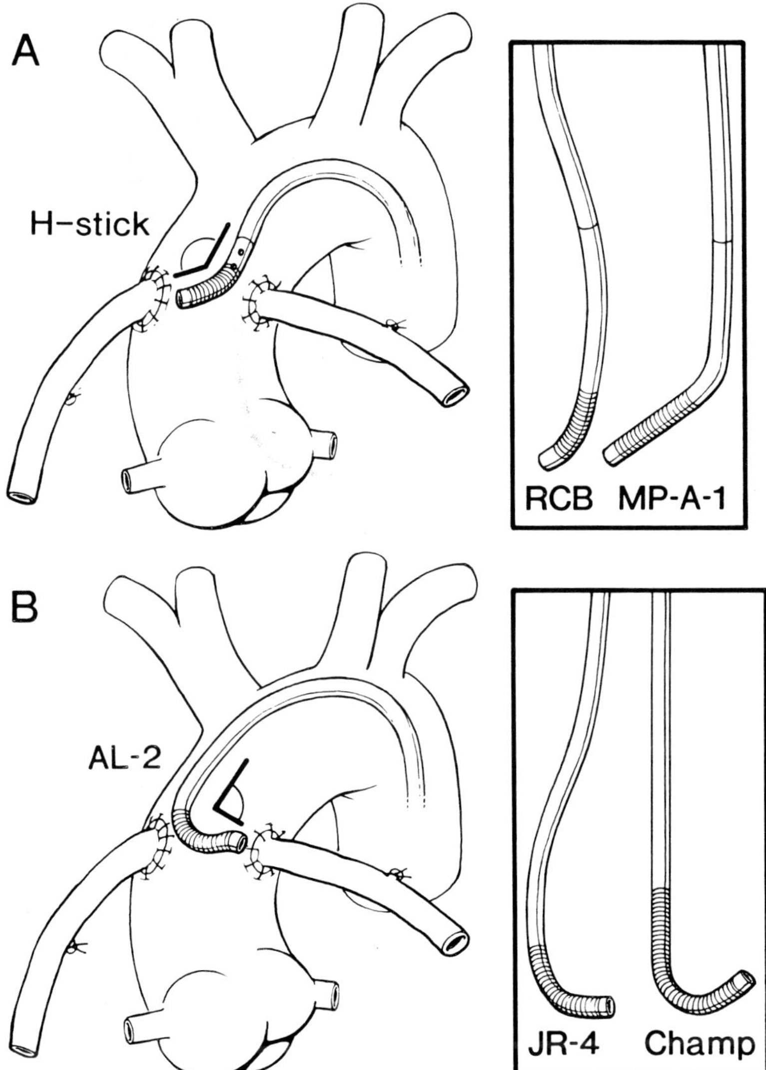

Figure 2 Engagement of bypass graft ostium with guide catheter. (A) Ostium arising from the right lateral aspect of the ascending aorta usually best approached with Judkins right, multi-purpose, hockey-stick, Amplatz, or right bypass catheters. Occasionally, less common catheters such as the El Gamal, Block, or Champ guide catheter provide greater stability. (B) Ostia arising from the lest or anterior aspect of the aorta are usually engaged with Judkins right, left bypass, Amplatz or Champ guide catheters.

suitable for use in vein grafts. Peripheral angioplasty balloons are available with 10-, 15-, 20-, 30-, and 40-mm balloon lengths mounted onto catheters made to track a 0.018-inch coronary guide wire. In most cases, overall catheter lengths are the same as traditional coronary angoplasty balloons (about 135 cm). Newer balloons can sustain moderate to high balloon inflation pressures (12–16 atm). Balloon diameters up to 8 mm are readily available.

Sequential saphenous vein grafts may present special challenges. Occlusion at the distal anastomosis of such a graft, or within the target vessels at the end of the graft, may not be within reach of a 135-cm angioplasty balloon catheter. Three options are available to remedy this problem. First, the guide catheter may be intentionally inserted into the proximal portion of the graft. Performed carefully, this maneuver can be safe and effective, but the risk of proximal graft injury cannot be eliminated. Relatively straight guide shapes, such as multipurpose catheters, are best for this. Second, angioplasty may be conducted from the brachial artery rather than the femoral artery, permitting use of shorter (80–90 cm) guide catheters, which will liberate greater balloon length for insertion into the graft [15]. Note that the transradial approach, which is gaining in popularity in the United States, is of no benefit here, since 90-cm catheters are too short to be used from the radial artery access site. Third, a shortened guide cathether may be used.

Special short guide catheters are available and should be considered when approaching distal lesions. If these special catheters are not immediately available, a standard-length catheter can be shortened to achieve the same purpose. We have described a technique for shortening femoral guide catheters [16]. The amount of guide catheter shortening to be undertaken can be determined by measuring the excess catheter length (from vascular access sheath hub to catheter proximal hub) using a diagnostic catheter seated in the vein graft ostium as a measuring template. With the guide catheter out of the body, the proximal portion of the guide catheter can be cut off using a number 11 scalpel or strong sterile scissors. Replacement hubs are available commercially. On rare occasion, the need to shorten the guide catheter may be realized only after the guide is in place. If the graft ostial engagement was problematic, it is possible to shorten the guide while it is in place. The process must be done quickly to avoid significant blood loss, but we have been successful in shortening guide catheters even with the coronary guide wire in place. If this is attempted, it is important to remove the balloon catheter completely to avoid accidentally nicking it with the scalpel blade while cutting the guide (scissors are *not* appropriate for this).

Although not the principal focus of this chapter, a few comments regarding the internal mammary artery angioplasty technique are germane. The chief difficulty with internal mammary artery angioplasty is access to the aterial ostium. If a free mammary artery graft is used, then the approach is identical to that for a saphenous vein bypass graft. With the more common in situ internal mammary graft, atherosclerosis or tortuosity around the aortic arch and great vessels may impede proper engagement. An internal mammary artery guide catheter with a sharply angulated tip is usually adequate for internal mammary artery angioplasty, but use of a less angulated catheter (such as a Judkins right catheter) may be necessary to gain initial access to the subclavian artery. When tortuosity in the great vessels makes movement of the guide catheter difficult, a 9 French Judkins right guide catheter may be situated with its distal tip at the base of the subclavian artery. This guide catheter should be shortened in the manner described earlier prior to insertion. Through the 9 French right Judkins guide catheter, a 7 French internal mammary artery guide catheter may be inserted. The support offered by the 9 French Judkins right guide catheter can make proper engagement of an internal mammary artery possible, even in very difficult and tortuous circumstances.

Since the internal mammary artery can be very long, balloon length issues germane to sequential saphenous vein bypass grafts may also apply. The same solutions can be employed to resolve the problem.

On occasion, extreme vascular tortuosity, high-grade atherosclerosis, or a very unusual origin for the internal mammary artery may make engagement of the vessel from the transfemoral root impossible. Under these circumstances, a brachial artery approach should be used [15]. Dorros has designed a series of guide catheters suited specifically for transbrachial angioplasty of the internal mammary artery [17]. This family of unique shapes, combined with other, standard angioplasty guide catheters, makes engagement of virtually every internal mammary ostium possible.

One additional issue is spasm of the origin of the internal mammary artery. Careful manipulation and placement of the guide can reduce the risk of this, and the use of smaller, 6F or 7F guide catheters may also be helpful, although reduced opacification may be a problem.

Once the graft ostium has been engaged securely, the conduct of balloon angioplasty does not differ substantially between native coronary arterial lesions and bypass graft lesions, except to the extent that some precautions may be necessary to minimize complications (see the next section). There are many belief systems that influence how angioplasty is done (varying balloon inflation pressures, inflation times, balloon length, use of adjunctive nonballoon devices, etc.), but there are no compelling data to support most practices.

III. PROCEDURAL AND EARLY COMPLICATIONS

Although vein graft angioplasty is performed frequently, the principal published literature reports on only about 3,000 patients (Table 1). Balloon angioplasty of vein grafts is subject to all the complications associated with balloon angio-

Table 1 Published Acute Results of Balloon Angioplasty in Saphenous Vein Bypass Grafts

Authors, year [Ref.]	Patients (no.)	Success (%)	AMI (no.)	CABG (no.)	Deaths (no.)
Gruentzig et al., 1979 [43]	5	60	nr	0	0
Ford et al., 1981 [44]	9	86	0	0	0
Jones et al., 1983 [45]	37	95	5	5	0
Douglas et al., 1983 [46]	62	94	1	1	0
El Gamal et al., 1984 [47]	44	93	2	0	0
Block et al., 1984 [48]	40	78	0	1	0
Dorros et al., 1984 [49]	33	79	nr	nr	0
Corbelli et al., 1985 [50]	47	92	nr	nr	0
Reeder et al., 1986 [51]	19	84	1	0	1
Douglas et al., 1986 [24]	235	92	16	3	0
Cote et al., 1987 [52]	101	85	1	1	0
Ernst et al., 1987 [53]	33	97	nr	nr	nr
Pinkerton et al., 1988 [54]	100	93	nr	nr	nr
Dorros et al., 1988 [18]	53	83	1	nr	1
Reed et al., 1989 [55]	52	90	0	nr	0
Cooper et al., 1989 [56]	24	75	nr	0	1
Plakto et al., 1989 [57]	101	92	12	4	4
Webb et al., 1990 [58]	158	84	4	1	0
Jost et al., 1991 [59]	41	93	0	0	0
Plokker et al., 1991 [60]	454	90	13	6	3
Reeves et al., 1991 [61]	57	84	9	2	2
Douglas et al., 1991 [62]	599	90	14	21	7
Meester et al., 1991 [63]	84	82	8	2	4
Danzi et al., 1992 [64]	25	83	1	2	1
Morrison et al., 1994 [28]	75	93	2	1	2
Avital et al., 1995 [65]	219	95	15	1	3
Abdel-Meguid et al., 1995 [27][a]	68	90	3	2	1
Abdel-Meguid et al., 1995 [27][b]	72	89	5	4	3
Total	2,847	89.6%	113 (3.9%)	57 (2.3%)	33 (1.2%)

AMI = acute myocardial infarction; nr = not reported.
[a]Ostial lesions only.
[b]Nonostial lesions only.
Patient characteristics and definitions for events varied between studies. The initial treatment was balloon angioplasty only; other devices used only when angioplasty unsuccessful. Some patients may have been counted in more than one study.

plasty of native coronary arteries. The most significant special risk of vein graft angioplasty is distal embolization of atheromatous or thrombotic material. Embolization has been reported to occur in up to 6% of treated patients [18], and is related to graft age [19]. In a 1993 meta-analysis of 16 published series, de Feyter et al. [7] found event rates after vein graft angioplasty to be similar to those reported for native coronary artery angioplasty, except for a higher risk of distal embolization (2%). Significant embolization is associated with the development of angina and a high rate of myocardial infarction. Indeed, some studies use a rise in creatine phosphokinase enzymes as evidence of distal embolization, even in the absence of angiographic evidence of the same.

Distal embolization may be appreciated angiographically as poor distal runoff and/or truncation of a distal vessel. The development of poor distal runoff, or "no reflow" after catheter-based therapy, is associated with a 10-fold increase in hospital mortality [20]. When it occurs, administration of intragraft urokinase may be helpful [18]. Some operators advocate the use of intracoronary heparin, although the efficacy of this has not been well studied. Intracoronary calcium antagonists attenuate myocardial ischemia under these conditions [21], and intracoronary verapamil in 100–250-μg boluses has been used effectively to promote capillary vasodilatation and improve blood flow. Many experienced operators share anecdotes regarding the utility of intracoronary verapamil for vein graft emboli, but this strategy has not been investigated rigorously.

Attempts at mechanical disruption of embolic material may also be helpful. When a significant distal branch is occluded with apparent embolic material, insertion and rotation of one or more coronary guide wires into that region may help to break up the embolus and enhance distal flow. For larger vessels, insertion of an angioplasty balloon into the occluded segment may serve the same purpose. Inflation of the balloon may not be necessary, but low-pressure, long-duration inflations are occasionally helpful.

Reports of abrupt closure rates have varied widely [7,19]. The mechanism of occlusion is presumed to be similar to that of native coronary arteries: the development of obstructive intimal flaps and dissection. However, the relatively small number of patients treated at any one institution (or group of institutions) is so small that analysis of associated characteristics is difficult and unreliable. Management of vein graft abrupt closure is more complicated in patients who have had prior thoracotomy, since emergency repeat bypass surgery in these patients is associated with a high incidence of morbid events and should be avoided whenever possible [22]. Use of prolonged balloon inflations and autoperfusion balloons may be successful; there is current interest in special low-pressure autoperfusion balloon catheters that can deliver drug locally without complete interruption of blood flow [23]. However, application of coronary stents has replaced most other methods as the best management strategy for vein graft abrupt closure.

Vein graft rupture is exceedingly uncommon. This rare event was first reported by Douglas [24], when a single case was seen in more than 200 patients. When it occurs, it can usually be managed conservatively. The mediastinal fibrotic reaction that follows thorocotomy will usually contain and limit extravasation of blood. Persistent bleeding may be controlled with use of an autoperfusion balloon catheter to tamponade the area. Reversal of heparin may be needed, but it is not necessary uniformly. An extensive injury resulting from a graft tear may evoke a robust proliferative response, so the long-term outcome of these injured grafts is likely to be poor.

IV. RESTENOSIS AND LATE ADVERSE EVENTS

Restenosis following balloon angioplasty of saphenous vein grafts varies according to the site of dilatation. A review of data from 12 published case series with angiographic follow-up indicated that the highest restenosis rate occurs when angioplasty is done at the aortoostium, where restenosis was found in 56% of patients [7], although rates as high as 80% have been seen in some series [19]. The reasons for this high rate of restenosis are unknown, but are probably related, in part, to the influence of elastin fibers at the aortoostium, which may contribute to recoil. Restenosis rates within the body of vein grafts are also high, averaging 52% in 12 published series [7]. Again, mechanisms are not known; presumably, excessive intimal hyperplasia is somehow triggered by the unusually friable, thrombotic, and cellular form of atherosclerosis that develops in vein grafts. Interestingly, restenosis at the distal anastomosis of a vein graft occurs at much lower rates (average of 26% patients), which approximates the incidence of restenosis seen after angioplasty of native coronary arteries. It is unclear why the restenosis rates are lower at distal anastomoses. The role of adverse remodeling, which seems to be very important in restenosis after angioplasty of native coronary arteries and peripheral arteries [25], has not been defined for saphenous vein graft lesions.

The most disappointing aspect of balloon angioplasty for vein graft disease has been the frequency of adverse clinical events after treatment. In one of the earliest reports on long-term follow-up, Douglas et al. [24] reported that 13% of 166 patients required at least one additional balloon angioplasty procedure and 21% required repeat bypass surgery (which was associated with an 11% mortality) during follow-up, ranging from 1 to 8 years. More recently, Dorros et al. [26] reported an unadjusted 5-year survival of only 59% among patients undergoing angioplasty of vein graft lesions, compared with 86% survival for patients having angioplasty of coronary arterial lesions. Workers at the Cleveland Clinic found that about 60% of patients undergoing angioplasty of ostial or proximal vein graft lesions experienced death, myocardial infarction, repeat coronary revascularization, or repeat cardiac-related hospital admission over a 2-year period [27]. At the Mayo Clinic, about 25% of patients treated between 1985 and 1995 were alive and free of severe angina or major adverse events 5 years after treatment (Figure 3); 35% had died and another 13% had suffered a new nonfatal myocardial infarction or required repeat bypass surgery, or both (unpublished data).

On the basis of these and similar data, a proposal has been made that balloon angioplasty only be offered to patients who are projected to have a low risk and a high likelihood of long-term benefit [7]. Patients with old grafts (older than 8 years), total occlusions, diffuse disease, or discrete disease with large plaque volume, and those with anatomical features that put the patient at high risk of cardiogenic shock in the event of abrupt closure or embolization (such as a sole remaining vein graft to a large myocardial territory), should be offered angioplasty only when alternative methods of therapy are not possible. While this strategy makes sense, a limiting consideration is the relatively high risk of adverse events faced by these patients when they are referred for repeat bypass surgery. A study by Morrison et al. [28] found a higher 30-day survival rate among 75 patients treated with coronary angioplasty compared retrospectively with a matched cohort of patients treated surgically (97% vs. 92%, $p <$ 0.05), although by 6 months there was no difference in adverse event rates, and by 5 years a trend toward better survival with surgery was seen. It does

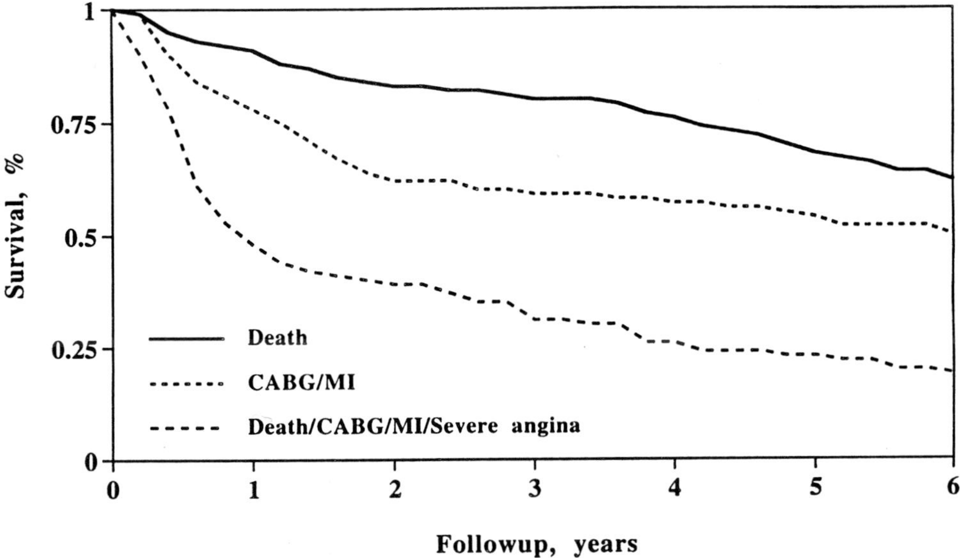

Figure 3 Event-free survival after balloon angioplasty of saphenous vein graft lesions at the Mayo Clinic, 1985 through 1995.

appear that patients who escape recurrent symptoms or adverse clinical events during the first 6 months after treatment are at lower risk thereafter [29]. Thus, balloon angioplasty may be considered a suitable alternative to repeat bypass surgery for at least some patients, but there are few data to support an argument that balloon angioplasty of vein graft lesions provides results that are superior to surgery, at least in the long term. Indeed, the adverse event rate is so substantial with both methods of treatment that they may both be considered palliative procedures.

V. ANGIOPLASTY OF NATIVE CORONARY ARTERIAL LESIONS IN PATIENTS WITH PRIOR BYPASS SURGERY

Whenever vein graft lesions are assessed, the native coronary arterial route leading to the bypassed vascular segment should be evaluated carefully to determine whether angioplasty of the native coronary artery might be possible. Diffuse disease or chronic total occlusions may make this approach untenable, but occasionally a difficult vein graft angioplasty may be avoided by choosing a more straightforward native coronary angioplasty approach. Data on the relative risks of this strategy are sparse, but in selected patients the strategy has been successful [30,31].

In addition, the long-term outlook for these patients seems more favorable. Dorros et al. [30] found, in patients with prior bypass surgery, that a strategy of treating both native coronary lesions and vein graft lesions in the same setting yielded a 5-year unadjusted mortality equivalent to that observed for patients undergoing angioplasty of native coronary artery lesions only (86%). The point of this study was to demonstrate the effectiveness of combining native and vein graft angioplasty, but it suggests that native artery treatment may confer greater benefits than treatment of vein graft lesions. Confidence in this conclusion would require analysis of a larger number of unselected patients, but the realities of clinical practice make it unlikely that enough patients suitable for randomization would ever be found for study in this fashion.

VI. ADJUNCTIVE MEDICAL THERAPIES

Since thrombus is thought to play a pivotal role in the development of atherosclerosis and acute clinical syndromes in vein graft lesions, it is reasonable to theorize that local application of thrombolytic drugs might have a beneficial effect. On the other hand, the pathophysiology of thrombus development and propagation may differ between diseased native coronary arteries and vein grafts, so it is possible that thrombolytic drugs may work differently in these two settings. Adjunctive intracoronary thrombolysis has not proven to be of benefit during angioplasty of complex lesions in native coronary arteries [32].

The best work with adjunctive intragraft thrombolysis has been reported by Hartmann and coworkers, who found that prolonged infusions of high-dose (up to 250,000 u/hr) urokinase (Abbott Laboratories, Abbott Park, IL) combined with balloon angioplasty were effective in recanalizing occluded vein grafts [33]. Early observational studies indicated that nearly 80% of occluded grafts could be opened with a 12-hour urokinase infusion followed by balloon angioplasty, and that patency was maintained for more than 2 years in about two-thirds of those grafts that opened initially. Distal occlusions, which allow good infusion-catheter engagement with the vein graft, recent occlusions, and good distal runoff were factors identified as having a favorable effect on this treatment strategy.

This work was followed by a multicenter study, the Recanalization of Chronically Occluded Aortocoronary Saphenous Vein Bypass Grafts with Long-term Low-Dose Direct Infusion of Urokinase Trial (ROBUST), designed to evaluate the effectiveness of prolonged low-dose (100,000 u/hr) intragraft urokinase infusion in 107 patients with vein graft total occlusions treated with balloon angioplasty [34]. Patients were treated with urokinase for an average of 25 hours. Initial patency was achieved in 74 patients (69%); balloon angioplasty was performed in 88% of these patients. Success rates varied with the complexity of the disease and the age of the graft. Distal embolization (rise in creatine kinase MB fraction without Q-wave development) occurred in 17% of patients. There were no deaths among patients with successful recanalization, but seven deaths among patients with failed treatment (overall death rate 6.5%). Six-month angiography was available in only 54% of treated patients, and the treated vessel was patent in only 40% of these patients. However, the frequency of recurrent severe angina was reduced from 71% with unsuccessful procedures to 22% with successful recanalization. Deviation from the stated protocol was common in this study and made interpretation of results difficult. Finally, cost was not addressed, but in view of the multiple catheterization procedures and the need to keep the patient in an intensive care environment, this appeared to be an expensive treatment strategy.

It should be emphasized that these data apply to patients with single occluded vein grafts, and not to the majority of patients seen with vein graft disease who have subtotal occlusions, often in more than one vascular territory. The efficacy and safety of low-dose thrombolysis in other patient subsets is untested.

With the advent of glycoprotein IIb:IIIa inhibitors, the role of intracoronary (and intragraft) thrombolysis is declining. Again, there are no sound studies to guide therapy. But some related basic research has been encouraging [35], and the experiences of those who use ReoPro™ (abciximab, Centocor [division of Eli Lilly], Indianapolis, Ind.) frequently have been so favorable that enthusiasm for prolonged intragraft thrombolytic infusions is falling.

Several platelet inhibitor compounds, both intravenous and oral agents, are under study currently.

At this point, it seems that adjunctive thrombolysis may be of value in selected patients, particularly patients with single subtotal vein graft stenoses, but it is unlikely to be so effective that it can be used reliably as independent therapy. It seems more likely that newer potent antiplatelet drugs will prove to be valuable adjuncts to graft angioplasty. Variants of current thrombolytic drugs, such as recombinant forms of urokinase, and novel thrombolytic drug combinations may influence future practice patterns. The addition of plasminogen to thrombolytic "cocktails" may improve their effectiveness. Newer methods of thrombolytic delivery may also have an effect. For example, use of a pulse-spray technique has been associated with increased thrombolytic efficacy in lower-extremity arterial recanalization, especially when the occlusion is relatively new [36].

VII. IMPACT OF NEW DEVICES

The roles of alternative devices in the management of vein graft disease are discussed elsewhere in this textbook. It is of interest that the perceived limitations of balloon angioplasty in saphenous vein grafts has led to great enthusiasm for nonballoon technologies in the management of this disease. Use of coronary or the larger peripheral stents has become very common, despite the lack of randomized data demonstrating the effectiveness of this approach. Indeed, investigators are so convinced of the benefit of coronary stent placement in vein graft disease that several have stated publicly their opposition to randomized trials because they were felt to be unethical. Nonetheless, at least one such trial has completed patient enrollment at this time (Stent Versus Balloon Angioplasty for Aortocoronary Saphenous Vein Bypass Graft Disease, or SAVED trial), which aims to compare complications (especially embolization rates) and restenosis rates between patients treated with conventional angioplasty and those treated with angioplasty plus Johnson & Johnson stent placement. An interim analysis for this study indicated that the restenosis benefit seen with stent placement in coronary artery lesions may be achievable in vein graft lesions as well [37]. At the Mayo clinic, we have observed that the risk of distal embolization is similar during balloon angioplasty with or without stent placement (unpublished data). Nonetheless, individual experiences have been favorable with stent use, while the limited published experience indicates low complication rates and improved treatment durability [8,38,39].

At the time of this writing, only one study has shown that a nonballoon device can provide some benefit over balloon angioplasty for vein graft disease. The Second Coronary Angioplasty Versus Excisional Atherectomy Trial (CAVEAT II) found a small restenosis benefit with directional atherectomy

(DVI, Redwood City, Calif.) over balloon angioplasty [40]. Initial hospital complications were greater, but late complications and the need for repeat interventions was lower among patients treated with directional atherectomy. Of the other two atherectomy devices approved for general use, the high-speed rotational atherectomy device (Rotablator, SciMed Life Systems [division of Boston Scientific], Minneapolis, Minn.) is poorly suited for treatment of vein graft lesions, with the exception of aortoostial disease [41], but the transluminal extraction endarterectomy device (TEC; Interventional Technologies, Inc., San Diego, Calif.) has proven very useful in this setting. A trial is underway currently (<u>TEC</u> <u>Be</u>fore <u>St</u>ent Study, or TEC BEST) to determine if pretreatment with TEC improves results of vein graft treatment involving stent placement. The excimer laser device has quite a good record in the treatment of vein graft disease, despite the low ratio of device diameter to vein graft diameter for many patients [42].

VIII. CONCLUSION

Dr. John Douglas wrote in 1990 of vein graft balloon angioplasty [19]:

> The thorny issues involving angioplasty of conduit lesions are atheroembolization and restenosis. Any major expansion of indications for angioplasty must await solutions to these problems. To avoid embolization, vein-graft atheroma must be removed completely (atherectomy), fragmented and removed (use of a disrupting force plus extraction of fragments), or ablated (laser technology). . . . Restenosis remains the major limiting factor in vein-graft angioplasty. Whether atherectomy, stent placement, or laser technology will have a significant impact on this problem remains to be determined. . . . The restenosis rate will not be reduced significantly until new pharmacologic approaches to this problem have been developed.

A few years later, these comments seem both in and out of phase. Embolization and restenosis remain the chief limitations to the technique. However, balloon angioplasty is an efficient, effective therapeutic choice in many patients, particularly those with discrete disease at the distal anastomosis of a graft. As is discussed elsewhere in this text, new devices have contributed substantially to improved outcomes with vein graft treatment, but neither atherectomy techniques nor laser therapies have reduced distal embolization rates to acceptable levels. The restenosis issue is still unsettled, but certainly the substantial advancements made in limiting native coronary artery restenosis through the use of stents should yield some useful information with respect to vein graft disease. With respect to adjunctive medical therapies, the hope offered by intragraft thrombolysis has not been realized, but the newer antiplatelet drugs have great promise.

We endeavor to practice evidence-based medicine, particularly when caring for high-risk patients such as those with prior coronary artery bypass surgery. Unfortunately, few studies have been done to define the ideal approach to patients with vein graft disease. Despite this, some general principles have been established. Revascularization of obstructive vein graft lesions is sensible because such therapy is associated with symptom relief and a mortality advantage in many patients, and balloon angioplasty is often preferable to surgical revascularization because of the technical complexities of repeat coronary bypass surgery and its attendant risks. Still, it must be acknowledged that catheter-based therapies cannot be considered definitive therapy for most patients with vein graft disease. Certainly, balloon angioplasty is a palliative procedure, having little effect on the natural history of advanced vein graft disease and with a majority of patients requiring additional treatment in the short term. New devices create optimism for better outcomes for this difficult patient group. But because of increased complexity and costs, new devices and drug regimens should be used cautiously until objective evidence of benefit has been provided. Ongoing clinical studies will soon clarify the usefulness of some of these newer approaches.

REFERENCES

1. Favaloro R. Saphenous vein autograft replacement of severe segmental coronary artery occlusion: operative technique. Ann Thorac Surg 1968; 5:334–339.
2. Dobell A. Arthur Vineberg and the internal mammary artery implantation procedure. Ann Thorac Surg 1992; 53:167–169.
3. Loop F, Lytle B, Cosgrove, D, Stewart RW, Goormastic M, Williams GW, Golding LA, Gill CC, Taylor PC, Sheldon WC, Proudfit WL. Influence of the internal-mammary-artery graft on 10-year survival and other cardiac events. N Engl J Med 1986; 314:1–6.
4. Ramstrom J, Lund O, Cadavid E, Thuren J, Oxelbark S, Henze A. Multiarterial coronary artery bypass grafting with special reference to small vessel disease and results in women. Eur Heart J 1993; 14:634–639.
5. Campeau L, Crochet D, Lesperance J, Bourassa M, Grondin C. Postoperative changes in aortocoronary saphenous vein grafts revisited: angiographic studies at two weeks and at one year in two series of consecutive patients. Circulation 1975; 52:369–377.
6. Bourassa M. Long-term vein graft patency. Curr Opin Cardiol 1994; 9:685–691.
7. de Feyter PJ, van Suylen RJ, de Jaegere PP, Topol EJ, Serruys PW. Balloon angioplasty for the treatment of lesions in saphenous vein bypass grafts. J Am Coll Cardiol 1993; 21:1539–1549.
8. de Jaegere P, van Domburg R, de Feyter P, Ruygrok PN, van der Grissen WJ, van den Brand MJ, Serruys PW. Long-term clinical outcome after stent placement in saphenous vein grafts. J Am Coll Cardiol 1996; 28:89–96.
9. Garratt KN, Edwards WD, Kaufmann UP, Vlietstra RE, Holmes D, Jr. Differential histopathology of primary atherosclerotic and restenotic lesions in coronary

arteries and saphenous vein bypass grafts: analysis of tissue obtained from 73 patients by directional atherectomy. J Am Coll Cardiol 1991; 17:442–448.

10. Bourassa M, Lesperance J, Campeau L, Grondin C. Serial angiographic studies after aortocoronary bypass surgery. Postoperative patency rates. In: Lichtlen P, ed. Coronary Angiography and Angina Pectoris. Stuttgart: Thieme, 1976:199–205.

11. Bourassa M, Enjalbert M, Campeau L, Lesperance J. Progression of coronary artery disease between 10 and 12 years after coronary artery bypass graft surgery. In: Roskamm H, ed. Prognosis of Heart Disease. Progression of Coronary Arteriosclerosis. Berlin: Springer Verlag, 1983:150.

12. Department of Health and Human Resources. National Statistics: Healthcare Cost and Utilization Project-3, 1992. Agency for Health Care Policy and Research, 1996: www.ahcpr.gov:80/data/.

13. Harris W, Mock M, Orszulak TO, Schaff H. Holmes DR, Jr. Use of coronary artery bypass surgical procedure and coronary angioplasty in treatment of coronary artery disease: changes during a 10-year period at Mayo Clinic Rochester. Mayo Clin Proc 1996; 71:927–935.

14. Loop F. The surgical treatment of atherosclerotic coronary heart disease. In: Schlant R, Alexander R, eds. The Heart (vol 8). New York: McGraw-Hill, 1994:1367–1380.

15. Garratt KN, Holmes DR Jr. Transbrachial, transaxillary, and transradial angioplasty. In: Ellis S, Holmes DJ, eds. Strategic Approaches in Coronary Intervention. Baltimore: Williams & Wilkins, 1996:578–597.

16. Chan R, Rihal C, Menke K, Winter S, Holmes DR Jr. Adaptor device for shortening guide catheters to access distal lesions in coronary angioplasty. Cathet Cardiovasc Diagn 1993; 30:249–251.

17. Garratt K, Menke K. Angioplasty Guiding Equipment. In: Vlietstra R, Holmes DR Jr, eds. Coronary Balloon Angioplasty. Cambridge: Blackwell Scientific Publications, 1994:20–81 (Vlietstra R, ed. Series in Interventional Cardiology).

18. Dorros G, Lewis RF, Mathiak LM, Johnson WD, Brenowitz J, Schmahl T, Tector A. Percutaneous transluminal coronary angioplasty in patients with two or more previous coronary artery bypass grafting operations. Am J Cardiol 1988; 61: 1243–1247.

19. Douglas JJ. Angioplasty of saphenous vein and internal mammary artery bypass grafts. In: Topol E, ed. Interventional Cardiology (vol 1). Philadelphia: WB Saunders, 1990:327–343.

20. Abbo K, Dooris M, Glazier S, et al. Features and outcome of no-reflow after percutaneous coronary intervention. Am J Cardiol 1995; 75:778–782.

21. Rauch B, Richardt G, Barth R, Zimmerman R, Tillmanns H, Schomig A, Kubler W, Neumann FJ. Intracoronary gallopamil during percutaneous transluminal coronary angioplasty. J Cardiovasc Pharmacol 1992; 20(suppl 7):S32–S39.

22. Craver J, Weintraub W, Jones E, Guyton R, Hatcher CR Jr. Emergency coronary artery bypass surgery for failed percutaneous coronary angioplasty. A 10-year experience. Ann Surg 1992; 215:425–433.

23. Mitchel J, Fram D, Palme DF III, Foster R, Hirst JA, Azrin MA, Bow LM, Eldin AM, Waters DD, McKay RG. Enhanced intracoronary thrombolysis with urokinase using a novel, local drug delivery system. In vitro, in vivo, and clinical studies. Circulation 1995; 91:785–793.

24. Douglas JJ, Robinson K, Schlumpf M. Percutaneous transluminal angioplasty in aortocoronary venous graft stenoses: immediate results and complications (abstr). Circulation 1986; 74(suppl II):II-281.

25. Currier J, Faxon D. Restenosis after percutaneous transluminal coronary angioplasty: have we been aiming at the wrong target? J Am Coll Cardiol 1995; 25:516–520.

26. Dorros G, Iyer S, Mathiak LM, Anderson AJ. The impact of balloon angioplasty of coronary artery and/or vein bypass graft lesion(s) upon the survival of patients > or = 5 years after their last bypass surgery. Eur Heart J 1993; 14:1354–1364.

27. Abdel-Meguid A, Whitlow P, Simpfendorfer C, Sapp SK, Franco I, Ellis SG, Topol EJ. Percutaneous revascularization of ostial saphenous vein graft stenoses. J Am Coll Cardiol 1995; 26:955–960.

28. Morrison DA, Crowley ST, Veerakul G, Barbiere CC, Grover F, Sacks J. Percutaneous transluminal angioplasty of saphenous vein grafts for medically refractory unstable angina. J Am Coll Cardiol 1994; 23:1066–1070.

29. Kolettis T, Miller H, De Bono D. Coronary angioplasty in patients with prior coronary artery bypass grafting. Intl J Cardiol 1990; 28:333–339.

30. Dorros G, Lewis R, Mathiak L. Coronary angioplasty in patients with prior coronary artery bypass surgery: all prior coronary artery bypass surgery patients and patients more than 5 years after coronary bypass surgery. Cardiol Clin 1989; 7: 791–803.

31. Unterberg C, Buchwald A, Wiegand V, Kreuzer H. Coronary angioplasty in patients with previous coronary artery bypass. Angiology 1992; 43:653–660.

32. Ambrose J, Almeida O, Sharma S, Torre SR, Marmur JD, Israel DH, Ratner DE, Weiss MB, Hjemdahl-Monsen CE, Myler RK, Moses J, Unterecker WJ, Grunwald AW, Garrett JS, Cowley MJ, Anwar A, Sobolski J. Adjunctive thrombolytic therapy during angioplasty for ischemic rest angina. Results of the TAUSA Trial. TAUSA Investigators. Thrombolysis and Angioplasty in Unstable Angina trial. Circulation 1994; 90:69–77.

33. Hartmann JR, McKeever LS, Stamato NJ, Bufalino VJ, Marek JC, Brown AS, Goodwin MJ, Cahill JM, Enger EL. Recanalization of chronically occluded aortocoronary saphenous vein bypass grafts by extended infusion of urokinase: initial results and short-term clinical follow-up. J Am Coll Cardiol 1991; 18:1517–1523.

34. Hartmann J, McKeever L, O'Neill W, White CJ, Whitlow PL, Gilmore PS, Doorey AJ, Galichia JP, Enger EL. Recanalization of chronically occluded aortocoronary saphaneous vein bypass grafts with long-term, low-dose direct infusion of urokinase (ROBUST): a serial trial. J Am Coll Cardiol 1996; 27:60–66.

35. Rubin B, McGraw D, Sicard G, Sa S. New RGD analogue inhibits human platelet adhesion and aggregation and eliminates platelet deposition on canine vascular grafts. J Vasc Surg 1992; 15:683–691.

36. Braithwaite B, Quinones-Baldrich W. Lower limb intraarterial thrombolysis as an adjunct to the management of arterial and graft occlusions. World J Surg 1996; 20:649–654.

37. Savage M, Douglas J, Fischman D, Fenton S, King S, Regine C, Bailey S, Overlie P, Werner J, Leon M, Henser R, Brinker J, Buchbinder M, Smalling R, Sueord D, Rake R, Gebhardt S, Kerensky R, Wargovich T, Goldberg S. Coronary stents versus balloon angioplasty for aorto-coronary saphenous vein bypass graft disease: interim results of a randomized trial (abstr). J Am Coll Cardiol 1995; 25:79A.

38. Garratt KN. Catheter-based therapy for saphenous vein bypass graft disease. J Invas Cardiol 1997; 9:61–70.

39. Eeckhout E, Kappenberger L, Goy J. Stents for intracoronary placement: current status and future directions. J Am Coll Cardiol 1996; 27:757–765.

40. Holmes D Jr, Topol EJ, Califf RM, Berdan LG, Leya F, Berger PB, Whitlow PL, Safian RD, Adelman AG, Kellett MA Jr, Talley JD, Shani J, Gottlieb RS, Pinkerton CA, Lee KL, Keeler GP, Ellis SG. A multicenter, randomized trial of coronary angioplasty versus directional atherectomy for patients with saphenous vein bypass graft lesions. CAVEAT-II Investigators. Circulation 1995; 91: 1966–1974.

41. Cardenas J, Strumpf R, Heuser R. Rotational atherectomy in restenotic lesions at the distal saphenous vein anastomosis. Cathet Cardiovasc Diagn 1995; 36:53–57.

42. Bittl JA, Sanborn TA, Yardley DE, Tcheng JE, Isner JM, Chokski SK, Strauss BH, Abela GS, Walter PD, Schmidhofer M, Power JA. Predictors of outcome of percutaneous excimer laser coronary angioplasty of saphenous vein bypass graft lesions. The Percutaneous Excimer Laser Coronary Angioplasty Registry. Am J Cardiol 1994; 74:144–148.

43. Greuntzig A, Senning A, Siegenthaler W. Nonoperative dilatation of coronary-artery stenosis. Percutaneous transluminal coronary angioplasty. N Engl J Med 1979; 301:61–68.

44. Ford W, Wholey M, Zikria E, Somandani S, Sullivan M. Percutaneous transluminal dilation of aortocoronary saphenous vein bypass grafts. Chest 1981; 79:529–535.

45. Jones E, Douglas J, Gruentzig A, Craver JM, King SB, Guyton RA, Hatcher CR. Percutaneous saphenous vein angioplasty to avoid reoperative bypass surgery. Ann Thorac Surg 1983; 36:389–395.

46. Douglass J, Gruentzig A, King SB III, Hollman J, Ischinger T, Meier B, Craver JM, Jones EL, Waller JL, Bone DK, Guyton R. Percutaneous transluminal coronary angioplasty in patients with prior coronary bypass surgery. J Am Coll Cardiol 1983; 2:745–754.

47. El Gamal M, Bonnier H, Michels R, Heijman J, Stassen E. Percutaneous transluminal angioplasty of stenosed aortocoronary bypass grafts. Br Heart J 1984; 52:617–620.

48. Block P, Cowley M, Kaltenbach M, Kent K, Simpson J. Percutaneous angioplasty of stenoses of bypass grafts or of bypass graft anastomotic sites. Am J Cardiol 1984; 53:666–668.

49. Dorros G. Johnson W, Tector A, Schmahl T, Kalush S, Janke L. Percutaneous transluminal coronary angioplasty in patients with prior coronary artery bypass grafting. J Thorac Cardiovasc Surg 1984; 87:17–26.

50. Corbelli J, Franco I, Hollman J, Simpfendorfer C, Galan K. Percutaneous transluminal coronary angioplasty after previous coronary artery bypass surgery. Am J Cardiol 1985; 56:398–403.

51. Reeder G, Bresnahan J, Holmes DR Jr, Mock MB, Orszulak TA, Smith HC, Vlietstra RE. Angioplasty for aortocoronary bypass graft stenosis. Mayo Clin Proc 1986; 61:14–19.

52. Cote G, Myler R, Stertzer S, Clark DA, Fishman-Rosen J, Murphy M, Shaw RE. Percutaneous transluminal angioplasty of stenotic coronary artery bypass grafts: 5 years' experience. J Am Coll Cardiol 1987; 9:8–17.

53. Ernst J, van der Feltz T, Ascoop C, Bal ET, Vermeulen FE, Knaepen PJ, van Bogeryen L, van den Berg EJ, Plokker HW. Percutaneous transluminal coronary angioplasty in patients with prior coronary artery bypass grafting. J Thorac Cardiovasc Surg 1987; 93:268–275.

54. Pinkerton C, Slack J, Orr C, Vantassel J, Smith M. Percutaneous transluminal angioplasty in patients with prior myocardial revascularization surgery. Am J Cardiol 1988; 61:15G–22G.

55. Reed D, Beller G, Nygaard T, Tedesco C, Watson D, Burwell L. The clinical efficacy and scintigraphic evaluation of post-coronary bypass patients undergoing percutaneous transluminal coronary angioplasty for recurrent angina pectoris. Am Heart J 1989; 117:60–71.

56. Cooper I, Ineson N, Demirtas E, Coltart J, Jenkins S, Webb-Peploe M. Role of angioplasty in patients with previous coronary artery bypass surgery. Cathet Cardiovasc Diagn 1989; 16:81–86.

57. Platko W, Hollman J, Whitlow P, Franco I. Percutaneous transluminal angioplasty of saphenous vein graft stenosis: long-term follow-up. J Am Coll Cardiol 1989; 14:1645–1650.

58. Webb J, Myler R, Shaw R, Anwar A, Mayo JR, Murphy MC, Cumberland DC, Stertzer SH. Coronary angioplasty after coronary bypass surgery: initial results and late outcome in 422 patients. J Am Coll Cardiol 1990; 16:821–820.

59. Jost S, Gulba D, Daniel W, Amende I, Simon R, Eckert S, Lichtlen PR. Percutaneous transluminal angioplasty of aortocoronary venous bypass grafts and effect of the caliber of the grafted coronary artery on graft stenosis. Am J Cardiol 1991; 68:27–30.

60. Plokker H, Meester B, Serruys P. The Dutch experience in percutaneous transluminal angioplasty of narrowed saphenous veins used for aortocoronary arterial bypass. Am J Cardiol 1991; 67:361–366.

61. Reeves F, Bonan R, Cote G, Crepeau J, de Guise P, Gosselin G, Campeau L, Lesperance J. Long-term angiographic follow-up after angioplasty of venous coronary bypass grafts. Am Heart J 1991; 122:620–627.

62. Douglas JJ, Weintraub W, Liberman H, Jenkins M, Cohen, C, Morris D. Update of saphenous vein graft (SVG) angioplasty: restenosis and long-term outcome (abstr). Circulation 1991; 84(II):II-249.

63. Meester B, Samson M, Suryapranata H, Bonsel G, van den Brand M, de Feyter PJ, Serruys PW. Long-term follow-up after attempted angioplasty of saphenous vein grafts: the Thoraxcenter experience 1981–1988. Eur Heart J 1991; 12:648–653.

64. Danzi G, Mauri L, Formentini A, Pirelli S, Campolo L. The PTCA of venous grafts: the immediate and long-term results. Giornale Ital Cardiol 1992; 22:1285–1291.

65. Avital S, Wacksman R, Rozenman Y, Mosseri M, Lotun C, Hasin Y, Gotsman MS. Angioplasty for vein grafts and native coronary arteries after previous coronary artery bypass grafting. Harefuah 1995; 129:96–99.

10

Atherectomy for Saphenous Vein Bypass Graft Disease

David R. Holmes, Jr.
Mayo Clinic, Rochester, Minnesota

The treatment of saphenous vein bypass graft disease occupies an increasing part of the practice of interventional cardiology [1–6]. While conventional percutaneous transluminal coronary angioplasty (PTCA) has been used in selected patient subsets, the results of therapy have been mixed, depending upon the specific location of the stenosis (e.g., aorto-ostial versus more diffuse disease), and the age of the graft. In general, the older the graft and the more diffuse the disease, the higher the complications with conventional PTCA and the greater the chance of a suboptimal initial or long-term result with increased restenosis [1–9]. Because of these problems, new, alternative approaches to the treatment of vein graft disease have been evaluated including atherectomy. Of the three specific atherectomy devices currently available for routine clinical practice, only directional coronary atherectomy (DCA) and transluminal extraction atherectomy (TEC) have been relatively widely used for the treatment of vein graft disease.

I. DIRECTIONAL ATHERECTOMY

Directional atherectomy, the first new device approved after conventional PTCA, has been widely used and evaluated in single-center experiences, registry studies, and, recently, a randomized clinical trial [10–16]. Although it was originally developed to optimize the initial result of therapy, early data suggested that it may also result in improved restenosis rates. Application for vein graft stenoses was an attractive concept, in that a large device (7 French or 7 French Ex) could be used to treat large grafts, and because the grafts themselves are not usually tortuous or calcified, the device could be delivered relatively easily. In the initial DCA observational series [10], approximately 15–20% of procedures involved treatment of saphenous vein grafts. Finally, removal of plaque was thought to decrease the chance of distal embolization as well as to improve the initial angiographic result and potentially to impact restenosis.

Cowley et al. [11] reported the multicenter experience of directional atherectomy for vein graft disease. Twenty-one centers performed 318 procedures and treated 363 vein graft stenoses from 1988 to 1990. Core laboratory assessment was not performed. The lesion location was ostial (18%), proximal (34%), midshaft (33%), or distal (13%). Angiographic success (residual stenosis <50%) was achieved in 86% of lesions attempted, and clinical success was achieved in 85% of all patients who were treated. Major complications were infrequent: Death occurred in 0.9%, urgent coronary bypass graft surgery in 0.9%, and new-Q-wave myocardial infarction in 1.3%. A major complication occurred in 2.5% of patients. Less severe complications were more frequent: Distal embolization was documented in 7.2%, non-Q-wave myocardial infarction in 4.4%, and acute occlusion in 1.9%. Vein graft perforation was very rare, being documented in only 0.6% of patients. Angiographic follow-up was incomplete and was performed in only 149 patients, usually for clinical indications. There was a marked difference in restenosis rates, depending upon whether the lesion had been previously treated or was a primary de novo lesion; for restenosis lesions, the repeat restenosis rate was 75%, compared with only 38% for primary de novo lesions ($p < .001$). This multicenter experience concluded that "directional atherectomy is a safe and effective therapy for selected saphenous vein graft disease." Furthermore, restenosis rates for primary de novo lesions appeared lower than previously documented with conventional PTCA [1,2,5,13].

These data, among others that documented a good initial outcome and relatively low restenosis rates when compared to cohorts of patients being treated with conventional PTCA, led to the formulation of the CAVEAT-II trial, which randomized patients with de novo bypass graft stenoses to either PTCA or DCA (Table 1) [14]. The assumptions for sample size calculations for these trials are very important. It was assumed that in older grafts with discrete stenoses, the restenosis rate with conventional PTCA would be 60%, compared with 40% for DCA. It was also assumed that 15% of procedures would either be unsuccessful or involve crossover and that 15% of patients would be lost to angiographic follow-up. Given these assumptions, using an alpha of .05 and 80% power, a trial of 300 patients was initiated in 54 centers in 1992 and enrolled 305 patients up to April 1993.

Table 1 CAVEAT-II

	DCA	PTCA
N	149	156
Male sex	123 (82.6%)	132 (84.6%)
Prior MI	109 (73.2%)	98 (62.8%)
Unstable angina	133 (89.3%)	138 (88.5%)
Congestive heart failure	23 (15.4%)	21 (13.5%)
Graft age (years)	9.5	9.9
Ejection fraction (%)	52	50
Type of graft:		
Single	131 (88.5%)	127 (81.9%)
Sequential	14 (9.5%)	21 (13.6%)
Y	3 (2.0)	7 (4.5%)

The average age of the vein graft to be treated in the 305 patients was 9.5 years for DCA and 9.9 years for PTCA. Eighty-nine percent of patients had unstable angina, including progressive angina, rest angina, and postinfarction angina. Comorbid conditions were common, but were more frequent in the DCA group (36.9% vs. 27.6%). The patients randomized to DCA had improved initial success rates (89.2% vs. 79.0%, $p = .019$) when assessed by the angiographic core laboratory (Table 2). The initial angiographic dimensions were also improved, with the target stenosis improving from 73.7% to

Table 2 Outcome Treatment

	DCA $n = 149$	PTCA $n = 156$	p
Angio success:			
Site assessment	144 (98.0%)	151 (97.4%)	
Core laboratory	124 (89.2%)	117 (79.0%)	.019
Residual stenosis	31.5%	37.6%	<.001
Complications:			
CABG	1 (0.67%)	2 (1.3%)	
Death in hospital	3 (2.0%)	3 (1.9%)	1.00
MI	26 (17.4%)	18 (11.5%)	.142
Non-Q-wave	24 (16.1%)	15 (9.6%)	.09
Q-wave	2 (1.3%)	3 (1.9%)	1.0
Acute closure	7 (4.7%)	4 (2.6%)	.369
Composite endpoint[a]	30 (20.1%)	19 (12.2%)	.059

[a]Death, infarction, emergency CABG, or acute closure.

Table 3 Qualitative Coronary Angiography Results

	DCA	PTCA	*p*
Restenosis (>50%):			
Site assessment	51 (43.2)	61 (52.1)	
Core laboratory assessment	47 (45.6)	48 (50.5)	.491
Preprocedure:			
Reference size (mm)	3.45 (3.04,3.82)	3.46 (2.97,3.98)	
MLD (mm)	0.92 (0.70,1.23)	1.03 (0.76.1.29)	
Diameter stenosis %	73.7 (65.6,80.4)	71.7 (63.8,79.2)	
Postprocedure:			
Reference size (mm)	3.44 (2.96,3.83)	3.38 (2.99,3.94)	
MLD (mm)	2.43 (1.99,2.95)	2.22 (1.82,2.62)	
Diameter stenosis %	31.5 (23.5,39.4)	37.6 (28.6,45.6)	<.001
6-month follow-up:			
Reference size (mm)	3.42 (2.96,3.88)	3.42 (2.98,3.93)	
MLD (mm)	1.78 (1.20,2.27)	1.61 (0.92,2.18)	
% DS	47.3 (37.2,67.9)	52.5 (40.2,74.0)	.100
Acute gain (mm)	1.45 (0.99,1.92)	1.12 (0.78,1.58)	<.001
Late loss (mm)	0.62 (0.24,1.40)	0.53 (0.10,1.16)	.564
Net gain (mm)	0.68 (0.20,1.24)	0.50 (−0.09,1.06)	.066
Loss index	0.40 (0.16,0.84)	0.53 (0.10,1.04)	.567

31.5% for DCA, compared with 71.7% to 37.6% for PTCA ($p < .001$). The minimal luminal diameter increased from 0.92 mm to 2.43 mm for DCA, also significantly better than seen with conventional PTCA (1.03 mm to 2.22 mm) (Table 3). There was no difference in hospital mortality, which was low in each group (2.0% DCA, 1.9% PTCA) or in emergency CABG (0.67% vs. 0.64%). There was, however, an increase in myocardial infarction in the patients treated with DCA. This was related to non-Q-wave myocardial infarctions, which were more common with DCA. The incidence of Q-wave infarction was low (1.3% DCA vs. 0.67% PTCA). These results were similar to those for CAVEAT-I, which also documented an increase in non-Q-wave infarctions in patients randomized to DCA.

Distal embolization, defined as angiographic cutoff of the distal branch or vessel or decreased flow in a distal vessel that was previously patent in the absence of an occlusion at the target lesion, occurred in 28 patients in the entire trial [18]: 20 patients assigned to directional atherectomy (13.4%) and 8 assigned to PTCA (5.1%) ($p = .011$). In patients with distal embolization, in-hospital adverse event rates were increased at 71% versus 20%, with an odds ratio of 9.87 (95% confidence interval 4.65, 20.94). In patients with distal embolization there were two deaths (7%) and 19 myocardial infarctions (68%), the majority of which were non-Q-wave. There was no difference in outcome, irrespective of whether the distal embolization was associated with directional atherectomy use or with conventional PTCA. During 12 months of follow-up of these patients, adverse event rates were also higher in the patients with distal embolization odds ratio 3.05 (1.95, 4.76; 95% confidence interval). Multivariate analysis identified factors associated with increased incidence of distal embolization and included use of directional atherectomy (71% in distal embolization patients compared to 47% in patients without distal embolization, $p = .011$) and presence of angiographically documented thrombus (39% in distal embolization vs. 14% in patients without distal embolization). With conventional PTCA, Liu et al. [7] found that diffusely diseased vein grafts with large plaque volume and presumed thrombus are also independently predictive of distal embolization. The importance of platelets in distal embolization has been emphasized in the EPIC trial results. In the patients in EPIC treated with directional atherectomy who received 7E3 (abciximab, ReoPro), the distal embolization rates were not increased compared with conventional PTCA [19].

The primary endpoint for CAVEAT-II was angiographic restenosis. As predicted from the projections used to plan the trial, the angiographic restenosis rate for patients randomized to DCA was 45.6%; the surprising finding was that the restenosis rate with conventional PTCA was only 50% in these 10-year-old vein grafts. This was not statistically significantly different from DCA. A similar direction of results was seen, irrespective of whether visual estimate or core angiographic laboratory readings were used. Given the restenosis rate with conventional PTCA, the trial appeared to be underpowered to identify a significant difference.

The discrete data points regarding minimal luminal diameter can be seen in Figure 1 and in Table 3. There was significantly more acute gain in the patients treated with atherectomy. While the net gain tended to remain higher (0.68 mm vs. 0.50 mm, DCA vs. PTCA), this was only a trend ($p = .06$).

Clinical follow-up was available for 300 patients for a median follow-up of 6.2 months (Table 4). There was no difference in survival, which was 95.3% for DCA and 92.3% for PTCA ($p = .415$) or Q-wave myocardial infarction. Patients randomized to DCA had significantly fewer repeat percutaneous interventions of the target, 13.2% compared with 22.4% of angioplasty patients ($p = .041$); the composite of death, infarction, repeat bypass surgery, and repeat intervention, however, was similar ($p = .199$).

The final conclusions from CAVEAT-II were that DCA resulted in a higher initial angiographic success rate, a larger initial improvement in vein graft dimensions, decreased performance of target vessel intervention, but no difference in angiographic restenosis. In addition, distal embolization rates

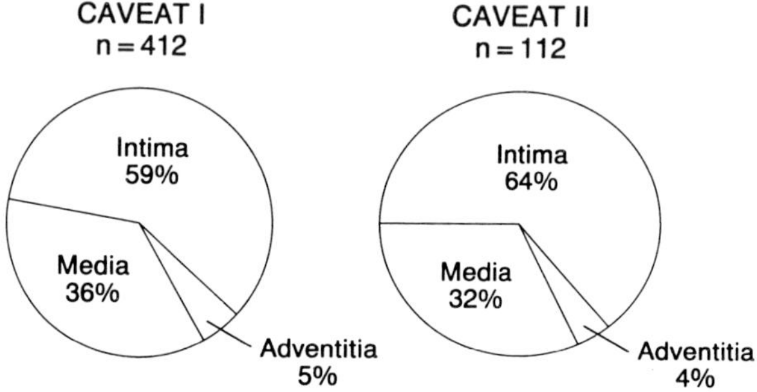

Figure 1 The majority of patients in both CAVEAT I and II had tissue samples that involved only the intima, and the distribution of samples among intima, media, and adventitia was similar in the two trials.

were increased with DCA. Finally, there was a difference in repeat percutaneous target lesion revascularization favoring DCA.

In an attempt to create an increasingly large lumen, the potential for deep tissue injury exists. CAVEAT-II [20] investigators evaluated the relationship between the depth of tissue resection and subsequent restenosis. This relationship was explored for both native as well as vein graft lesions treated with DCA.

Table 4 Six-Month Event-Free Survival Analysis

Event	Six-month event-free survival rate		Log rank
	DCA	PTCA	p
Death	0.953	0.923	.415
MI (site	0.798	0.837	.466
Q-wave MI (site)	0.972	0.960	.389
CABG	0.944	0.953	.935
Stroke	0.987	0.993	.975
Recath	0.463	0.458	.357
Any intervention	0.758	0.711	.144
Target intervention	0.874	0.796	.067
Percutaneous intervention	0.811	0.750	.078
Hospitalization	0.543	0.514	.788
Angina	0.616	0.638	.902
CHC > 1	0.682	0.641	.734
Composite event (death, MI, CABG, percutaneous intervention)	0.599	0.579	.291

In CAVEAT-II, 113 patients had vein graft tissue available. Subintimal deep wall resection was seen in 40 (35%); this finding was not associated with adverse early outcome success, or early complications (Table 5). Six month restenosis rates varied; when resection was limited to the intima, a restenosis rate of 40.4% was found whereas in patients with subintimal resection, the restenosis rate was 57.12%. This difference was not statistically significant; this could relate to the sample size involved.

Selection of treatment modalities for saphenous vein bypass graft disease should take into account single-center and multicenter experiences as well as the results of randomized trials. In addition, treatment for saphenous vein bypass graft disease must take into account the widespread use of a variety of stents, which have been reported in single-center and multicenter experiences to be as positive as directional atherectomy was prior to CAVEAT-II.

At the present time, directional atherectomy is still used to treat vein graft disease. The goal is to optimize the initial result and thereby hopefully improve longer-term results. Lesions that are suitable include aorto-ostial vein graft lesions (Figure 2) [15,16] and bulky lesions in the body or shaft of vein grafts (Figure 3). Ostial lesions are very difficult to treat with conventional PTCA and even with stents. Directional atherectomy may also be difficult because of guide catheter position, but can be very effective in debulking lesions (Figure 2). This can be followed by stenting if appropriate. Stephan et al. [15] analyzed 158 patients undergoing DCA of 160 ostial lesions. These lesions included 30 left main coronary artery or right coronary artery, 73 left anterior descending or circumflex, and 57 vein graft ostial stenoses. Overall procedural success (angiographic residual stenosis <50% and no death, Q-wave myocardial infarction, or urgent coronary bypass graft surgery) was achieved in 87%; major complications were infrequent, with no deaths or Q-wave myocardial infarctions and only one urgent bypass operation. In the 57 vein graft ostial lesion subset, procedural success was achieved in 88.6% of

Table 5 CAVEAT II Acute Outcome

	Intimal resection	Subintimal resection	p
N	73	40	
Procedural success (%)	93	100	.168
CABG (%)	0	0	
MI[a] (%)	20.6	12.5	.284
QMI	2.7	0	.539
non-QMI	17.8	12.5	.461
Death (%)	1.4	.0	

[a]Clinical site documentation.

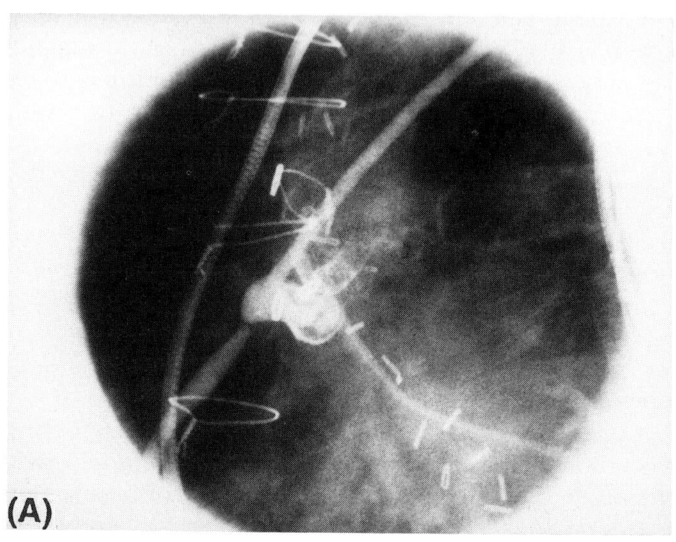

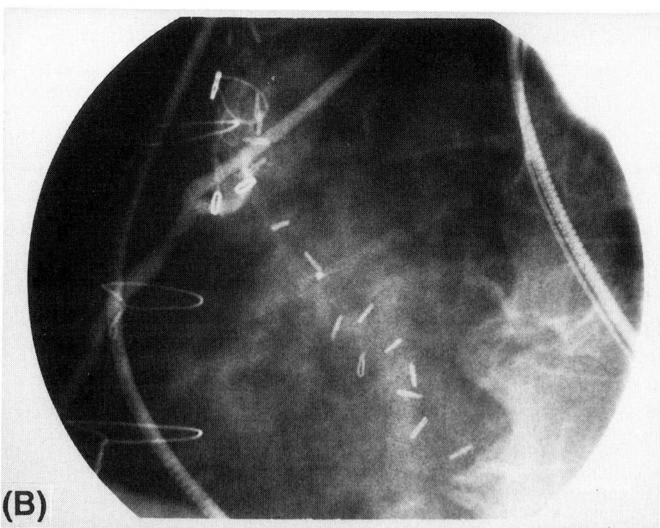

Figure 2 Left anterior oblique view of ostial stenosis of right coronary vein graft (A); directional atherectomy results in significant debulking (B); This is followed by biliary stent implantation (C) leaving an excellent final result (D).

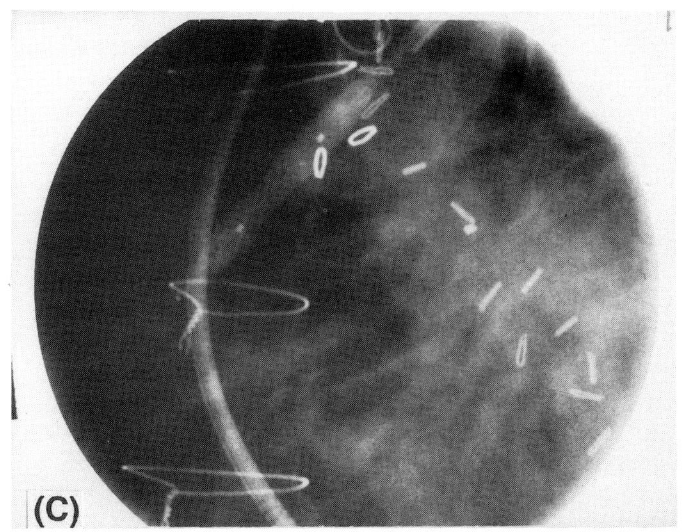

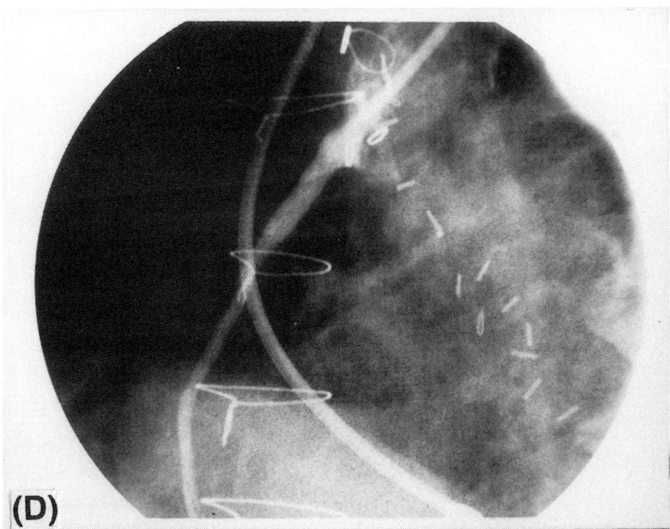

Figure 2 Continued.

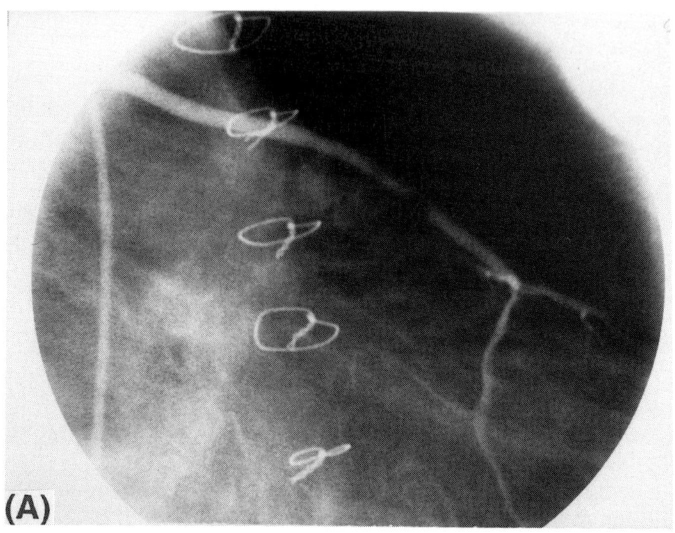

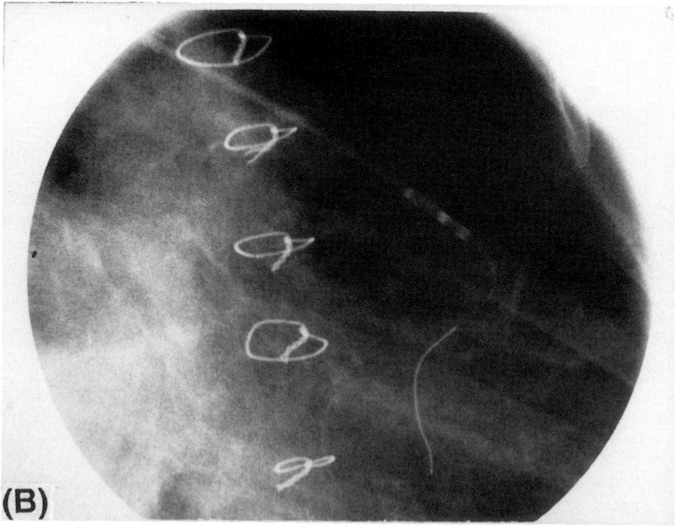

Figure 3   Directional coronary atherectomy of a single discrete lesion (A) in the shaft of a sequential vein graft. Device is easily positioned (B). After multiple cuts, adjunctive balloon dilatation is used to optimize result (C).

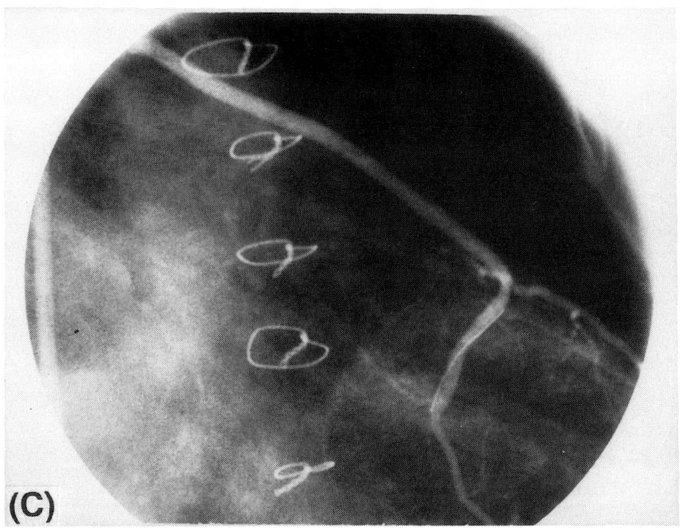

Figure 3 Continued.

de novo lesions and 81.8% of restenotic lesions. In these patients treated for vein graft stenoses, there were no deaths, Q-wave infarctions, or emergency surgical procedures. Non-Q-wave myocardial infarctions were documented in six patients (11%) and distal embolization in four (7%). In this series, repeat angiography was performed in only 90 of 138 patients with initially successful DCA. The restenosis rate for de novo ostial vein graft lesions was 47%; this contrasts with restenotic ostial vein graft lesions, in whom repeat restenosis occurred in 93%.

Bulky lesions in the body or shaft of vein grafts may respond poorly to conventional PTCA. In approaching these lesions, DCA can be used to debulk the lesion; often this is followed by stent implantation. Whether this approach is superior to optimal DCA alone or to stent implantation alone remains to be determined. If this approach is selected, it must be remembered that CAVEAT-II indicates that distal embolization rates are increased. As has been mentioned, distal embolization appears to be related to platelet debris. Intensive antiplatelet regimens, e.g., GP IIb/IIIa receptor antagonist drugs, may decrease the incidence of this complication.

For other lesions, e.g., long diffuse disease or distal anastomoses, DCA has a very limited role, either because it is not effective or has increased complication (the former) or because it is not usually needed because conventional PTCA works so well (the latter). If directional atherectomy is chosen

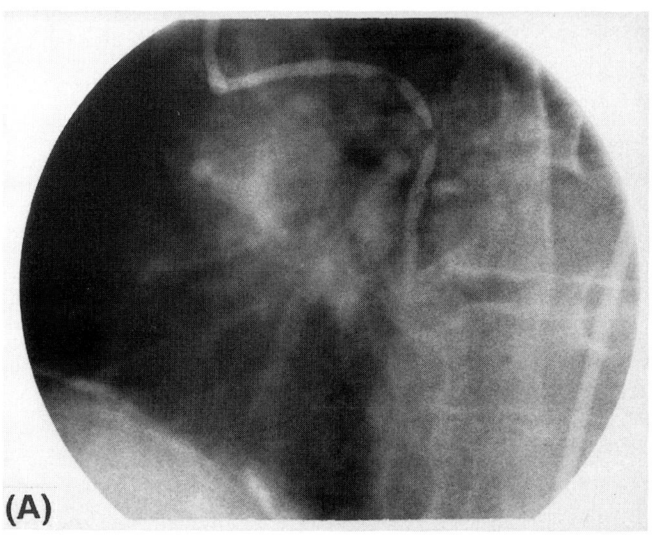

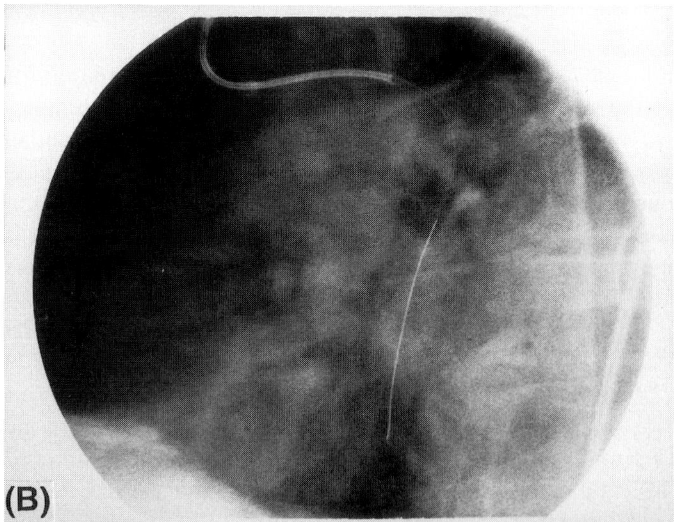

Figure 4 Left anterior oblique of vein graft to LAD with multiple filling defects and complete occlusion (A). TEC atherectomy of the entire graft (B) results in restoration of flow. Following dilitation, an excellent improvement (C).

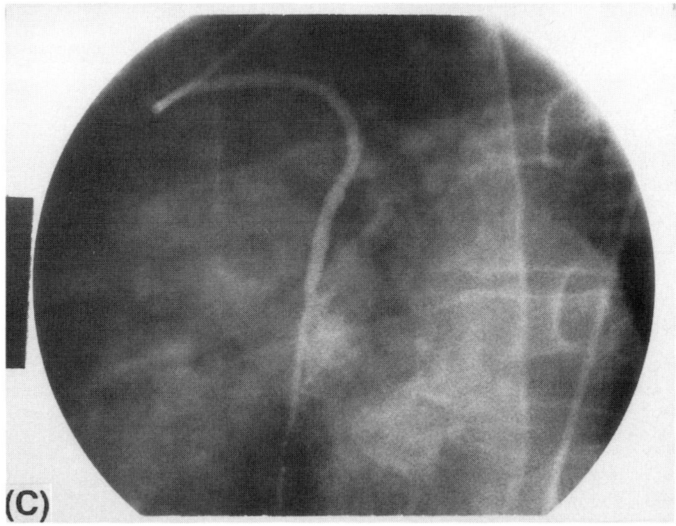

Figure 4 Continued.

for discrete lesions, the approach should be to optimize the initial results by using post-DCA adjunctive PTCA or stenting if needed. The same principles of a bigger initial result being associated with a better long-term result appear to be equally applicable for vein grafts as for the native coronary arteries.

II. TRANSLUMINAL EXTRACTION

While directional atherectomy is ideally suited for discrete lesions, transluminal extraction (TEC) has been more commonly used in more diffuse disease or even in occluded vein grafts. The treatment of these anatomic subsets of patients using conventional PTCA techniques alone or in combination with local administration of thrombolytic therapy has been characterized by increased complications, particularly distal embolization and late reocclusion. TEC has been used in these patients to optimize the initial results either alone (Figure 4) or in combination with stents (Figure 5).

A multicenter registry experience has recently reported on the outcome of TEC on 650 vein graft lesions in 538 patients [21]. The majority of patients (79.6%) had severe angina, either Canadian Cardiovascular Society class III or IV, and 13.8% were hospitalized with acute myocardial infarction. The grafts were usually old and had complex disease: The mean age was 8.3 years, and

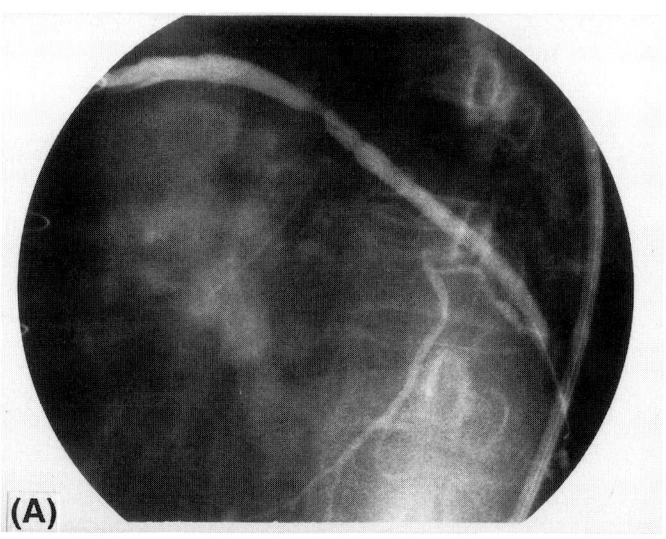

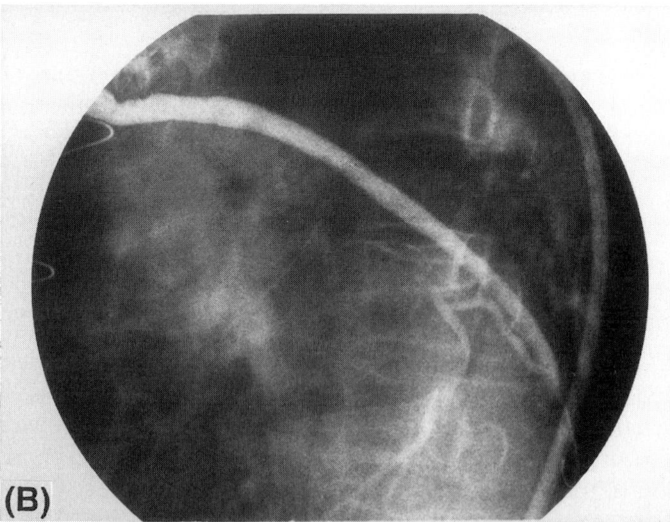

Figure 5 Left anterior oblique view of the obtuse marginal graft prior to treatment with TEC atherectomy (A) and following biliary stent implantation (B).

85% were over 3 years of age; the lesions were eccentric (50%), contained angiographically apparent thrombus (28%), or were ulcerated (13%). In this high-risk group of lesions, the overall lesion success rate ($\geq$20% improvement in stenosis or $\leq$50% residual stenosis) was 93% (606 of 650 lesions). Clinical success, defined as angiographic success without death, emergency surgery, or Q-wave myocardial infarction, was achieved in 89%. In-hospital complications were relatively uncommon: 23 patients (4.3%) had a major complication, including in-hospital mortality (3.2%), nonfatal Q-wave myocardial infarction (0.7%), and emergency coronary bypass graft surgery (two patients, 0.4%). In-hospital complications were higher in the patients who had presented with acute myocardial infarction at the time of their index hospitalization. Other complications were more frequent and included distal embolization (3.7%), non-Q-wave myocardial infarction (1.8%), and acute closure (3.2%). Perforation occurred in only two patients. The effect of lesion morphology on outcome was assessed. Long lesions greater than 20 mm had decreased success rates (85% vs. 96%, $p <$ .05), as did total occlusions (75% success vs. 96%, $p <$ .05).

In other series, distal embolization has been more problematic, particularly with friable lesions. In the NACI registry [22], TEC atherectomy was used to treat 240 lesions, many of which were vein graft disease. In this NACI experience distal embolization occurred in 7% with TEC. Hong et al. [23] evaluated distal embolization after TEC atherectomy in 86 high-risk vein graft lesions. Distal embolization occurred in 11 (12.8%), often after adjunct PTCA; however, when distal embolization occurred it markedly affected outcome—major in-hospital complications of death, coronary bypass graft surgery, or Q-wave infarction occurred in 46% of this subset, versus only 2% of patients without distal embolization. The procedural success in patients with distal embolization was only 55%, versus 91% of patients without embolization. Correlates of distal embolization included angiographic evidence of thrombus. In another single-center series, Safian et al. [24] documented distal embolization in 11.9% of 158 treated vein graft lesions and no reflow in 8.8%. The strongest independent clinical correlate of a severe clinical complication, defined as in-hospital death, emergency CABG, or infarction, was no reflow, distal embolization, or acute closure.

More recently, Misumi et al. [25] evaluated 163 consecutive nonrandomized patients undergoing treatment for vein graft disease. TEC was used in 103 and conventional PTCA in 60 patients. Success rates ranged from 90.3% for TEC to 83.3% for PTCA but were not statistically different. However, patients treated with TEC had a lower incidence of distal embolization (3.9% versus 16.7%, $p =$ .005). Even in vein grafts with angiographic evidence of thrombus, TEC had less distal embolization (5.6% versus 31.8%, $p =$ .004).

In the multicenter registry experience [21], angiographic follow-up at 6 months was limited and voluntary. Two hundred twenty-seven patients with

268 lesions underwent angiography for a variety of reasons, some by protocol design, others for recurrent symptoms. In this selected group of patients with angiographic follow-up, the restenosis rate was 60%. Other angiographic follow-up studies are also limited. Safian et al. [24] reported on 158 vein graft lesions in 146 consecutive patients treated at a single center. At least some of these patients were also reported in the previously mentioned registry experience. In this single-center experience, complete clinical follow-up was available in 118 (92%) of 128 eligible patients at 6.0 ± 2.5 months. Late cardiac death occurred in 7%, Q-wave myocardial infarction in 4%, repeat CABG in 5%, and repeat target vessel intervention in 26%. Angiographic follow-up documented a restenosis rate of 69%; this included 29% of lesions that were totally occluded at follow-up. Other, smaller series have also documented high restenosis rates.

III. ROTATIONAL ATHERECTOMY

Rotational atherectomy is infrequently used for the treatment of saphenous vein bypass graft stenoses [26,27]. This lack of application is related to the underlying pathophysiology with soft friable lesions. Rotational atherectomy, however, has been reported in selected lesions, including discrete fibrotic or calcific aorto-ostial lesions [26,27] and fibrotic distal anastomoses, although the latter usually respond favorably to conventional PTCA.

IV. CONCLUSION

Treatment of vein graft disease remains problematic for percutaneous treatment strategies, with an increased potential for acute complications, particularly distal embolization and/or non-Q-wave myocardial infarction, as well as for longer-term problems with increased restenosis rates and decreased event-free survival. Atherectomy plays an important role in selected patients, based upon the specific lesion.

Directional atherectomy remains an excellent alternative to conventional PTCA for discrete stenoses either at the aorto-ostial location or within the shaft of the graft. Initial angiographic results are improved compared with conventional PTCA; distal embolization is increased, probably related to device size. This may be platelet-mediated and may be able to be affected by GP IIb/IIIa receptor blockers. If these are to be used, it is prudent to treat prophylactically rather than wait until the complication has occurred. Follow-up restenosis rates are similar to those for conventional PTCA in the only randomized trial reported to date, although repeat target lesion revascularization is less common after DCA. Future studies will evaluate the role of debulking lesions with DCA and stent implantation to optimize results.

Transluminal extraction catheter is used more commonly for higher-risk lesions, i.e., longer diffuse disease with greater thrombus burden. While there are no randomized trials reported, single-center and multicenter experiences with these high-risk lesions document good outcome; however, distal embolization rates are increased and are usually associated with markedly increased complications. Restenosis rates remain high, as do clinical events. There is a current randomized trial evaluating a combination of TEC followed by stenting, either with or without the use of a IIb/IIIa inhibitor.

To optimize further the approach to vein graft disease, devices that incorporate debulking, thrombus removal, and surface passivation are being tested. These include rheolytic thrombectomy systems which provide rapid fragmentation and aspiration of fresh thrombus and are being evaluated in current ongoing trials.

REFERENCES

1. deFeyter PJ, van Suylen RJ, de Jaegere PPT, Topol EJ, Serruys PW. Balloon angioplasty for the treatment of lesions in saphenous vein bypass grafts. J Am Coll Cardiol 1993; 21:1539–1549.
2. Platko WP, Hollman J, Whitlow PL, Franco J. Percutaneous transluminal coronary angioplasty of saphenous vein graft stenosis: long term follow-up. J Am Coll Cardiol 1989; 14:1645–1650.
3. Reeder GS, Bresnahan JF, Holmes DR Jr, Mock MB, Orszulak TA, Smith HC, Vlietstra RE. Angioplasty for aortocoronary bypass graft stenosis. Mayo Clinic Proc 1986; 61:14–19.
4. Cote G, Myler RK, Stertzer JH, Clark DA, Fishman-Rosen J, Murphy M, Shaw RE. Percutaneous transluminal angioplasty of stenotic coronary artery bypass grafts: 5 years' experience. J Am Coll Cardiol 1987; 9:8–17.
5. Douglas JS Jr, Gruentzig AR, King SB III, Hollman J, Ischinger T, Meier B, Craver JM, Jones EL, Waller JL, Bone DK, Guyton R. Percutaneous transluminal coronary angioplasty in patients with prior coronary bypass surgery. J Am Coll Cardiol 1983; 2:745–754.
6. Webb JG, Myler RK, Shaw RE, Anwar A, Mayo JR, Murphy MC, Cumberland DC, Stertz SH. Coronary angioplasty after coronary bypass surgery: initial results and late outcome in 422 patients. J Am Coll Cardiol 1990; 16:812–820.
7. Liu MW, Douglas JS Jr, Lembo NJ, King SB III. Angiographic predictors of a rise in serum creatine kinase (distal embolization) after balloon angioplasty of saphenous vein coronary artery bypass grafts. Am J Cardiol 1993; 72:514–517.
8. Trono R, Sutton C, Hollman J, Suit P, Ratliff NB. Multiple myocardial infarctions associated with atheromatous emboli after PTCA of saphenous vein grafts. A clinicopathologic correlation. Cleveland Clinic J Med 1989; 56:581–584.

9. Saber RS, Edwards WB, Holmes DR Jr. Balloon angioplasty of aortocoronary saphenous vein bypass grafts: a histopathologic study of six grafts from five patients with emphasis on restenosis and embolic complications. J Am Coll Cardiol 1988; 12:1501–1509.

10. Baim DS, Hinohara T, Holmes DR, Topol E, Pinkerton C, King SB III, Whitlow P, Kereiakes D, Farley B, Simpson JB. Results of directional coronary atherectomy during multicenter preapproved testing. Am J Cardiol 1993; 72:6E–11E.

11. Cowley MJ, Whitlow PL, Baim DS. Directional coronary atherectomy of saphenous vein graft narrowings: multicenter investigational experience. Am J Cardiol 1993; 72:30E–35E.

12. Kaufmann UP, Garratt KN, Vlietstra RE, Holmes DR. Transluminal atherectomy of saphenous vein aortocoronary bypass grafts. Am J Cardiol 1990; 65:1430–1433.

13. Cowley MJ, DiSciascio G. Directional coronary atherectomy for saphenous vein graft disease. Cathet Cardiovasc Diagn 1993; 1:10–16.

14. Holmes DR Jr, Topol EJ, Califf RM, Berdan LG, Leya F, Berger PB, Whitlow PL, Safian RD, Adelman AG, Kellett MA Jr, Talley JD III, Shani J, Gottlieb RS, Pinkerton CA, Lee KL, Keeler GP, Ellis SG; the CAVEAT-II Investigators. A multicenter, randomized trial of coronary angioplasty versus directional atherectomy for patients with saphenous vein bypass graft lesions. Circulation 1995; 91: 1966–1974.

15. Stephan WJ, Bates ER, Garratt KN, Hinohara T, Muller DW. Directional coronary atherectomy of coronary and saphenous vein graft ostial stenoses. Am J Cardiol 1995; 75:1015–1018.

16. Kerwin PM, McKeever LS, Marek JC, Hartman JR, Enger EL. Directional atherectomy of aortoostial stenoses. Cathet Cardiovasc Diagn 1993; Suppl 1: 17–25.

17. Rabbani RR, Bell MR, Grill DE, et al. Clinical follow-up after successful percutaneous coronary angioplasty of saphenous vein graft disease and the importance of long term assessment. In press.

18. Lefkovitz J, Holmes DR, Califf RM, Safian RD, Pieperk, Keeler G, Topol EJ. Predictors and sequelae of distal embolization during saphenous vein graft intervention from the CAVEAT-II trial. Circulation 1995; 92:734–740.

19. Challapal RM, Eisenberg MJ, Sigmon K, Lemberger J. Platelet glycoprotein IIb/IIIa monoclonal antibody (c7E3) reduces distal embolization during percutaneous intervention of saphenous vein grafts (abstr). Circulation 1995; 92:I–607.

20. Holmes DR Jr, Garratt KN, Isner JM, Kearney M, Bearden LG, Schwartz RS, Califf RM, Topol EJ, for the CAVEAT I and II Investigators. Effect of subintimal resection on initial outcome and restenosis for native coronary lesions and saphenous vein graft disease treated by directional coronary atherectomy: A report from the CAVEAT I and II investigators. J Am Coll Cardiol 1996; 28:645–651.

21. Meany TB, Leon MB, Kramer BL, Margolis JR, Matthews RV, Whitlow PL, Moses JW, Knopf WD, Tommaso CL, Sketch MH Jr, O'Neill WW. Transluminal extraction catheter for the treatment of diseased saphenous vein grafts. A multicenter experience. Cathet Cardiovasc Diagn 1995; 34:112–120.

22. NACI Registry. Unpublished data.

23. Hong MK, Popma JJ, Pichard AD. Clinical significance of distal embolization after transluminal extraction atherectomy in diffusely diseased saphenous vein grafts. Am Heart J 1994; 127:1496–1503.
24. Safian RD, Grines CL, May MA, Lichtenberg A, Juran N, Schreiber TL, Pavlides G, Meany TB, Savas V, O'Neill WW. Clinical and angiographic results of transluminal extraction coronary atherectomy in saphenous vein bypass grafts. Circulation 1994; 89:302–312.
25. Misumi K, Matthews RV, Sun GW, et al. Reduced distal embolization with transluminal extraction atherectomy compared to balloon angioplasty for saphenous vein graft disease. Cathet Cardiovasc Diagn 1996; 39:246–251.
26. Cardenas JR, Strumpf RK, Heuser RR. Rotational atherectomy in restenotic lesions at the distal saphenous vein graft anastomosis. Cathet Cardiovasc Diagn 1995; 36:53–57.
27. Abhyankar AD, Vaidya KA, Bernstein L. Rotational atherectomy of calcified ostial saphenous vein graft lesions with long term follow-up: a case report. Int J Cardiol 1995; 52:11–12.

11
Stenting for Saphenous Vein Graft Disease

David R. Holmes, Jr.
Mayo Clinic, Rochester, Minnesota

The treatment of saphenous vein graft disease has changed rapidly. Multiple observational series have documented that the results of treatment with conventional PTCA have been suboptimal because of the problem of distal embolization, non-Q-wave infarction, inadequate initial dilatation, and restenosis. These recalcitrant problems have focused emphasis on new, alternative approaches. As each new approach has been evaluated, initial enthusiasm has been high, only to be tempered by results of more scientifically controlled trials with longer follow-up. This has been exemplified by the changing pattern of directional coronary atherectomy for treatment of vein graft disease since the publication of CAVEAT-II (see Chapter 11). At the present time, stenting for vein graft disease is widely practiced and is considered by some to be the treatment of choice. There are, however, limited controlled data. Stenting for vein graft disease involves consideration of the specific lesion to be treated, the indication for stenting, and the specific stent configuration available. The lesions that have been most problematic with conventional PTCA have included (a) aorto-ostial lesions, which have been found to respond poorly to conventional PTCA, with high restenosis rates and elastic recoil, (b) body of shaft vein graft lesions, particularly more diffuse disease, which have resulted in increased acute complications as well as increased restenosis, and (c) restenotic lesions, which have high rates of recurrent restenosis. Distal anastomotic lesions usually respond well to conventional PTCA, with excellent initial success rates and low restenosis rates. Stenting has been used to approach all of these lesion groups.

I. JOHNSON & JOHNSON INTERVENTIONAL SYSTEMS (JJIS) CORONARY STENT

An increasingly large experience has been developed with the JJIS coronary stent. A multicenter experience including patient recruitment from 20 sites has been presented in 589 consecutive patients undergoing treatment of saphenous vein graft bypass lesions from 1990 to 1992 [1]. Consecutive patients meeting the selection criteria were enrolled in this study. Angiographic exclusions included true aorto-ostial lesions, distal anastomotic lesions, diffuse disease, lesions containing intracoronary thrombus, and vein grafts either <3 mm or >5 mm in diameter. These exclusions were aimed at optimizing the potential success rates of stenting, because these characteristics have been previously documented to be associated with increased complications. The average age of the vein graft treated was 8.9 ± 4.2 years; the majority were over 4 years old (Table 1). Sixty-one percent were de novo lesions.

There was successful stent deployment in 582 patients (98.8%). The majority of patients (82.7%) received a single stent. The remainder of the patients had multiple stents implanted, usually nonoverlapping, for the treatment of separate discrete lesions. The complication profile in these old grafts was very favorable (Table 2). Of the 582 patients with successful stent implantation, major in-hospital complications occurred in 17 (2.9%). These included death in 10 (1.7%), Q-wave myocardial infarction in 2 (0.3%), and urgent coronary bypass graft surgery in 5 (0.9%). Non-Q-wave myocardial infarction was documented in 28 (4.8%). Distal embolization was uncommon, being seen in only 11 (1.9%), and was associated with poststent evidence of conduit stent thrombus formation despite the intense anticoagulation regimen, which included

Table 1   Multicenter U.S. Palmaz-Schatz Stent Experience

Mean age (years)	66 ± 9
Saphenous vein graft age (years)	8.9 ± 4.2
Saphenous vein graft target (%)	
Left anterior descending	31
Circumflex	30
Right coronary artery	21
Other	18
Prior angioplasty of target lesion (%)	39
Unstable angina (%)	72
High surgical risk (%)	49
Mean lesion length (mm)	7.6 ± 4.9

n = 582.
From Ref. 1.

Table 2 Acute Outcome

Stent	Author [Ref.]	Study period	No. of patients	Success rate (%)	Early closure (%)	Infarction (%)	Emergency CABG (%)	Death (%)	Distal embolization (%)	Restenosis (%)
JJIS cor	Wong [1]	'90–'92	589	99	1.4	0.3	0.9	1.7	1.9	30
JJIS cor	Pomerantz [2]	'88–'91	69	99	—	10[a]	0	0	1.4	25
JJIS cor	Maiello [3]	'90–'93	43	94	0	4.6	2.3	2.3	—	11
JJIS cor	Wong [4]	'90–'93	108	95	0	16.9[a]	0	1.9	2	—
JJIS cor	Strumpf [5]	'90–'91	26	100	3.8	3.8	0	0	—	13
JJIS cor	Carrozza [6]	'88–'91	84	100	0.4	4	—	0	—	25
JJIS cor	Fenton [7]	'90–'91	198	98.5	0.5	—	—	—	—	34
JJIS cor & biliary	Piana [8]	'88–'93	150	98.5	0.6	7.9[a]	0	0.6	—	17
JJIS biliary	Wong [14]	'90–'93	123	95	0	11.0[a]	0.8	0.8	3	—
JJIS biliary	White [15]	—	11	100	0	0	0	0	0	—
Wiktor	Fortuna [18]	'91–'93	101	95	2	3	1	1	—	—
Gianturco-Roubin	Dorros [19]	'91–'93	96	96	1	8	0	3	—	—
Wallstent	Urban [20]	'86–'88	13	100	0	0	0	0	7.7	20
Wallstent	deScheerder [21]	'88–'90	69	100	10	7.2	5.8	4.3	—	47
Wallstent	Strauss [22]	'86–'90	145	100	7	—	—	—	—	48
Wallstent	Eeckhart [23]	'86–'93	40	100	2	2	2	0	—	35

JJIS = Johnson & Johnson Interventional Systems; cor = coronary.
[a]Q- and non-Q-wave myocardial infarction.

aspirin, dipyridamole, warfarin, dextran, and heparin. Stent thrombosis was very uncommon, being documented in only 8 patients (1.4%).

The most common complication was bleeding, which occurred in 14.3% of patients. This bleeding was typically related to vascular access; treatment, however, required transfusion in 6.3% of patients and surgical intervention in an additional 8%. Two patients died with retroperitoneal hemorrhage.

Clinical follow-up was available in all patients, for a mean of 8.4 ± 4.0 months (Figure 1). Prior to stent implantation, 87% of patients were Canadian Cardiovascular Society Class III or IV, while at follow-up only 16% had these severe symptoms. As can be seen, nonfatal Q- or non-Q-wave myocardial infarctions were infrequent. Seventy-six patients underwent repeat revascularization of the target lesion, with either PTCA ($n = 45$) or coronary bypass graft surgery ($n = 31$). Death occurred in 28 patients (4.9%). Although the etiology of the mortality is difficult to determine, of the 28 deaths that occurred following discharge, Wong et al. [1] felt that only 5 were definitely related to the stent.

Angiographic follow-up was incomplete, available in only 66% of eligible patients. Based on a dichotomous definition (≥50% diameter stenosis), restenosis occurred in 29.7%. Multivariable logistic regression analysis identified four factors that were independent predictors of restenosis, including treatment of a restenotic lesion (odds ratio 3.50, $p < .001$), reference vessel diameter,

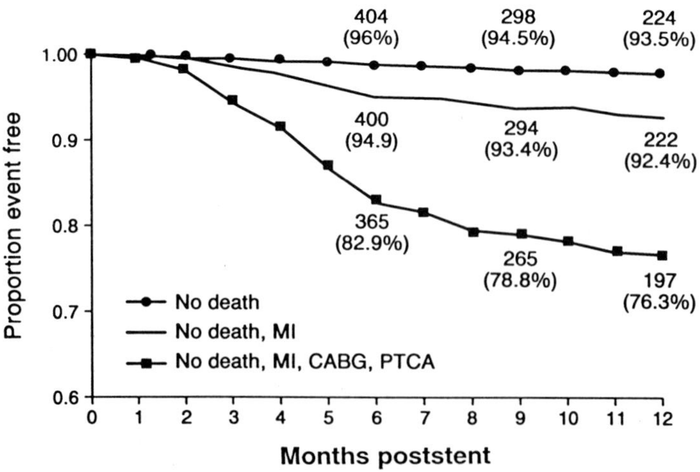

Figure 1 Event free survival curves following JJIS stent implantation. At 12 months, there is a progressive decrease in the combined event free survival of death, MI, CABG, and PTCA.

diabetes mellitus, and the final percent diameter stenosis. Patients with prior angioplasty had a restenosis rate of 46.1%, versus 18.3% in patients in whom a de novo lesion was treated.

This multicenter registry experience is the largest available for the Johnson & Johnson Interventional Systems (JJIS) coronary stent. Smaller series, using standard 15-mm or shorter 7-mm stents, have also been reported (Table 2) [2–8]. In these series, success rates for the treatment of focal lesions have also been excellent (approximately 95%), with low complication rates, including very low rates of subacute closure (Figures 2 and 3). The results in these selected patient series cannot be generalized to higher-risk lesions—aorto-ostial location, diffuse or friable disease, or lesions containing large thrombus burden, all of which are at higher risk of inadequate initial results, increased complications acutely, and a higher incidence of restenosis. These caveats notwithstanding, the results appear very encouraging, with a low restenosis rate (particularly when de novo lesions are treated), a low initial cardiac complication rate, and good 6-month clinical follow-up, and they have solidified the view of at least some active investigators that, in appropriate lesions, this specific stent is one of the treatments of choice.

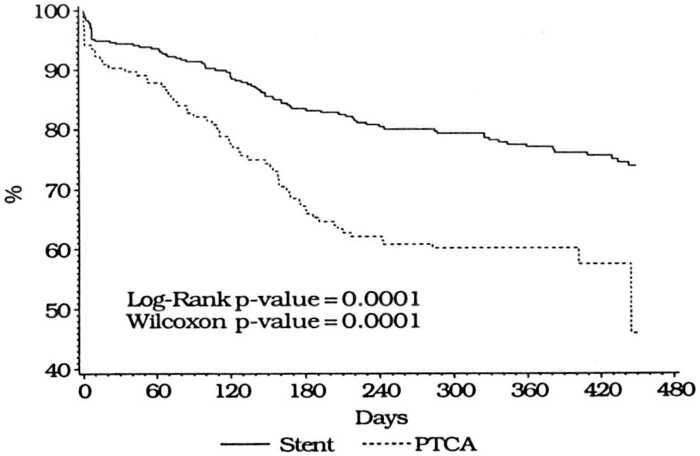

Figure 2 Patients treated either with stent (___) or conventional PTCA (——) have a progressive decline in event free survival with the combined endpoint of death, QMI, and repeat revascularization but this is significantly improved after stent implantation.

Table 3 Late Clinical Follow-Up on Multicenter JJIS Experience

Event (%)	Actuarial follow-up events		
	6 Months	12 Months	24 Months
Death	5	8	14
Infarction	7	8	8
Coronary surgery	7	9	12
PTCA	6	8	12
Free of death, MI, CABG, or PTCA	75	67	55

661 patients, 775 vein graft lesions.
From Ref. 11.

Brener et al. [9] compared the one year outcome of patients in the Palmaz-Schatz vein graft stent registry with patients in the coronary angioplasty arm of the CAVEAT-II trial. There were 377 patients with de novo graft lesions in the JJIS registry and 156 in CAVEAT-II. The patients were similar with respect to age, gender, and other baseline characteristics with the exception of the fact that patients treated in CAVEAT-II had more unstable angina (88% vs. 71%, $p < .01$). The mean graft age was 9 ± 4 years. Procedural failure with a residual stenosis >50% was slightly more common in PTCA patients, 2.6% vs. 0.8%, but this was not statistically significant ($p = .63$). The final mean residual stenosis was much less for stent patients, $6 \pm 10\%$ vs. $37 \pm 14\%$ ($p < .001$). There was no significant difference in hospital outcome (Table 3). At one year of follow-up, the incidence of mortality was similar, 8% PTCA and 6% stent. Patients treated with stents had a significant improvement in the composite endpoint of death, QMI, or repeat revascularization, 19% vs. 43% (Figure 4). Angiographic restenosis was significantly less frequent with stents, 18% vs. 52% ($p < .001$). Although there are limitations to this type of cross registry comparison, the results are encouraging.

A single randomized trial of stenting versus conventional PTCA for de novo vein graft lesions using the Palmaz-Schatz™ coronary stent has been finished [10]. The trial focused on good-risk lesions, i.e., short (requiring ≤2 stents), large vessels (3.0–5.0 mm), nonostial, and not containing angiographically apparent thrombus; in addition, patients with abnormal depressed left ventricular function were excluded. The mean graft age was 10 years. Initial outcomes were improved in the patients randomized to stenting: angiographic success rate (95% vs. 75%, $p < .0001$), clinical success rate (92% vs. 69%, $p < .0001$), improved postprocedural maximal lumen diameter (2.81 mm vs. 2.16 mm, $p < .0001$), and a trend toward decreased non-Q-wave infarction rates. The combined endpoint of Q-wave myocardial infarction, death, or need for bypass surgery was similar between stented and dilated patients. Follow-up

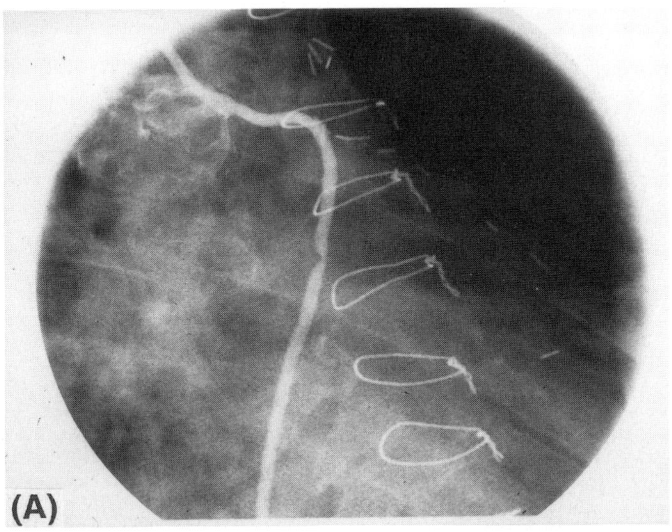

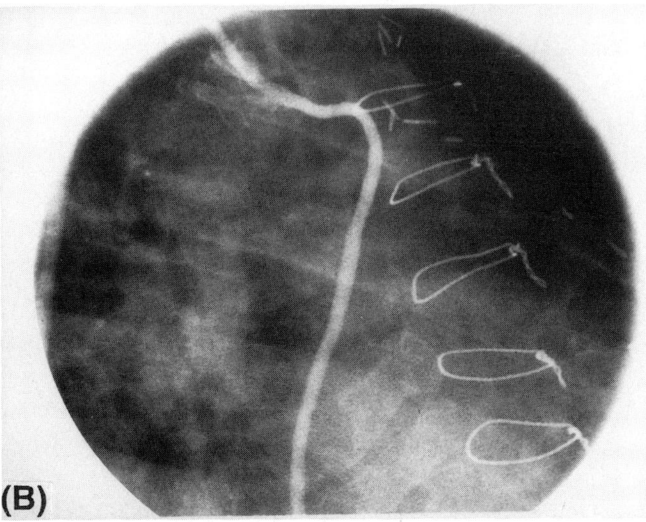

Figure 3 (A) Stent implantation for treatment of focal lesion in an obtuse marginal graft base, (B) post stent implantation.

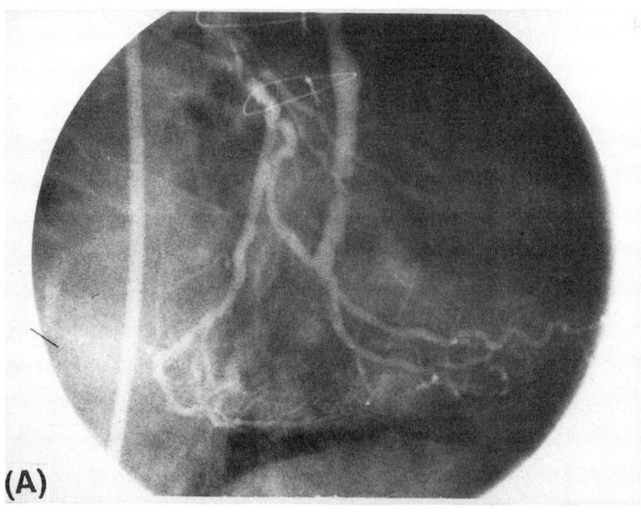

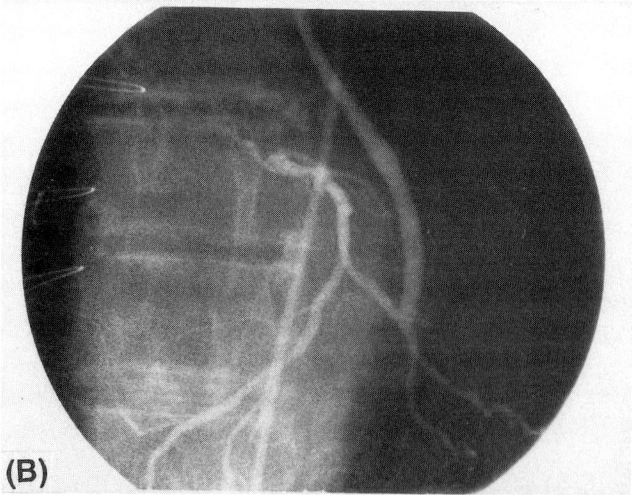

Figure 4 Pre- (A) and post- (B) JJIS coronary stent implantation with an excellent angiography result.

angiography at 6 months documented that late loss was greater in the stented group, but net gain overall remained greater in the stented group. A modest reduction in the combined endpoint of death, infarction, and need for repeat revascularization was seen in the stented group (26% vs. 38%, p = .05).

Despite early favorable results with this specific stent, the long-term follow-up of patients with vein graft disease remains of concern. With conventional PTCA, there is progressive deterioration, with adverse clinical events that continue to occur over time, in contrast to the treatment of native coronary arterial lesions, in which adverse events are usually limited to the first year [11]. Similarly, Sketch et al. [12] have reported on the long-term outcome of stent placement in saphenous vein bypass graft stenoses (Table 3). In the multicenter JJIS experience with clinical follow-up data on 661 consecutive patients with 775 lesions, there was progressive attrition. At 12 months, the incidence of event-free survival was 67%, but it fell to 55% at 2 years (Table 3). Piana et al. [8] documented a 14% mortality at 15.5 months in 150 patients being treated with either a Johnson & Johnson coronary or biliary stent, and Pomerantz et al. [2] documented a 10% mortality at 1 year in patients treated with a Johnson & Johnson coronary stent. Finally, deJaegere et al. [13] evaluated the long-term follow-up in 62 patients treated with stent implantation in vein grafts. The median age of the grafts was 7.7 years. Initial angiographic success was achieved in 98%; in hospital, however, nine major cardiac events occurred, thus only 89% of patients had a clinical success. During follow-up, adverse events were frequent. As can be seen in Figure 4, survival at 5 years was 83 ± 5%, whereas survival free of myocardial infarction was only 61 ± 6%.

II. JOHNSON & JOHNSON BILIARY STENT

There has been considerable interest in the Johnson & Johnson biliary stent for treatment of discrete vein graft stenoses [8,14,15]. This stent has the advantage that it is of variable size, from 4 to 9 mm, and thus can be used for the larger vein grafts. It also comes in variable lengths and configurations, from 10 mm to 40 mm. An articulated 20-mm stent is perhaps the most widely used (PS 204). In addition to variable lengths and sizes, this stent has the ability of being more radiodense than the coronary version.

These stents have been widely used (Figure 5), although there is only a modest amount of published data and no controlled randomized trials (Table 4). Most of the data on acute outcomes is available in abstract series, although some is in manuscript form. Wong et al. [14] reported a single-center experience of 188 biliary stents in 124 patients with 163 saphenous vein graft lesions. In 82.8%, a single stent was placed, usually a PS 204 (20-mm) design. Stent

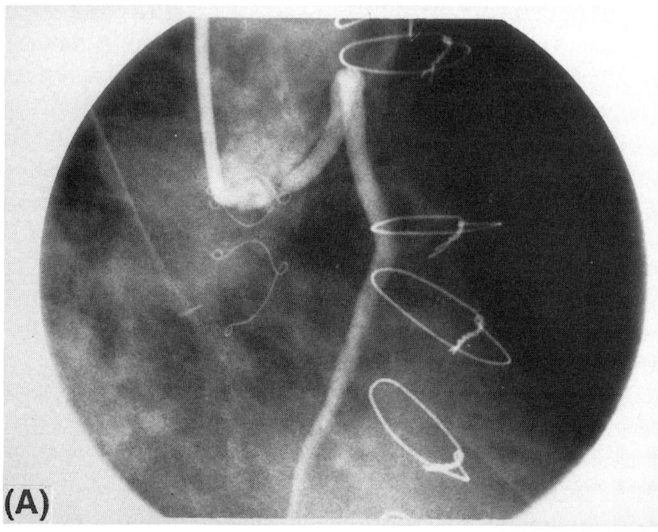

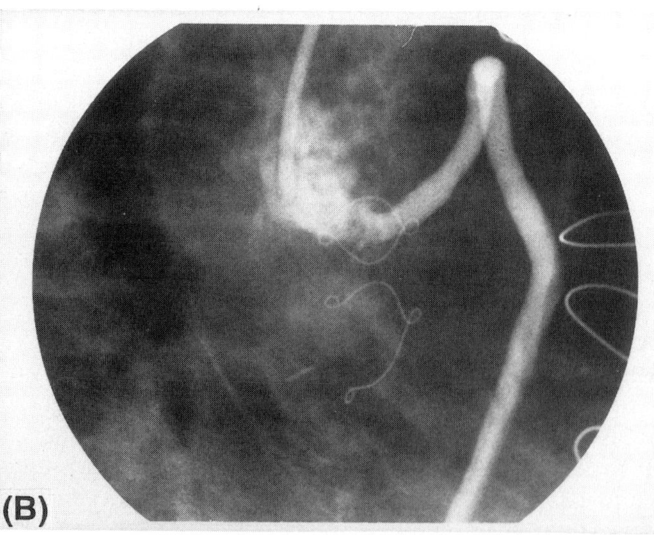

Figure 5　Right anterior oblique of vein graft to first obtuse marginal pre- (A) and postbiliary stent implantation (B).

Table 4 Late Clinical Follow-Up Multicenter JJIS Experience*

Event (%)	Actuarial follow-up events		
	6 Month	12 Month	24 Month
Death	5	8	14
Infarction	7	8	8
Coronary surgery	7	9	12
PTCA	6	8	12
Free of death, MI, CABG or PTCA	75	67	55

*661 patients, 775 vein graft lesions.
From Ref. 13.

implantation was successful in 161 of 163 lesions (98.8%) in 123 patients. Major complications were infrequent, being seen in only 2 (1.6%), and included death in 1 patient, emergency coronary bypass graft surgery in 1 patient, and non-Q-wave myocardial infarction in 13 patients (11%). No Q-wave myocardial infarctions were documented. Subacute thrombosis was seen in only 2 (1.7%). None of these complication rates were any different than those in 108 patients treated by these same authors for vein graft disease using the Johnson & Johnson coronary stent. Vascular complications were common, with vascular repair required in 10.1% and a transfusion in 27% of patients. These were probably affected by the intense antiplatelet/anticoagulant regimens utilized. At the present time, these intense regimens are no longer used.

These results are similar to those reported earlier by Piana et al. [8], who reported on stent placement in 208 (8.7 ± 4-year-old) saphenous vein bypass graft lesions with 146 coronary Johnson & Johnson stents and 54 biliary stents. In this group, the results of both stent types were analyzed together. Stent deployment was successful in 197 attempts (98.5%), with only one death and no Q-wave myocardial infarction or emergency surgery. As was true in the series by Wong et al. [13], non-Q-wave infarction rates were relatively high (7.3%), as were peripheral vascular complications, requiring surgery in 8.5% and transfusion alone in 14.0%.

There is limited longer-term follow-up of patients undergoing biliary stent implantation for vein graft disease. During a mean follow-up of 142 ± 75 days in 115 patients, Wong et al. [14] documented a 6-month event-free survival of 80%, with two deaths, one Q-wave myocardial infarction, four repeat surgical procedures (4%), and 12 repeat vein graft dilatations. Given the large size of these grafts with a final minimal luminal diameter of 3.18 ± 0.65 mm, and the known relationship between restenosis and final minimal luminal diameter, whether other devices would give comparable results remains to be determined.

Despite the advantages of the biliary stent, there are also major potential disadvantages, including the lack of a delivery system, the large size, and the need to hand-mount the stent on a peripheral balloon, with the potential for distal embolization. A delivery system can be fabricated using a 7 French straight delivery tube within a 9 French guiding catheter [16]. This can help, particularly for tortuous vein grafts or vein grafts that arise from the aorta with significant angulation, for example, the obtuse marginal vein grafts. If a delivery system is not used, the stent must be securely crimped on the delivery balloon—in general, hand-crimping is performed, although mechanical devices are available. The stent is positioned in the center of the balloon and crimped. Excessive force should be avoided, for it can rupture the balloon or damage the stent. After crimping, the stent should be secure enough that it will not migrate with gentle manual pressure. This decreases the likelihood that the stent will migrate on the balloon during delivery. During delivery of the stent, inflation of the balloon to 1/4 or 1/2 atmosphere decreases the chance of inadvertent movement of the stent.

III. DELIVERY PROBLEMS

During delivery, the rigid, inflexible stent may have trouble tracking around severe angulation. Gently curved guiding catheters with excellent support are extremely important. For the right coronary artery and left anterior descending, a multipurpose guiding catheter is excellent and probably the catheter of choice. For obtuse marginal or higher-arising grafts, Amplatz catheters may be required, although they are more angulated, with the potential for problems with deployment. If during attempts to pass the stent out of the guiding catheter the stent is seen to move proximally on the delivery balloon, the whole system should be withdrawn enbloc to prevent embolization. If movement is seen, a sheath system may be required. If after delivery of the stent to the vein graft the stent moves, attempts to withdraw it into the guiding catheter should be avoided, to prevent distal embolization. The stent may have to be deployed in the location where it is dislodged, which is usually proximal to the lesion. The target lesion may, therefore, need to be treated after this. If during balloon inflation the delivery balloon is found to be ruptured (usually related to excessive manual crimping), the stent can still be delivered using an angiographic power injector set to deliver 5 cc of 50% contrast at 20 cc/sec, with a maximum PSI of 400 [17]. With increasing experience, these problems become uncommon. Following stent implantation, high-pressure balloon inflation should be performed, although with large peripheral balloons, high pressures are limited.

IV. OTHER STENT DESIGNS

There is less information on other stent designs used for the treatment of vein graft disease (Table 2) [18–23].

A. Coiled Wire Stents

Wiktor Stent

The Wiktor stent has also been used to treat patients with saphenous vein bypass graft disease. The multicenter registry experience includes 101 patients [18]. In these patients, the stents were implanted for a number of different indications, including threatened closure (31%), acute closure (2%), and suboptimal result after PTCA (9%); in the remaining patients (51%), stent placement was elective. The procedural success rate in this mixed group of patients and lesions was 90%, and the residual final diameter stenosis was 12%. Despite the variable indications, complication patterns and rates were low—mortality 1%, Q-wave myocardial infarction 3%, and emergency coronary bypass graft surgery 1%. Subacute closure occurred in only 2% of patients. Intermediate-term follow-up in these patients documented a mortality of 6%, myocardial infarction in 2%, and target lesion revascularization in 10%.

Gianturco-Roubin

Dorros et al. [19] reported on the use of the original Gianturco-Roubin metallic coiled stent in 96 patients with 101 saphenous vein graft lesions. The mean age of the graft was 8.5 ± 1.8 years. The indication for treatment varied but was usually threatened closure (84%); in the remaining patients, abrupt closure was the indication. Therefore, these patients were at higher risk of subsequent events. In this selected group, procedural success was achieved in 96%. In-hospital complications included mortality in three (3%), Q-wave myocardial infarction in two (2%), and non-Q-wave myocardial infarction in six (6%). During the time in which these stents were placed, the typical anticoagulation regimen included dipyridamole, aspirin, dextran, and Coumadin. As has been documented with other series during this time, bleeding was a substantial issue and occurred in 22% of patients. Predismissal vein graft angiography was performed in 96% of eligible patients and confirmed stent and vein graft patency in 99%. From this experience it can be concluded that

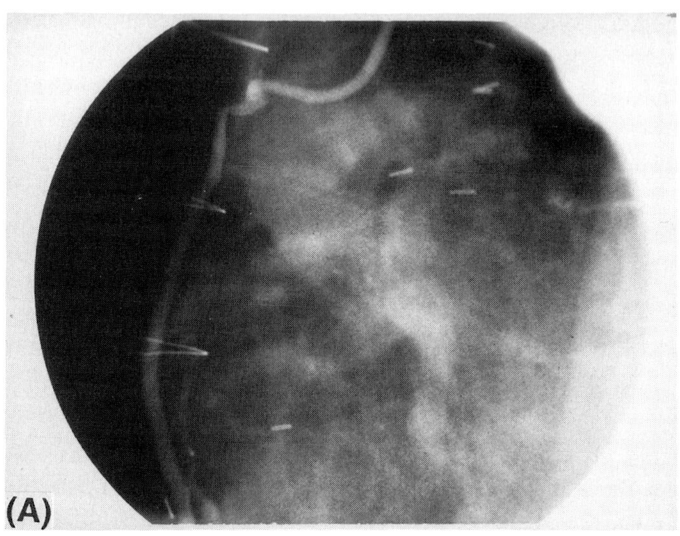

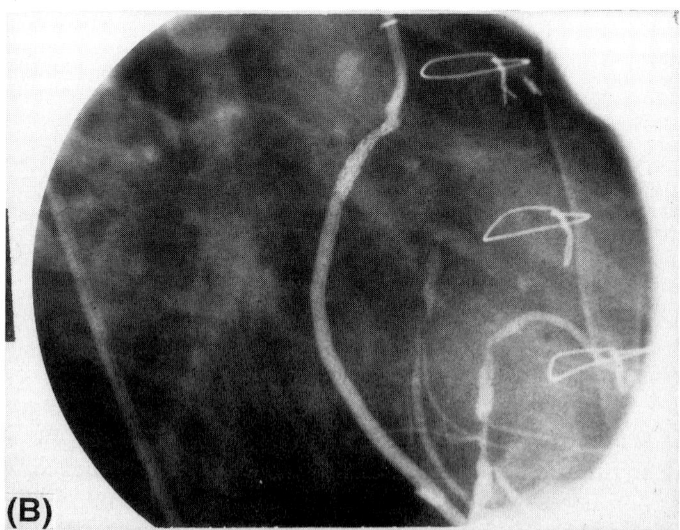

Figure 6 Left anterior oblique view of ostial stenosis of RCA vein graft (A). A Wiktor (TM) stent is implanted (B). During attempts at post dilatation, the stent is dislodged (C).

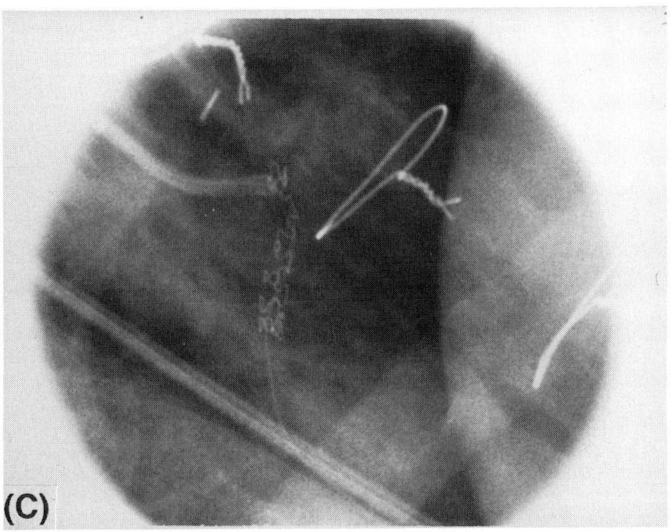

Figure 6 Continued

this particular stent design can be effectively used to treat acute or threatened closure of vein grafts following conventional PTCA.

Metallic wire coil stents have specific advantages. They are more flexible and can be positioned in tortuous vessels. This is facilitated by the lack of a delivery system, since these stents are crimped on a bare balloon. This is also a disadvantage in that the stents are fragile and can be deformed during placement or even embolized (Figure 6). In addition, recrossing these stents for postdeployment can damage the stent or displace it. Because of these problems, aortoostial lesions are not usually treated with these specific stent configurations. The other disadvantage is the specific design, which can allow friable tissue that is often present in degenerated vein grafts to prolapse between the coils. Newer iterations—for example, shorter-weave coils—may make these issues less problematic.

Self-Expanding Stents [20–23]

The self-expanding wire-mesh Wallstent has generated substantial interest for the treatment of saphenous vein graft disease because of its ability to seal off friable atheromatous plaque, which is the typical feature of degenerating vein grafts (Figures 7 and 8). Although this first stent used clinically has been used

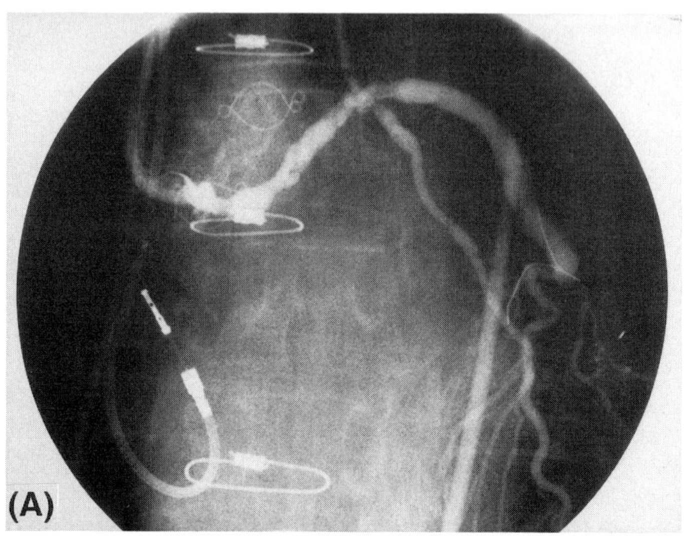

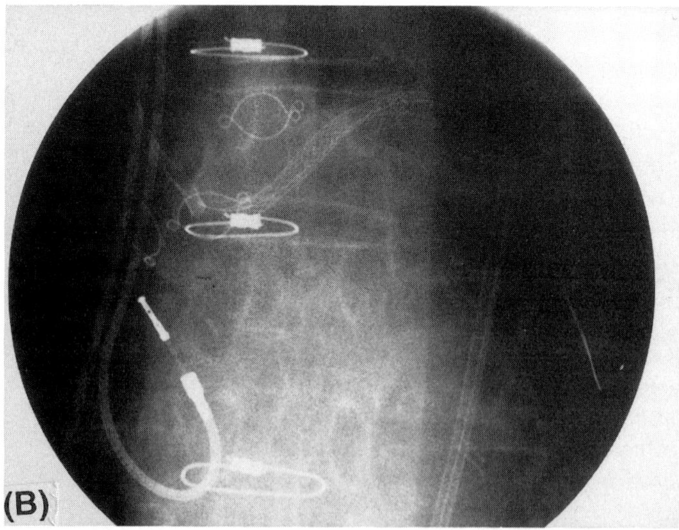

Figure 7 Implantation of Wallstent at the ostium of an old irregular vein graft (A). Stent deployment guided by the ring markers used for marking the grafts (B) then high pressure deployment (C). A residual filling defect remains.

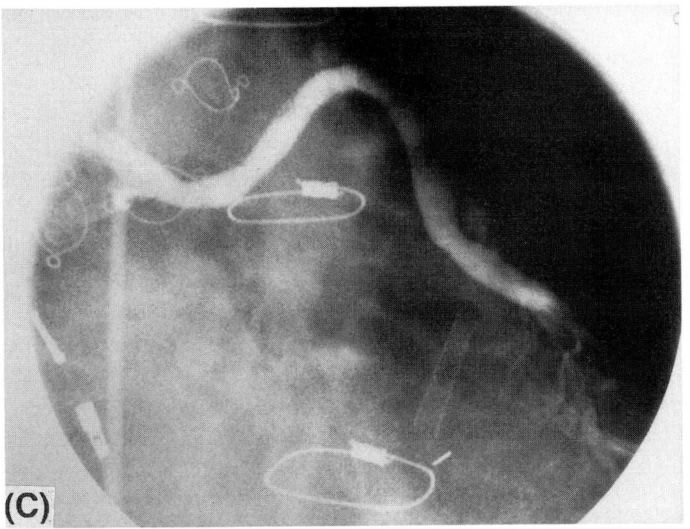

Figure 7 Continued

intermittently since 1986, there is still relatively limited published experience about either acute or long-term outcomes. It has recently become avaialble in the United States and is being evaluated in a multicenter randomized trial versus conventional PTCA. In the published series, success rates have been 100%. The largest published series includes 145 patients treated from 1986 to 1990 [22]. The majority of these stents were placed electively (92%), and most of the lesions were de novo (80%). The lesion characteristics were often unfavorable and included long lesions and degenerating vein grafts. Angiographic follow-up was available in 82% of patients and documented restenosis rates of 34%. In other, smaller series of patients, restenosis rates have ranged from 20% to 47%. Clinical follow-up at an average of 20 months documented a mortality of 9%.

This particular stent, with its variable length and size, is an attractive option for the treatment of saphenous vein graft disease. Implantation is easier in vein grafts than in native coronary arteries because side branches are usually not a problem unless the graft is sequential. For the treatment of ostial stenoses, this stent is more difficult to use because of its tendency for relatively

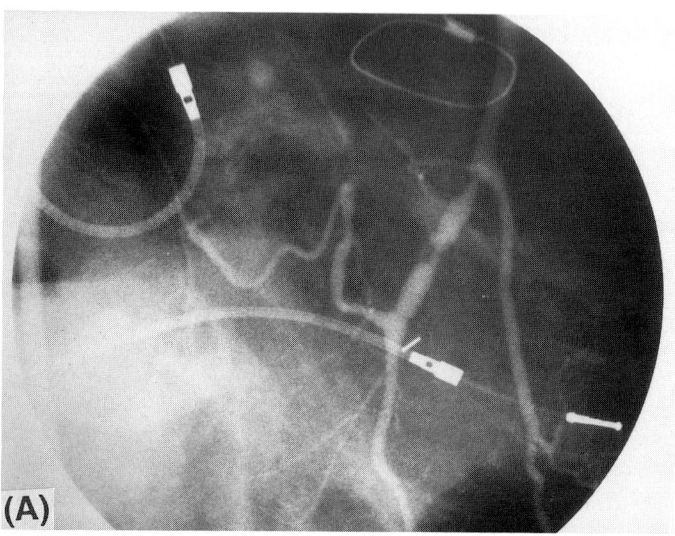

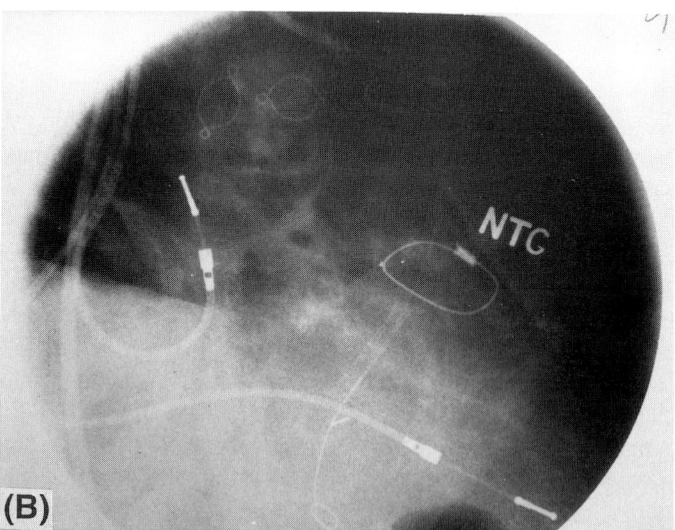

Figure 8 Right anterior oblique view of sequential vein graft to circumflex marginal. Prior to treatment there are tandem lesions (A). A Wallstent is implanted (B) and then post dilated giving an excellent result (C).

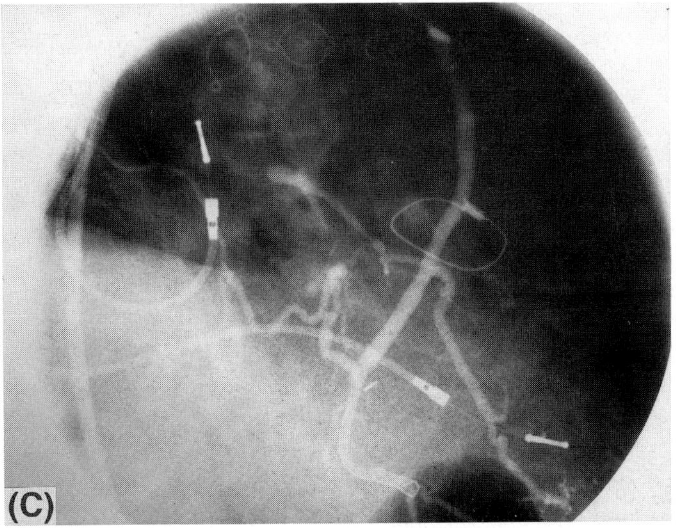

Figure 8 Continued

unpredictable shortening. More advanced iterations have improved this undesirable characteristic but have not eliminated it.

V. CONCLUSION

Stents for the treatment of vein graft disease are extremely promising and in many practices have become a treatment of choice. This change in practice is based primarily upon the results of observational series, not well-controlled scientific studies, although the latter are now being performed. The initial results of these prior studies were excellent, even in higher-risk patient subsets, and appear to be improved compared with conventional PTCA. These excellent initial results were obtained despite what we now believe to be suboptimal stent implantation—without high-pressure poststent deployment inflation, without intravascular ultrasound guidance, and with very intense anticoagulant regimens. This last circumstance is the cause of the high incidence of vascular complications, particularly bleeding, which has been documented in

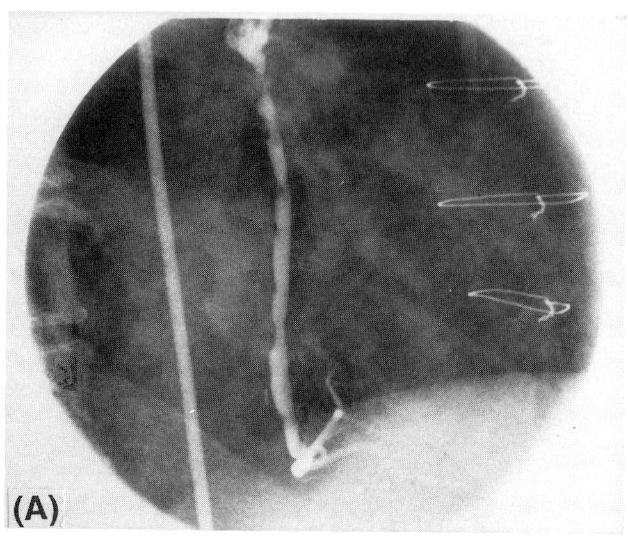

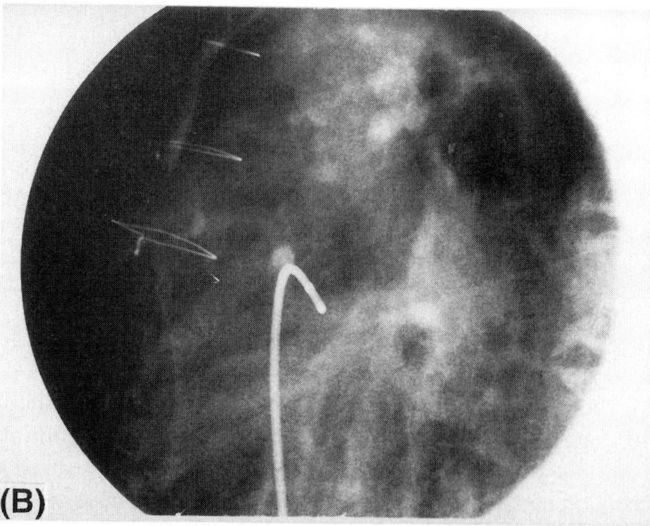

Figure 9 (A) Right oblique view of RCA vein graft with diffuse disease. (B) Following implantation of an ostial stent there is no reflow.

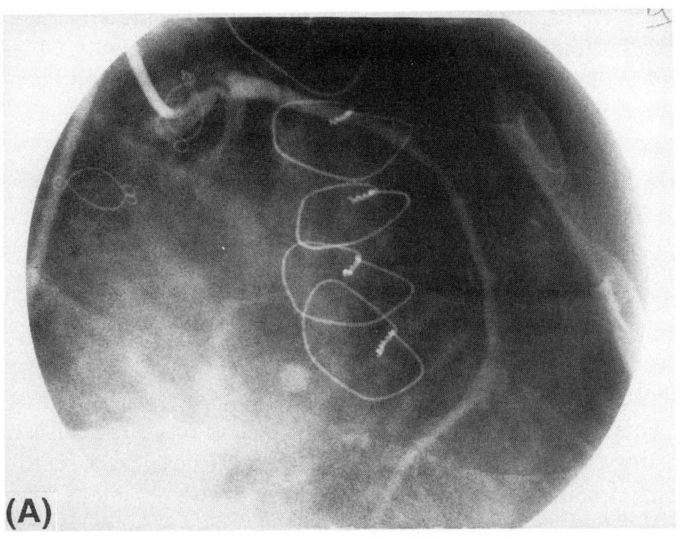

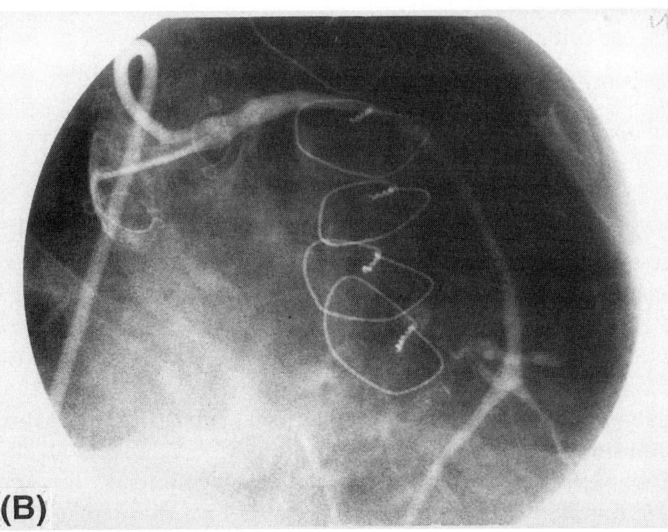

Figure 10 Pre- (A) and postbiliary stent implantation for an ostial stenosis. An articulation artifact is still present even after high pressure deployment (B).

the observational series. With the current use of aspirin and ticlopidine alone, these bleeding complications can be expected to decrease significantly. Subacute closure rates for the vein graft stent series have been very low and can be expected to remain low.

Despite these promising results, many questions remain unanswered. There are, however, several principles that apply to the treatment of vein graft disease.

1. Treatment of de novo lesions results in lower restenosis rates compared with the treatment of restenotic lesions. This finding has been true irrespective of which device has been used, i.e., conventional PTCA, directional coronary atherectomy, or stent. This has important implications for treatment selection; i.e., the initial device/treatment should be the optimal device/treatment, because it has the best chance to succeed in the long term.

2. Distal embolization rates are increased in the treatment of vein graft disease (Figure 9). This is particularly true with older vein grafts, more diffuse disease, and preexisting thrombus. This embolization may occur during predilatation, during stent implantation, or, less likely, during postdeployment dilatation. When embolization occurs, irrespective of the cause, adverse event rates are increased both acutely and in the long term. The increasingly widespread use of GP IIB/IIIA platelet receptor antagonists may be very important to prevent distal embolization.

3. Diffuse disease remains a problem because of the underlying pathophysiology. Long stents, particularly the Wallstent, may be more suitable for treatment in this setting. Covered stents have been described either using composite autologous veins or synthetic material. In the future, covered stents may become the treatment of choice.

4. Discrete isolated shaft/body lesions respond very favorably to slotted tubular designs. In some patients, delivery of these to the site may be difficult. They can also be treated with metallic coil stents, although coverage of friable material may be problematic.

5. Aorto-ostial lesions remain difficult to treat, due to recoil problems, the need for precise placement, and increased restenosis (Figure 10). Care should be taken to avoid having stents protrude into the aorta, because of the problem of reengagement or the potential concern for embolization. In this location, metallic coil stents are difficult to place and may be damaged during recrossing. Debulking of these lesions prior to stent implantation may be very effective. Slotted tubular stents are most commonly used for these anatomic situations [24].

6. For distal anastomotic lesions, stents may not be required, because the results of conventional PTCA are often excellent. If a stent is required, the taper between the vein graft and the distal vessel must be kept in mind. A coiled stent design that can be adapted to the taper or the self-expanding Wallstent may be the treatment of choice.

7. Subacute closure of vein grafts after stenting is uncommon [25]. This is currently being tested with the use of aspirin and ticlopidine in a randomized trial. It is anticipated that the results will remain very low because of the large size of these vessels.

8. Perhaps the most fundamental concern is the long-term follow-up of these patients. Published data to date document that there is continued attrition of these higher-risk patients [12,13]. Careful follow-up for identification of adverse events and prompt treatment, or hopefully, prevention of these adverse events will be required. Newer stent designs and newer approaches to vein graft disease may help obviate this concern.

REFERENCES

1. Wong SC, Baim DS, Schatz RA, Teirstein PS, King SB 3rd, Curry RC Jr, Heuser RR, Ellis SG, Cleman MW, Overlie P, Hirshfeld JW, Walker CM, Litvack F, Fish D, Brinker JA, Buchbinder M, Goldberg S, Chuang YC, Leon MB. Immediate results and late outcomes after stent implantation in saphenous vein graft lesions: the multicenter U.S.A. Palmaz-Schatz stent experience. J Am Coll Cardiol 1995; 26:704–712.
2. Pomerantz RM, Kuntz RE, Carrozza JP, Fishman RF, Mansour M, Schnitt SJ, Safian RD, Baim DS. Acute and long-term outcome of narrowed saphenous venous grafts treated by endoluminal stenting and directional atherectomy. Am J Cardiol 1992; 70:161–167.
3. Maiello L, Colombo A, Gianrossi R, Goldenberg S, Martini G, Finci L. Favourable results of treatment of narrowed saphenous vein grafts with Palmaz-Schatz stent implantation. Eur Heart J 1994; 15:1212–1216.
4. Wong SC, Popma JJ, Kent KM, Prichard AD, Satler LF, Mintz GS, Leon MB. Clinical experience with stent implantation in the treatment of saphenous vein graft lesions. J Inter Cardiol 1994; 7:565–573.
5. Strumpf RK, Mehta SS, Ponder R, Heuser RR. Palmaz-Schatz stent implantation in stenosed saphenous vein grafts: clinical and angiographic follow-up. Am Heart J 1992; 123:1329–1336.
6. Carrozza JP, Kuntz RE, Levine MJ, Pomerantz RM, Fishman RF, Mansour M, Gibson CM, Senerchia CC, Diver DJ, Safian RD, Baim DS. Angiographic and clinical outcome of intracoronary stenting: immediate and long-term results from a large single-center experience. J Am Coll Cardiol 1992; 20:328–337.
7. Fenton SH, Fischman DL, Savage MP, Schatz RA, Leon MB, Baim DS, King SB, Heuser RR, Curry RC Jr, Rake RC, Goldberg S. Long-term angiographic and clinical outcome after implantation of balloon-expandable stents in aortocoronary saphenous vein grafts. Am J Cardiol 1994; 74:1187–1191.
8. Piana RN, Moscucci M, Cohen DJ, Kugelmass AD, Senerchia C, Kuntz RE, Baim DS, Carrozza JP Jr. Palmaz-Schatz stenting for treatment of focal vein graft stenosis: immediate results and long-term outcome. J Am Coll Cardiol 1994; 23: 1296–1304.

9. Bremer SJ, Ellis SG, Apperson-Hansen C, et al. Comparison of stenting and balloon angioplasty for narrowings in aortocoronary saphenous vein conduits in place for more than five years. Am J Cardiol 1997; 79:13–18.

10. Douglas JS, Savage MP, Bailey ST, et al. Randomized trial of coronary stent and balloon angioplasty in the treatment of saphenous vein graft stenosis. J Am Coll Cardiol 1996. In press.

11. Rabbani RR, Bell MR, Grill DE, Simari RD, Holmes DR Jr. Clinical follow-up after successful percutaneous coronary angioplasty of saphenous vein graft disease and the importance of long-term assessment. Mayo Clin Proc. In press.

12. Sketch MH, Wong SC, Chuang YC, Phillips HR, Heuser R, Savage M, Stack RS, Baim DS, Schatz RA, Leon MB. Progressive deterioration in late (2-year) clinical outcomes after stent implantation in saphenous vein grafts: the multicenter JJIS experience. J Am Coll Cardiol 1995; 25:79. (Abstract)

13. de Jaegere PP, Van Domberg RT, de Feyter PJ, Ruygrok PM, van der Giessen WJ, van den Brand MJ, Serruys PW. Long-term clinical outcome after stent implantation in saphenous vein grafts. J Am Coll Cardiol 1996; 28:89–97.

14. Wong SC, Popma JJ, Pichard AD, Kent KM, Satler LF, Mintz GS, Chuang YC, Hong MK, Ditrano CJ, Leon MB. Comparison of clinical and angiographic outcomes after saphenous vein graft angioplasty using coronary versus "biliary" tubular slotted stents. Circulation 1995; 91:339–350.

15. White CJ, Ramee SR, Collins TJ, Escobar A, Jain SP. Placement of biliary stents in saphenous vein coronary bypass grafts. Cathet Cardiovasc Diagn 1993; 30:91–95.

16. Nunez BD, Simari RD, Keelan ET, Menke KK, Garratt KN, Holmes DR Jr. A novel approach to the placement of Palmaz-Schatz biliary stents in saphenous vein grafts. Cathet Cardiovasc Diagn 1995; 35:350–353.

17. Keelan ET, Nunez BD, Berger PB, Holmes DR Jr, Garratt KM. Management of balloon rupture during rigid stent deployment. Cathet Cardiovasc Diagn 1995; 35:211–215.

18. Fortuna R, Heuser RR, Garratt KN, Schwartz R, Buchbinder M. Wiktor intracoronary stent: experience in the first 101 graft patients (abstr). Circulation 1993; 88(suppl I):309.

19. Dorros G, Bates MC, Iyer S, Kumar K, King JF, Palmer L, Dufek C, Mathiak L. The use of Gianturco-Roubin flexible metallic coronary stents in old saphenous vein grafts: in-hospital outcome and 7-day angiographic patency. Eur Heart J 1994; 15:1456–1462.

20. Urban P, Sigwart U, Golf S, Kaufmann U, Sadeghi H, Kappenberger L. Intravascular stenting for stenosis of aortocoronary venous bypass grafts. J Am Coll Cardiol 1989; 13:1085–1091.

21. de Scheerder IK, Strauss BH, de Feyter PJ, Beatt KJ, Baur LH, Wijns W, Heydrix GR, Suryapranata H, van den Brand M, Buis B, Serruys PW. Stenting of venous bypass grafts: a new treatment modality of patients who are poor candidates for reintervention. Am Heart J 1992; 123:1046–1054.

22. Strauss BH, Serruys PW, Bertrand ME, Puel J, Meier B, Goy JJ, Kappenberger L, Rickards AF, Sigwart U. Qualitative angiographic follow-up of the coronary Wallstent in native vessel and bypass grafts. Am J Cardiol 1992; 69:475–481.

23. Eeckhout E, Goy JJ, Stauffer JC, Vogt P, Kappenberger L. Endoluminal stenting of narrowed saphenous vein grafts: long-term clinical and angiographic follow-up. Cathet Cardiovasc Diagn 1994; 32:139–146.
24. Nordrehaug JE, Priestley K, Chronos N, Buller N, Sigwart U. Implantation of half Palmaz-Schatz stents in short aorto-ostial lesions of saphenous vein grafts. Cathet Cardiovasc Diagn 1993; 29:141–143.
25. Itoh A, Hall P, Maiello L. Intracoronary stent implantation in native coronary arteries and saphenous vein grafts. A consecutive experience with six types of stents without prolonged anticoagulation. Cathet Cardiovasc Diagn.

12
Excimer Laser Angioplasty for Saphenous Vein Graft Lesions

John A. Bittl*
*Brigham and Women's Hospital, and Harvard Medical School,
Boston, Massachusetts*

Although excimer laser angioplasty has been advocated for several types of complex lesions in native coronary arteries [1,2], this treatment has the unique trait among interventional devices of achieving higher success rates in saphenous vein grafts than in native vessels [3,4]. In spite of its unique capability for saphenous vein graft lesions, excimer laser angioplasty is not widely endorsed as a first-line device for this indication because of concerns about embolization or inadequate dilation. Recent studies suggest [3,4], however, that the risk of embolization with excimer laser angioplasty in saphenous vein grafts is very low and, though restenosis rates after adjunctive balloon angioplasty alone may be higher than ideal [5,6], adjunctive therapy after excimer treatment with directional atherectomy or stenting may result in more favorable long-term outcome [7,8]. This chapter reviews the subject of excimer laser angioplasty for saphenous vein graft lesions, presents an analysis of predictors of clinical outcome, and discusses the importance of adjunctive interventional therapies.

I. EXCIMER LASER ANGIOPLASTY

The technology of excimer lasers is based on the formation and dissociation of an excited dimer ("excimer") of xenon chloride, which emits energy at a wavelength of 308 nm in the ultraviolet portion of the electromagnetic

---

**Current affiliation*: Ocala Heart Institute, Ocala, Florida.

spectrum. Atherosclerotic plaque is vaporized by laser light at 308 nm at a threshold energy density (fluence) of approximately 30 mJ/mm^2 [9]. Each pulse at this fluence produces a crater about 40 μm deep. Thus, 25 pulses delivered over 1 second will ablate approximately 1.0 mm of atherosclerotic plaque.

The catheters for excimer laser angioplasty are available in diameters ranging from 1.3 to 2.0 mm, carry a lumen for guide wire positioning, and contain either a concentric or an eccentric densely packed array of 50–61-μm optical fibers. Although three XeCl excimer laser systems have been developed for angioplasty, only the Spectranetics–Advanced Interventional Systems are available for clinical use at the current time.

II. COMPARISON WITH NATIVE VESSEL ANGIOPLASTY

A. Clinical Success

Since 1989, several efforts have been made to use excimer laser angioplasty to treat lesions in saphenous vein grafts [10]. Recent studies have shown that clinical success with excimer laser angioplasty can be achieved in 90–94% of patients with saphenous vein grafts lesions, where clinical success is defined as less than 50% residual stenosis and absence of major in-hospital complications [2,4]. The success rate for lesions in saphenous vein grafts is significantly higher than that for lesions in native vessels (odds ratio [OR] = 2.0 [95% confidence interval 1.0, 5.5; P = .05]) [4].

B. Vessel Dissection

A limitation of excimer laser angioplasty for native vessel disease is the incidence of vessel dissection, which occurs in as many as 20% of patients [2,3, 11–13]. While most of these dissections are not flow limiting, major ischemic complications or flow impairment occur in about 5% of patients [2,3,11,12]. Fortunately, saphenous vein graft lesions are associated with a lower risk of dissection than lesions in native vessels (OR = 0.3 [0.1, 0.8], P = .01) [13].

C. Perforation

Vessel perforation occurs during excimer laser angioplasty in 1–2% of patients [12,14–16]. A detailed analysis of predictors of vessel perforation has revealed that saphenous vein graft lesions are associated with a trend toward lower rates of perforation than are lesions in native vessels (OR = 0.5 [0.1, 1.2]; P = .30) [14].

D. Restenosis

Although excimer laser angioplasty was initially developed to reduce restenosis by ablating atheromatous plaque without injuring the normal components of the arterial wall, lesion recurrence has been reported in approximately 50% of patients [17]. In an early study involving 200 patients undergoing excimer laser angioplasty for lesions in native coronary vessels and in saphenous vein grafts with a clinical follow-up rate of 99% and an angiographic follow-up rate of 83%, the incidence of clinical restenosis (recurrence of angina, positive exercise treadmill test, myocardial infarction, or the need for repeat revascularization) was 31%, and the overall 6-month incidence of angiographic restenosis was 47% [3]. In the subgroup of 15 patients with saphenous vein graft lesions, the angiographic restenosis rate of 20% was significantly lower than that for patients with native vessel disease [3]. An explanation for this finding was identified later in a formal geometric analysis of lumen narrowing, which defined the relation between vessel diameter and the likelihood of restenosis and suggested that larger vessels such as bypass grafts were less likely than smaller vessels to be associated with angiographic evidence of lumen narrowing at 6 months [17]. In the larger Percutaneous Excimer Laser Coronary Angioplasty Registry, the incidence of clinical restenosis was 46% [4]. Multivariable predictors of restenosis were lesion length $\geq$10 mm and stand-alone laser angioplasty (i.e., laser without adjunctive balloon angioplasty).

III. PREDICTORS OF OUTCOME FOR SAPHENOUS VEIN GRAFT LESIONS

In a series of 495 patients with saphenous vein graft lesions treated with excimer laser angioplasty, the clinical success rates ranged from 84% to 96% and were influenced by several clinical and angiographic variables (Figure 1) [4]. Patients with ostial lesions or lesions in the body of smaller saphenous vein grafts had superior success rates. The incidence of major complications in the cohort of 495 patients included death in 1.0%, emergency bypass surgery in 0.6%, and Q-wave myocardial infarction in 2.4%. Angiographic complications included embolization in 3.3%, perforations in 1.3%, and dissections in 8.8% [6]. The low rate of embolization was striking in view of the degree of degeneration involving several of the grafts in this series (Figure 2). A lower incidence of complications was seen for ostial lesions than for lesions in the body of the saphenous vein graft, for discrete lesions than for long lesions, and for lesions in vein grafts less than 3.0 mm in diameter than for lesions in large grafts (Figure 3). The overall angiographic restenosis rate for saphenous vein

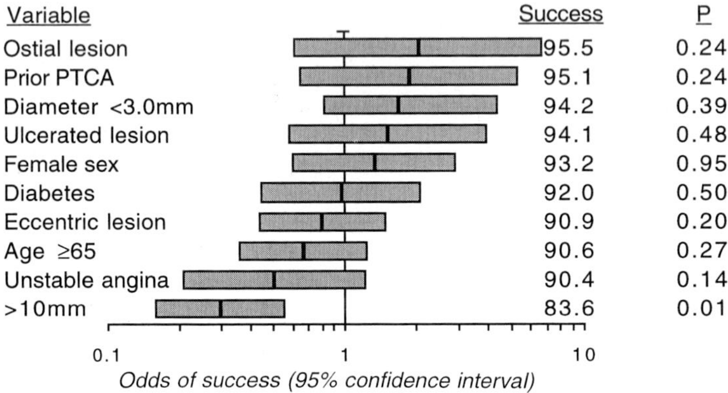

Figure 1 Predictors of success for excimer laser angioplasty of saphenous vein graft lesions: The likelihood of clinical success for a series of variables is given by the raw success rates, odds ratios, and univariable *P* values obtained by logistic regression analysis. The statistical reliability of the odds ratio is given by the 95% confidence intervals. Diameter <3.0 mm refers to graft reference diameter, and >10 mm denotes lesion length greater than 10 mm. (Adapted with permission from Ref. 4.)

graft lesions was approximately 55%, but was lower for discrete lesions in saphenous vein grafts greater than 3.0 mm in diameter (Figure 4).

Other studies have suggested that certain types of lesions in saphenous vein grafts should not be treated with excimer laser angioplasty. The presence of filling defects in saphenous vein grafts significantly reduces the success rate after excimer laser angioplasty and increases the risk of embolization and myocardial infarction (Figure 5) [18]. Thus, angiographic evidence of a large amount of thrombus in saphenous vein grafts should be considered a relative contraindication to excimer laser angioplasty.

IV. TECHNIQUES FOR SAPHENOUS VEIN GRAFT LESIONS

A. Guiding Catheters

Conventional guiding catheters can be used for excimer laser angioplasty of saphenous vein graft lesions. Coaxial alignment is important but not critical, because firm guide support is generally not needed to advance the activated laser catheter through the relatively soft lesion within a saphenous vein graft.

For excimer laser angioplasty of lesions lying within left-sided saphenous vein bypass grafts, left bypass guides or hockey stick–shaped guides are useful. For left saphenous vein graft bypass grafts with a severe initial upward course,

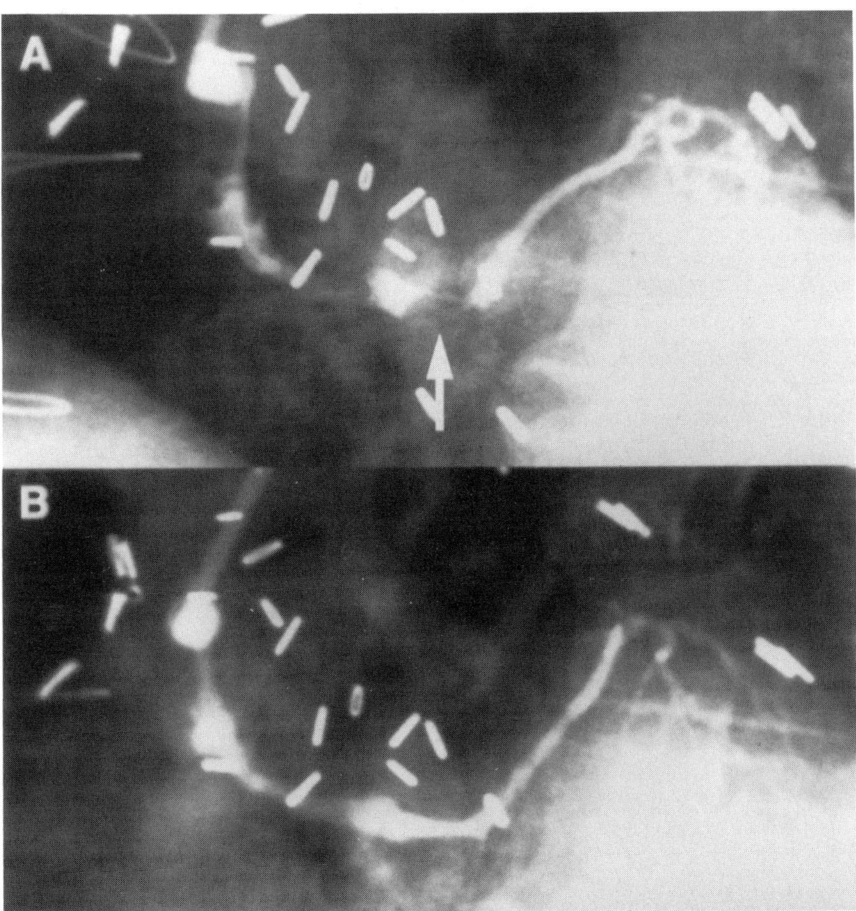

Figure 2 Excimer laser and adjunctive balloon angioplasty: An 82-year-old man presented with unstable angina associated with anterior ST depression and a subtotal occlusion (A, arrow) within the distal portion of a degenerated bypass graft to the left anterior descending artery. A 1.7-mm laser catheter was advanced through the lesion, followed by balloon dilatation with a 2.5-mm balloon, leaving an adequate residual lumen (B) and providing complete relief of chest pain without clinical, angiographic, or enzymatic evidence of distal embolization.

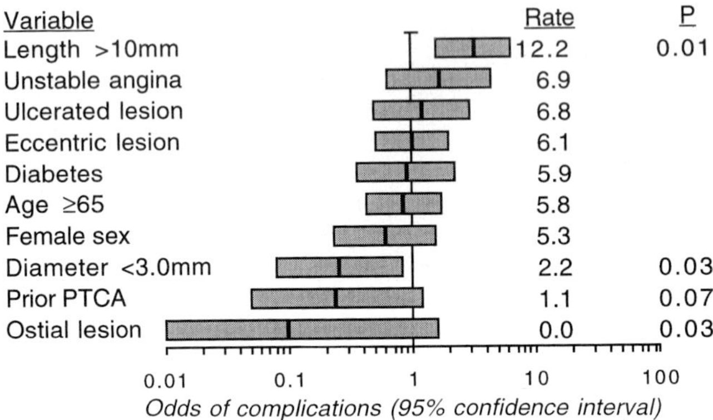

Figure 3 Predictors of major complications from excimer laser angioplasty for saphenous vein graft lesions: The likelihood of death, myocardial infarction, or urgent bypass surgery for a series of variables is given by the raw complication rates, odds ratios, and multivariable *P* values obtained by logistic regression analysis. The statistical reliability of the odds ratios is given by the 95% confidence intervals ($P < 0.05$ by univariate analysis if the confidence interval does not intersect the value 1.0). Diameter <3.0 mm refers to graft reference diameter, and length >10 mm denotes lesion length greater than 10 mm. (Adapted with permission from Ref. 4.)

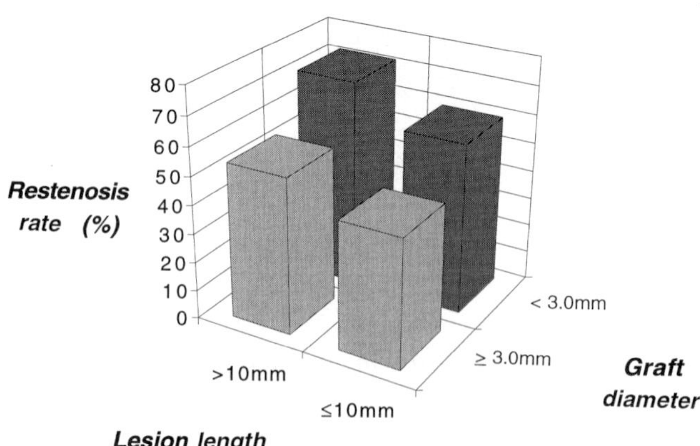

Figure 4 Predictors of restenosis: Restenosis rates are presented as a function of both lesion length and graft diameter. (Adapted with permission from Ref. 4.)

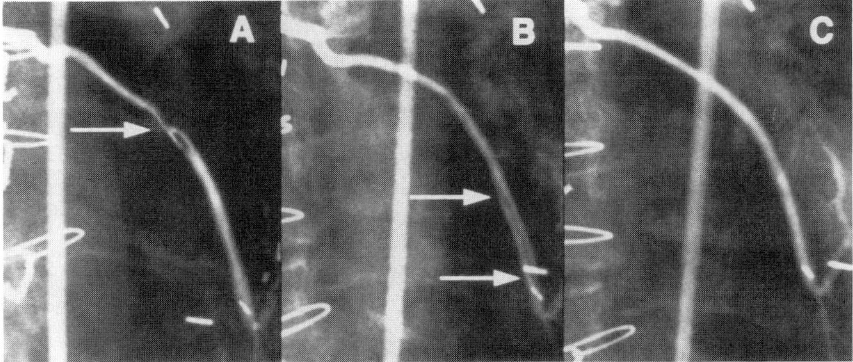

Figure 5 Filling defects and risk of embolization: This 56-year-old woman presented with unstable angina associated with a complex lesion with filling defects (A, arrow) in a small saphenous vein graft supplying the left anterior descending artery. After successful laser passage, adjunctive balloon angioplasty resulted in embolization of a large linear filling defect (B, arrows) that was successfully treated with intragraft urokinase and repeat balloon inflations (C).

internal mammary guides can provide ideal coaxial alignment (Figure 6). For left saphenous vein bypass grafts with an initial horizontal or downward course, left or right Amplatz or right Judkins guides are useful. For right saphenous vein bypass grafts with a downward course, either a multipurpose guide, right Judkins guide, or right Amplatz guide can be used.

Seven French guide catheters may be used for smaller 1.3 or 1.4 mm laser catheters, while 8 Fr. guide catheters are required for 1.6- or 1.7-mm laser catheters, and 9 Fr. guide catheters are required for 2.0-mm laser catheters.

B. Laser Catheters

To maximize the likelihood of a safe outcome and reduce the risk of vessel perforation with excimer laser angioplasty, it is important to select a laser catheter with a diameter smaller than the reference diameter of the target vessel. The laser catheter should be at least 1.0 mm smaller than the reference diameter of the vessel [14], to allow for a 1.0-mm "margin of safety." An alternative scheme for sizing the laser catheter is to use the "rule of two-thirds"; that is, the size of the laser catheter should be no bigger than two-thirds that of the reference diameter of the target vessel [15]. Both approaches would suggest that the 2.0-mm laser catheter would be appropriately sized for treating lesions in 3.0-mm saphenous vein grafts. Currently, it is recommended to limit ablation to one pass of a laser catheter per lesions.

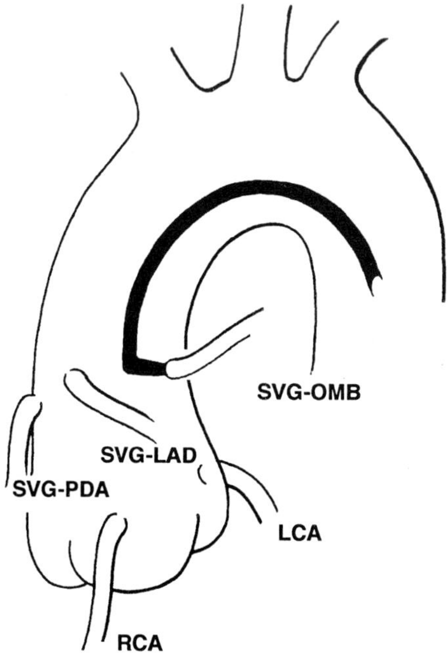

Figure 6 Guiding catheter selection for saphenous vein bypass grafts: Bypass grafts anastomosing to the obtuse marginal branches (SVG-OMG) are characteristically the most leftward and superior of the grafts and often have an initial upward course, for which the internal mammary guiding catheter frequently provides ideal coaxial alignment. (Figure modified from Ref. 23 by permission from McGraw-Hill Book Co.)

C. Guide Wires

For the 1.6- and 2.0-mm catheters, guide wires up to 0.018-in. diameter can be used. For the 1.3- and 1.4-mm laser catheters, an 0.014-in. guide wire is required, although an extra support wire may help in cases involving proximal vessel tortuosity.

D. Laser Technique

After the target lesion is crossed with the guide wire, the laser catheter is advanced to lie at the proximal end of the lesion. This catheter position should be documented on cine. Before activating the laser and beginning ablation of the lesion, every effort must be made to first remove all contrast medium from the target vessel by flushing the guide catheter with at least 30 mL of saline. During advancement of the laser catheter, saline should be flushed continuously through the guide catheter at a rate of 1–2 mL/sec. This is important, because the interaction between excimer laser radiation and retained contrast medium or blood may increase the generation of shock waves, with disruption of adjacent tissue planes [19,20].

During pulsed excimer laser angioplasty, laser energy is delivered at a fluence of 40–70 mJ/mm^2 at a frequency of 20–25 Hz for a duration of 1–5 seconds as the end of the catheter is advanced through the lesion. For soft lesions such as saphenous vein graft lesions, laser ablation may commence at a fluence of 40 mJ/mm^2. As the laser is activated, the catheter is advanced slowly under fluoroscopic guidance through the lesion at an average rate of 0.5–1.0 mm/sec. Faster rates of advancement may exceed the rate (40 μm per pulse) at which excimer laser irradiation can ablate atheromatous plaque [9]. After each train of laser pulses lasting 1–5 seconds, the laser catheter should not be activated for 10 seconds, to allow reversal of potential attenuation of energy transmission through the optical fibers. If the laser catheter meets resistance and cannot pass through the lesion at the initial fluence, the energy output should be increased by increments of 10mJ/mm^2 to a maximum of 60 or 70 mJ/mm^2. Once the laser catheter has been advanced completely through the stenotic segment, adjunctive posttreatment will be required in about 95% of laser angioplasty procedures, to reduce the residual stenosis below 10% (see later) [2,4].

E. Management of Complications

If dissection occurs, it should be managed like dissection after balloon angioplasty, using either prolonged perfusion balloon inflation, coronary stenting, or salvage directional atherectomy. If perforation occurs, a perfusion balloon catheter should be advanced over the guide wire and inflated at the perforation site to seal the leak in the vessel. In many cases, small perforations that present as localized contrast extravasation can be usccessfully treated with prolonged balloon inflation alone. A free perforation communicating with the mediastinal space that does not seal with prolonged balloon inflation alone may do so after reversal of anticoagulation; otherwise, emergency bypass surgery with oversewing of the perforation site is indicated.

F. Ostial Lesions

Because of the likelihood of elastic recoil after balloon dilatation of ostial lesions alone, these stenoses often require an ablative therapy such as excimer laser angioplasty for successful outcome (Figure 7). In a total of 65 patients

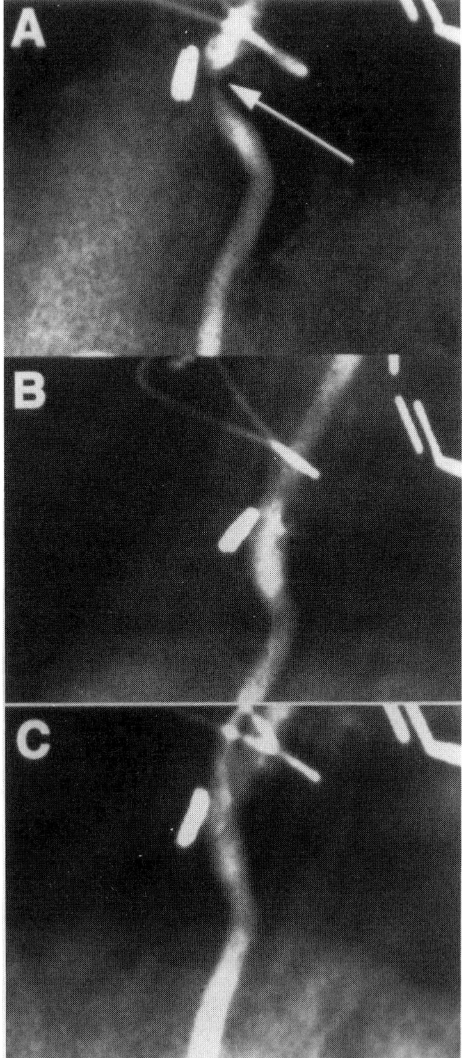

Figure 7   Excimer laser and adjunctive directional atherectomy: A 58-year-old woman developed gradually worsening angina 8 years after bypass surgery associated with an ostial lesion in the saphenous vein graft to the posterior descending artery (A). After treatment with the 2-mm laser catheter, improvement was seen (B). Adjunctive directional atherectomy resulted in less than 0% residual stenosis (C).

with ostial stenoses treated with excimer laser angioplasty, angiographic success was achieved in 62 (95%) [6]. No patient died or experienced myocardial infarction or urgent bypass surgery (Fig. 2). The success of excimer laser angioplasty for ostial vein graft stenoses is ensured by attention to coaxial alignment of guiding catheters.

G. Anastomotic Lesions

Lesions at the anastomotic site involving the connection between saphenous vein grafts and native coronary vessels inherently involved angulation and are very amenable to balloon angioplasty [21,22]. Excimer laser angioplasty is not generally recommended for angulated anastomotic lesions.

H. Adjunctive Therapy

For most lesions in grafts >3.0 mm in diameter, adjunctive balloon dilatation is recommended to achieve a successful result. The balloon should be selected to match the reference diameter of the graft. For lesions in grafts >2.75 mm in diameter, adjunctive atherectomy may be used to achieve an ideal result (Figure 7). If this is planned, it is important to use a 10 Fr femoral sheath and the appropriate 10 Fr guide catheter. Because excimer laser angioplasty is associated with a low rate of embolization and no reflow, this is an ideal pretreatment method for graft stenting (Figure 8). In addition, excimer laser angioplasty can be used successfully to treat in-stent restenosis.

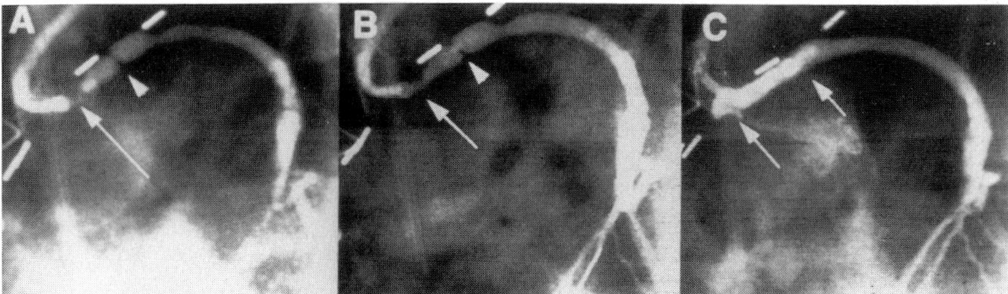

Figure 8 Excimer laser and adjunctive stenting. This 52-year-old gentleman developed unstable angina associated with anterior ST-segment changes and a complex lesion (A, arrows) in a large graft to the left anterior descending artery. After passage of a 2-mm laser catheter without any clinical or angiographic evidence of embolization, the site is improved (B). Placement of two tandem Palmaz-Schatz stents resulted in no residual stenosis (C).

V. CONCLUSION

The superior success of excimer laser angioplasty for lesions in saphenous vein grafts, as compared with that for lesions in native vessels, is explained by the reduced likelihood of vessel dissection, perforation, and major complications. The problem of restenosis continues to limit the usefulness of excimer laser angioplasty and adjunctive balloon angioplasty, but the use of excimer laser angioplasty along with stenting or directional atherectomy is a promising combination of therapies associated with low risk of embolization and reduced potential for restenosis.

REFERENCES

1. Cook SL, Eigler NL, Shefer A, Goldenberg T, Forrester JS, Litvack F. Percutaneous excimer laser coronary angioplasty of lesions not ideal for balloon angioplasty. Circulation 1991; 84:632–643.
2. Litvack F, Eigler N, Margolis J, Rothbaum D, Bresnahan JF, Holmes D, Untereker W, Leon M, Kent K, Pichard A, King S, Ghazzal Z, Cummins F, Krauthamer D, Palacios I, Block P, Hartzler GO, O'Neill W, Cowley W, Roubin G, Klein LW, Frankel PS, Adams C, Goldenberg T, Laudenslager J, Grundfest W, Forrester JS. Percutaneous excimer laser coronary angioplasty: results in the first consecutive 3,000 patients. J Am Coll Cardiol 1994; 23:323–329.
3. Bittl JA, Sanborn TA. Excimer laser-facilitated coronary angioplasty: relative risk analysis of acute and follow-up results in 200 patients. Circulation 1992; 86:71–80.
4. Bittl JA, Sanborn TA, Tcheng JE, Siegel RM, Ellis SG. Clinical success, complications and restenosis rates with excimer laser coronary angioplasty. Am J Cardiol 1992; 70:1533–1539.
5. Strauss BH, Natarajan MK, Yardley DE, Bittl JA, Batchelor WB, Sanborn TA, Power JA, Watson LE, Moothart R, Tcheng JE, Chishold RJ. Early and late quantitative angiographic results of vein graft lesions treated with excimer laser angioplasty. Circulation 1995; 92:348–356.
6. Bittl JA, Sanborn TA, Yardley DE, Tcheng JE, Isner JM, Chokshi SK, Strauss BH, Abela GS, Walter PD, Schmidhofer M, Power JA. Predictors of outcome of percutaneous excimer laser coronary angioplasty of saphenous vein bypass graft lesions. Am J Cardiol 1994; 74:144–148.
7. Holmes DR Jr, Topol EJ, Califf RM, Berdan LG, Leya F, Berger PB, Whitlow PL, Safian RD, Adelman AG, Kellett MJ, et al. A multicenter, randomized trial of coronary angioplasty versus directional atherectomy for patients with saphenous vein bypass graft lesions. CAVEAT-II Investigators. Circulation 1995; 91:1966–1974.
8. Piana RN, Moscucci M, Cohen DJ, Kuglemass AD, Snerchia C, Kuntz RE, Baim DS, Carrozza JP Jr. Palmaz-Schatz stenting for treatment of focal vein graft stenosis: immediate results and long-term outcome. J Am Coll Cardiol 1994; 23:1296–1304.
9. Grundfest WS, Litvack F, Forrester JS, Goldenberg T, Swan HJC, Morgenstern L, Fishbein M, McDermid JS, Rider DM, Pacala TJ. Laser ablation of human

atherosclerotic plaque without adjacent tissue injury. J Am Coll Cardiol 1985; 5:929–933.

10. Litvack F, Grundfest WS, Goldenberg T, Laudenslager J, Forrester JS. Percutaneous excimer laser angioplasty of aortocoronary saphenous vein grafts. J Am Coll Cardiol 1989; 14:803–808.

11. Bittl JA, Brinker JA, Isner JM, Sanborn TA, Tcheng JE. The changing profile of patient selection, techniques, and outcomes in excimer laser angioplasty. J Intervent Cardiol 1995; 8:653–660.

12. Baumbach A, Bittl JA, Fleck E, Geschwind HJ, Sanborn TA, Tcheng JE, Karsch KR. Acute complications of coronary excimer laser angioplasty: analysis of two multicenter registries. J Am Coll Cardiol 1994; 23:1305–1313.

13. Bittl JA, Estella P, Abela GS. Complications of laser coronary angioplasty. In: Lutz J, ed. Complications of Interventional Procedures. New York: Igaku-Shoin, 1995: 186–207.

14. Bittl JA, Ryan TJ Jr, Keaney JF Jr, Tcheng JE, Ellis SE, Isner JM, Sanborn TA. Coronary artery perforation during excimer laser coronary angioplasty. Journal name here 1993; 21:1158–1165.

15. Holmes DR Jr, Reeder GS, Ghazzal ZMB, Bresnahan JR, King SB III, Leon MB, Litvack F. Coronary perforation after excimer laser coronary angioplasty: the Excimer Laser Coronary Angioplasty Registry Experience. J Am Coll Cardiol 1994; 23:330–335.

16. Parker JD, Ganz P, Selwyn AP, Bittl JA. Successful treatment of an excimer laser-associated coronary artery perforation with the Stack perfusion catheter. Cath Cardiovasc Diagn 1991; 22:118–123.

17. Bittl JA, Kuntz RE, Estella P, Sanborn TA, Baim DS. Analysis of luminal narrowing after excimer laser coronary angioplasty. J Am Coll Cardiol 1994; 23:1314–1320.

18. Estella P, Ryan TJ Jr, Landzberg JS, Bittl JA. Excimer laser-assisted angioplasty for lesions containing thrombus. J Am Coll Cardiol 1993; 21:1550–1556.

19. Deckelbaum LI, Strauss BH, Bittl JA, Rohlfs K, Scott J. Effect of intracoronary saline on dissection during excimer laser angioplasty: a randomized trial. J Am Coll Cardiol 1995; 26:1264–1269.

20. Tcheng JE, Wells LD, Phillips HR, Deckelbaum LI, Golobic RA. Development of a new technique for reducing pressure pulse generation during 308 nm excimer laser coronary angioplasty. Cath Cardiovasc Diagn 1994; 34:15–32.

21. de Feyter PJ, van Suylen RJ, de Jaegere PPT, Topol EJ, Serruys PW. Balloon angioplasty for the treatment of lesions in saphenous vein bypass grafts. J Am Coll Cardiol 1993; 21:1539–1549.

22. Douglas JS Jr, Weintraub WS, Liberman HA, Jenkins M, Cohen CL, Morris DC. Update of saphenous vein graft angioplasty: restenosis and long-term outcome (abstr). Circulation 1991; 84(suppl II):II-249.

23. King SB III. Coronary arteriography and left ventriculography: multipurpose technique. In: King SB III, Douglas JS Jr, eds. Coronary Arteriography and Angioplasty. Philadelphia: McGraw-Hill, 1985:239–274.

13
Percutaneous Balloon Angioplasty of Saphenous Vein Bypass Grafts: Clinical–Morphologic Correlation

Bruce F. Waller
*Indiana University Medical School, St. Vincent Hospital, and
Nasser, Smith and Pinkerton Cardiology, Inc., Indianapolis, Indiana*

Cass A. Pinkerton, Charles M. Orr, and Edward T. A. Fry
*Nasser, Smith and Pinkerton Cardiology, Inc., The Indiana Heart Institute,
and St. Vincent Hospital, Indianapolis, Indiana*

Percutaneous balloon angioplasty (PBA) has demonstrated its usefulness in nonoperative treatment of obstructed coronary arteries. PBA has also been useful in dilating obstructed aortocoronary saphenous vein bypass grafts and narrowed internal mammary arteries used as bypass conduits. This chapter will focus on the anatomic basis for and pathologic changes resulting from saphenous vein balloon angioplasty [1–13].

I. MORPHOLOGIC RESULTS OF BALLOON ANGIOPLASTY OF SAPHENOUS VEIN BYPASS GRAFTS

Morphologic changes following angioplasty in saphenous vein grafts can be divided into those occurring in "young" and in "old" saphenous vein grafts. Operatively excised segments of saphenous vein bypass grafts from two patients undergoing PBA of the bypass graft early ($\leq$1 year) and late ($>$1 year) after aortocoronary bypass surgery served as the basis of this review [9]. Clinical and morphologic data from the two patients are summarized in Table 1 and Figures 1–9.

Table 1 Clinical and Morphologic Data in Two Patients Who Underwent PBA of Stenotic SVBGs Early (≤1 year) and Late (>1 year) After Aortocoronary Bypass Operation

Observation	Early graft (63-yr-old man)	Late graft (42-yr-old man)	
		Dilation procedure	
		#1	#2
Age of SV graft (months)	3	56	
Interval from bypass operation to PTA (months)	2	52	54
Interval from PTA to SV graft excision (months)	1	4	2
Angiography-angioplasty data:			
Maximal SV graft narrowing (%DR) (location) before PTA	95 (proximal)	95 (mid)	95 (mid)
Maximal SV graft narrowing (%DR) after PTA (total)	10 (85%)	25 (70%)	10 (85%)
Mean intragraft pressure (mm Hg) before and after PTA (total)	37 4 (33)	60 15 (45)	60 10 (50)
Number of balloon inflations	Multiple	4	8
Maximal balloon inflation pressure (atm)	12	9	10
Duration (sec) balloon inflation	60	90	90
Dilating catheter(s)	S25-30	G20-30	G20-20 G20-30 S37-25
Angiographic "dissection" or "splint"	0	0	+
Maximal SV graft narrowing (%DR) prior to SV excision	85		95
Morphologic data:			
Maximal SV graft narrowing (% XSA)	76–100		76–100
Graft narrowing (% XSA) at site of PTA	76–100		76–100
Cause of graft narrowing	IFT		IFT + AP
Calcific deposits	0		+
Evidence of PTA	+[a]		+[b]

[a]Loss of endothelial lining in area of balloon dilation but no tears, breaks, or cracks.
[b]Healing intimal separation (intimal flap).
AP = atherosclerotic plaque; DR = diameter reduction; IFT = intimal fibrous thickening; PTA = percutaneous transluminal angioplasty; SV = saphenous vein; XSA = cross-sectional area.

II. ANGIOPLASTY OF SAPHENOUS VEIN GRAFT EARLY AFTER BYPASS SURGERY ("YOUNG GRAFTS")

A. Clinical Features

A 63-year-old man (Table 1) with angina pectoris underwent PBA of the left anterior descending coronary artery [9]. Approximately 30 minutes after successful dilation, the left anterior descending coronary artery suddenly closed, and the patient became hypotensive and developed ventricular tachycardia and fibrillation. An angioplasty balloon was inserted, the vessel was successfully reopened, and the patient was stabilized. Despite multiple balloon inflations, the left anterior descending coronary continued to reclose, and the patient underwent aortocoronary saphenous vein bypass grafting to the left anterior descending coronary artery.

Seven weeks after bypass surgery, the patient had recurrent angina pectoris. Cardiac catheterization disclosed 95% symmetric diameter reduction of the saphenous vein bypass graft at the proximal (aortic) anastomotic site (Figure 1). The vein graft was dilated with a steerable 25-30 balloon, with multiple inflations of up to 60 seconds' duration, resulting in a marked increase in graft luminal diameter (Figure 1).

Four weeks after successful bypass graft angioplasty (3 months after graft insertion), the patient had recurrent angina. Repeat angiography disclosed

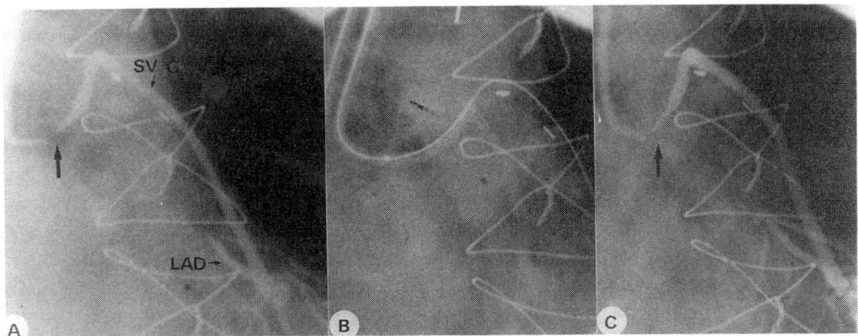

Figure 1 Angiographic frames of a saphenous vein bypass graft (SVBG) before and after transluminal balloon angioplasty 1 month before graft excision and 2 months after graft insertion. A: Severe luminal narrowing of the bypass graft near the aortic anastomotic site (arrow). B: Inflated angioplasty balloon located within the proximal saphenous vein graft. C: Marked increase in luminal diameter of saphenous vein graft following angioplasty (arrow). (LAD = left anterior descending coronary artery). (From Ref. 9, with permission.)

severe graft narrowing (restenosis) at the previous dilation site. This time, however, the stenotic segment was not smooth and symmetric but irregular and asymmetric. Because of the angiographic appearance of the stenotic segment and the rapid recurrence of stenosis, the patient underwent repeat bypass grafting. The proximal portion of the graft was excised at operation.

B. Morphologic Features

The operatively excised portion of saphenous vein graft (Figure 2) measured 40 mm in length and was free of calcific deposits. The excised segment included the site of maximal balloon inflation and a short distal portion in which the catheter and guide wire had passed but in which balloon inflation did not occur. The external diameter (about 7 mm) of the proximal 30 mm of graft (the portion subjected to angioplasty) was slightly wider compared with the external diameter (about 5 mm) of the distal nondilated segment (Figure 2). The entire specimen was cut transversely into eight 5-mm segments, numbered 1 to 8. Segments 1 to 6 were from areas of previous PBA, and segments 7 and 8 were from nondilated areas.

III. ANGIOPLASTY OF SAPHENOUS VEIN GRAFT LATE AFTER BYPASS SURGERY ("OLD GRAFTS")

A. Clinical Features

A 42-year-old man (Table 1) was hospitalized with acute myocardial infarction [9]. Continued chest pain prompted coronary angiography and subsequent double aortocoronary saphenous vein bypass grafting to the left circumflex coronary artery (margin branch and distal left circumflex). About 1 year later, he had recurrent chest pain, which worsened over the next 2 years. Repeat angiography 3 years later disclosed total occlusion of the graft to the distal left circumflex coronary artery and 50% diameter reduction in the midportion of the graft to the distal left circumflex marginal branch. Two years later, a third coronary angiogram disclosed progressive narrowing of all three major coronary artery systems and 50% diameter reduction of the bypass graft to the marginal branch of the left circumflex coronary artery.

The patient underwent repeat aortocoronary bypass operation with insertion of new grafts to the left anterior descending and right coronary systems. Two months later, angina pectoris recurred. Repeat angiography showed that the graft to the right coronary artery was open, the graft to the left anterior descending system was closed, and the graft to the left circumflex marginal branch now was narrowed 95% in diameter (Figure 3).

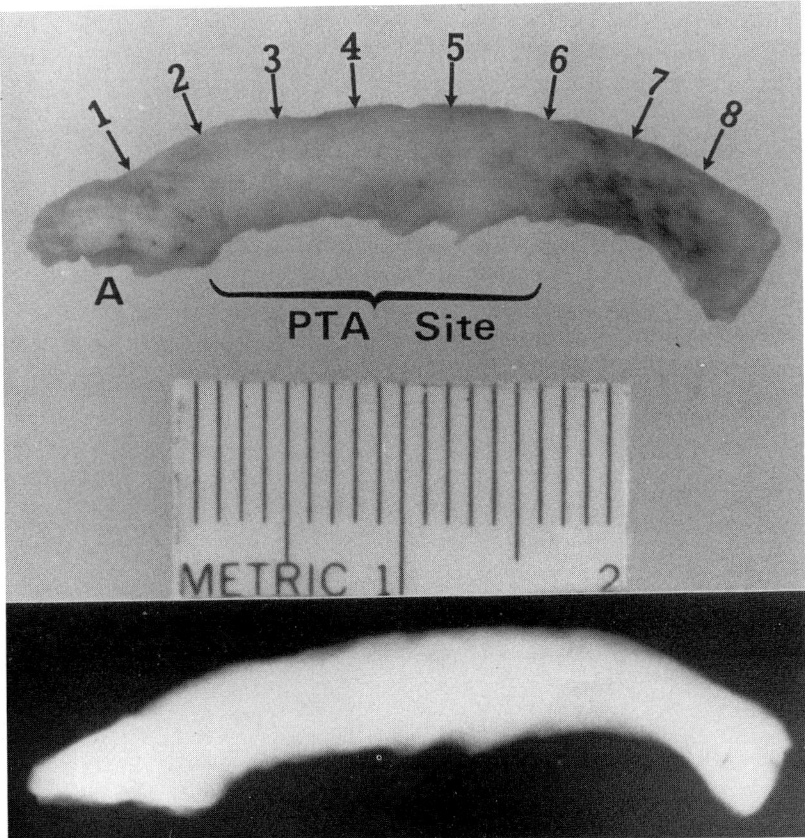

Figure 2 Operatively excised portion of a 3-month-old saphenous vein graft. *Upper*: The diameter of the proximal portion (aortic anastomotic and) (A) subjected to transluminal balloon angioplasty (PTA) is slightly wider than the diameter of the distal, nondilated segment. The numbers represent sites of transverse sections appearing in Figure 5. *Lower*: Radiograph of specimen discloses *no* calcific deposits. (From Ref. 9, with permission.)

The patient underwent PBA of the left circumflex graft (52 months after graft insertion) (Table 1), resulting in decreased graft luminal narrowing (from 95% to 20%) and decreased transstenotic mean pressure gradient (from 60 mm Hg to 15 mm Hg). Two months later, he had recurrent angina. Repeat angiography disclosed luminal irregularities of the right graft and 95% diameter narrowing of the left circumflex graft at the site of previous PBA (Figure 3).

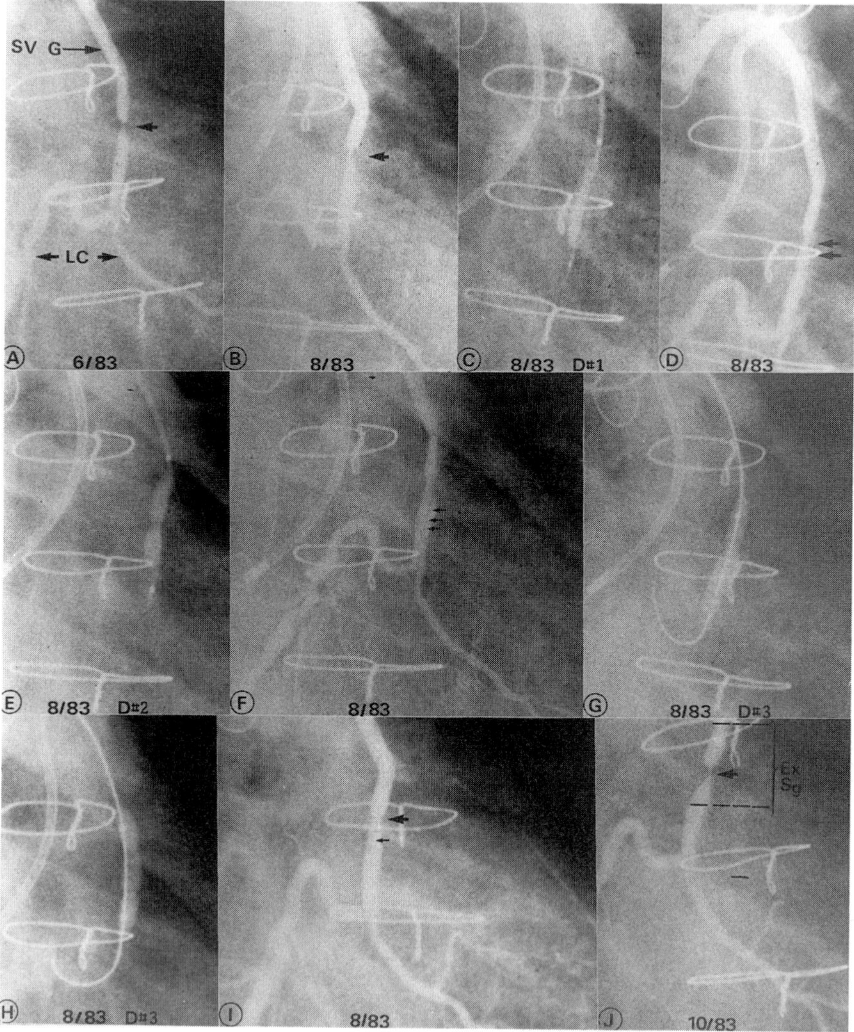

Figure 3 Serial angiographic frames of a saphenous vein bypass graft (SVBG) before and after two transluminal balloon angioplasty (TBA) procedures. A: Severe luminal narrowing in the mid portion of the SVBG (arrow) 52 months after insertion. TBA (not shown) resulted in decreased luminal narrowing (from 95 per cent to 20 per cent). (LC = left circumflex coronary artery). B: Restenosis at graft 2 months later at previous TBA site (arrow). C to I: Second TBA (54 months after insertion) involved serial dilations (D#1 to D#3) using progressively larger balloons, variable inflation pressures, and inflation durations. F and I show a localized "break," "fracture," or "dissection"

(continues)

The patient underwent a second angioplasty of the left circumflex graft (Figure 3). Serial dilations using progressively larger balloons, variable inflation pressure (6–9 atm), and balloon inflation durations (10–90 sec) (Table 1) resulted in decreased graft luminal narrowing (from 95% to 10%) and decreased mean transstenotic pressure gradient (from 60 mm Hg to 10 mm Hg). Furthermore, graft angiograms disclosed a localized dissection ("break," "crack," "fracture") at the angioplasty site (Figure 3).

The patient had recurrent angina 2 months later, when the sixth coronary angiogram disclosed restenosis (95% diameter reduction) of the graft to the left circumflex marginal branch (Figure 3) and total occlusion of the right graft. The patient underwent a third aortocoronary bypass operation. The midportion of the left circumflex conduit was excised at operation, and despite successful regrafting, the patient died at operation.

B. Morphologic Features

The operatively excised portiion of saphenous graft (Figure 4) measured 42 mm in length and had foci of calcific deposits in the area of dilation. The entire specimen was cut transversely into eight 5-mm-long segments, numbered 1 to 8. Segments 4 to 6 were from the site of maximal balloon inflation. The area of the angioplasty dissection noted angiographically (Figure 3) was specifically localized on the excised saphenous vein specimen (Figure 4, segments 4 to 6).

IV. MORPHOLOGIC OBSERVATIONS IN THE EARLY SAPHENOUS VEIN GRAFT

The lumen of each of the eight 5-mm saphenous vein segments was narrowed more than 75% in cross-secitonal area by intimal thickening (Figure 5). Histologically, the diffuse intimal thickening of both dilated and nondilated segments consisted of cellular fibrocollagenous tissue without foam cells or cholesterol clefts (intimal "fibrous hyperplasia," "fibrous proliferation").

---

line at the site of TBA (small arrows). The second TBA resulted in decreased luminal narrowing (from 95 per cent to 10 per cent). J: Restenosis of the graft 2 months later (56 months after insertion) at the previous TBA sites. The boxed area indicates the operatively excised segment (Ex Sg) of the saphenous vein graft. Numbers in each frame indicate month and year. (From Waller B.F., et al. Morphologic observations following percutaneous transluminal balloon angioplasty of early and late aortocoronary saphenous vein bypass grafts. J Am Coll Cardiol 1984; 4:784–92, with permission.)

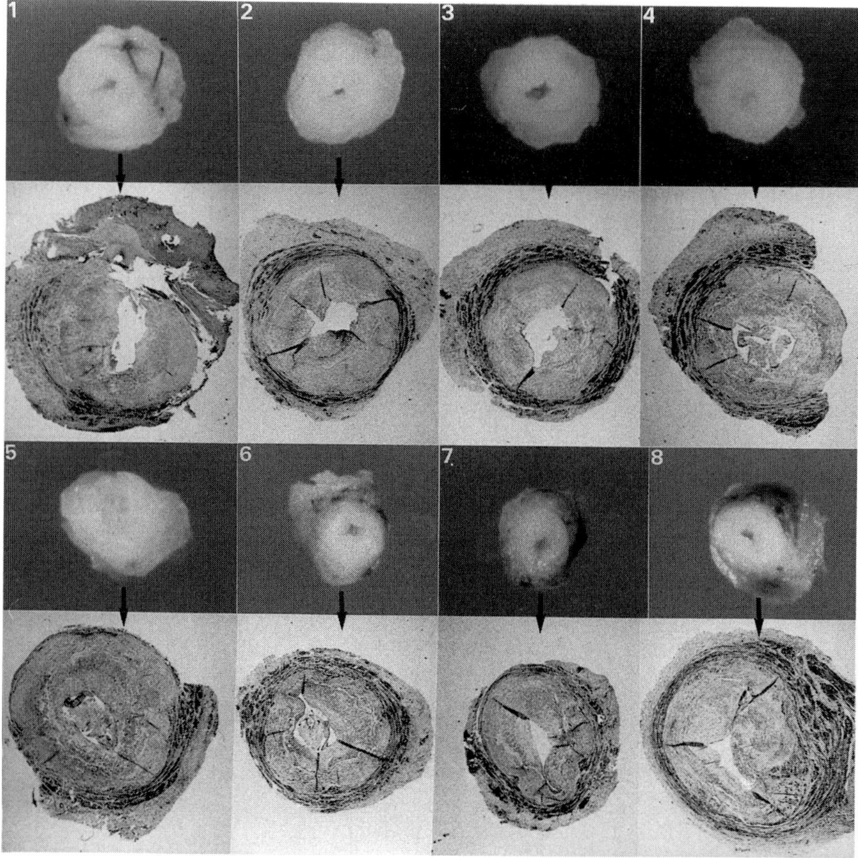

Figure 4 Morphologic and histologic photographs of the eight segments of saphenous vein graft corresponding to the sites labeled in Figure 2. Segments 1 through 6 are from the area of balloon inflation and dilation, and segments 7 and 8 are from nondilated portions of the graft (i.e., "controls"). Each of the eight segments had diffuse and severe cross-sectional area luminal narrowing by intimal thickening consisting of fibrocollagenous tissue. No segments contained atherosclerotic plaque or calcium deposits. No distinctive histologic changes were observed in the segments subjected to transluminal balloon angioplasty compared with control segments (elastic stains, ×6). (From Ref. 9, with permission.)

Segments 1 to 6 were serially sectioned at 10u intervals to search for sites of "splits," "tears," or "cracks" or other morphologic evidence of previous PBA. Control segments 7 and 8 were also sectioned in a similar fashion. Histologic assessment by light microscopy did not disclose any distinctive morphologic

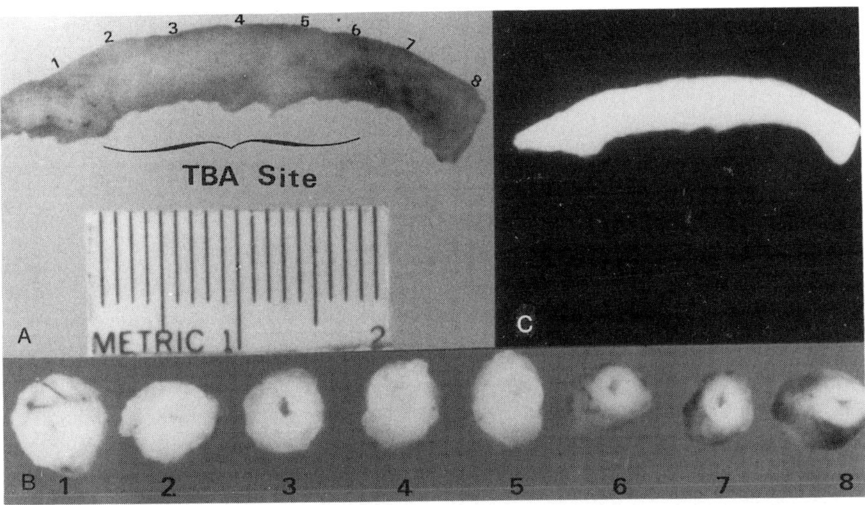

Figure 5 Operatively excised portion of a 56-month-old saphenous vein graft. *Upper*: The brackets indicate the site of two TBA procedures located in the mid-portion of the graft. (P = proximal end). The numbers represent sites of transverse sections appearing in Figure 7. *Lower*: Radiograph of transverse section discloses foci of calcific (Ca^{2+}) deposits. (From Ref. 9, with permission.)

lesion(s) in the intimal, medial, or adventitial layers of dilated or nondilated segments of the saphenous vein graft.

Ultrastructural evaluation of segments 2 (dilated) and 6 (nondilated) (Figure 6) disclosed the absence of endothelial luminal cells in the dilated segment compared with their presence in the nondilated segment. Cells lining the graft lumen in the *dilated* segment had features of myofibroblasts (cytoplasmic filaments with focal condensations and abundant rough endoplasmic reticulum). Fibrinlike extracellular material (possibly representing residual basement membrane) condensed along the luminal border of these myofibroblasts. The endothelial cells lining the lumen of the distal *nondilated* segment had luminal and abluminal micropinocytotic vesicles and well-formed intercellular junctions (Figure 6). No distinctive differences in myofibroblasts or collagen fibrils were noted between segments 2 and 8.

V. MORPHOLOGIC OBSERVATIONS IN THE LATE SAPHENOUS VEIN GRAFT

The lumen of each of the eight 5-mm saphenous vein segments had diffuse but variable degrees of intimal thickening (Figure 7). The maximal cross-sectional

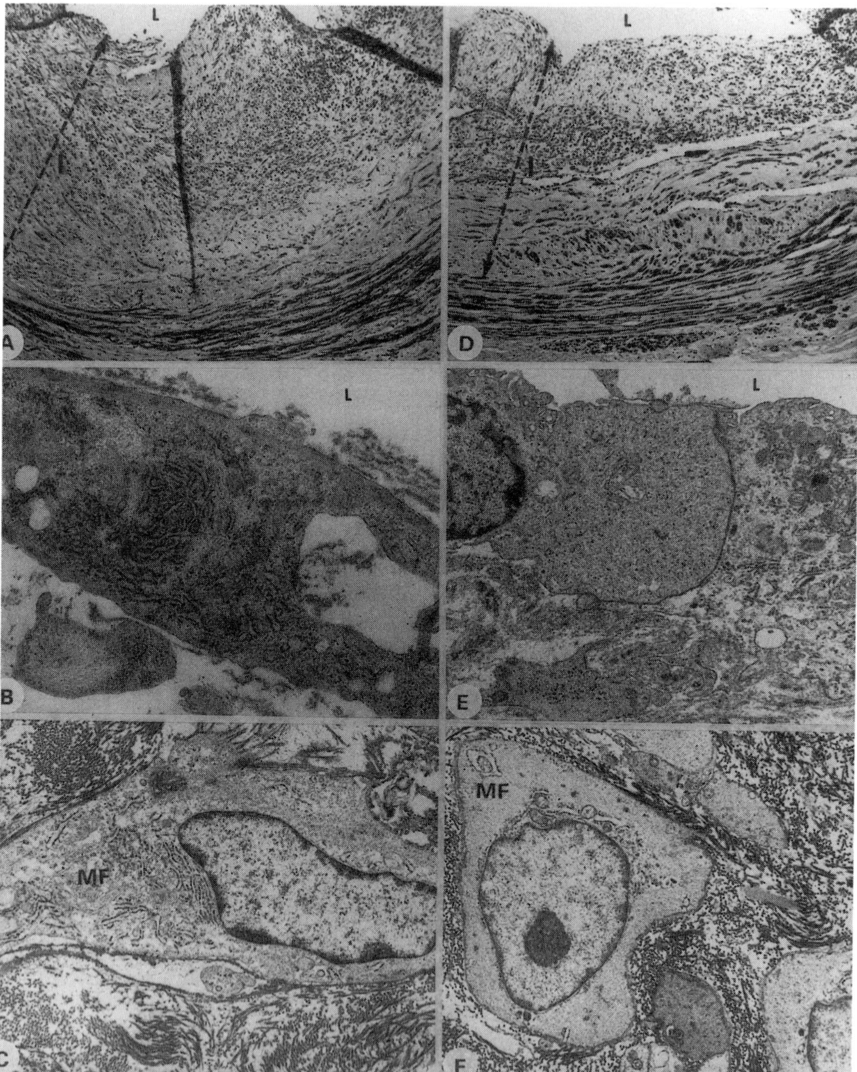

Figure 6 Light and electron micrographs of dilated (A, B, and C [segment 2 from Figure 5]) and nondilated (D, E, and F [segment 8 from Figure 5]) portions of the saphenous vein graft. A and D: Light micrographs of dilated (A) and nondilated (D) segments show that both segments have marked intimal thickening composed of smooth muscle cells and fibrocollagenous tissue (elastic stains, ×40). B and E: Electron micrographs at the luminal border of dilated (B) and nondilated (E)

(continues)

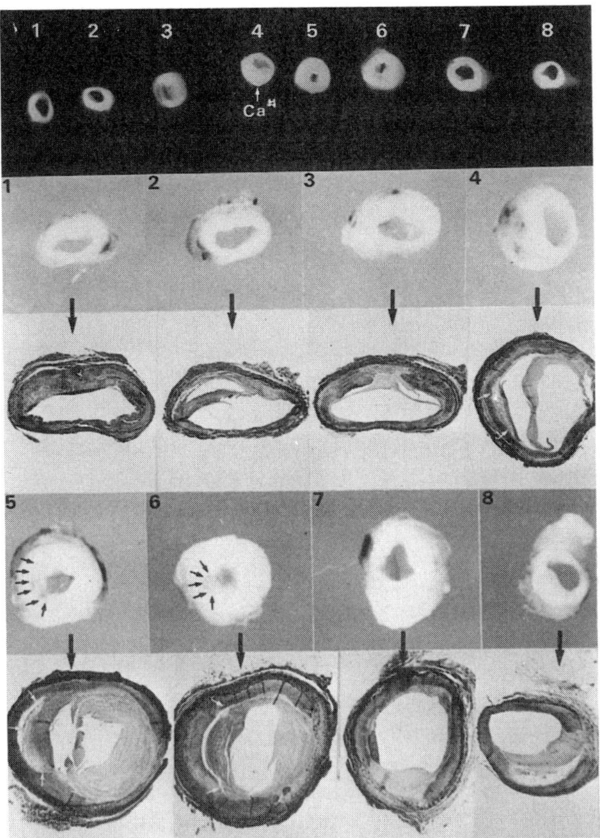

Figure 7 Radiographs (upper panel) and photographs (lower panel) of morphologic and histologic segments of saphenous vein graft corresponding to the sites labeled in Figure 4. Each of the segments show diffuse but variable degrees of intimal thickening composed of atherosclerotic plaque. The segment with the most severe luminal narrowing (5) corresponds to the area of previous transluminal balloon angioplasty procedures (small arrows). (From Ref. 9, with permission.)

segments show a loss of endothelial cells, with micropinocytotic vesicles bordering the lumen in E. A short segment of basement membrane is visible at the lower right (×8300). C and F: Electron micrographs from deeper portions of the intimal thickening of the dilated (C) and nondilated (F) segments show similar types of myofibroblastic cells (MF) and dense bundles of collagen fibrils (×8300). (From Ref. 9, with permission.)

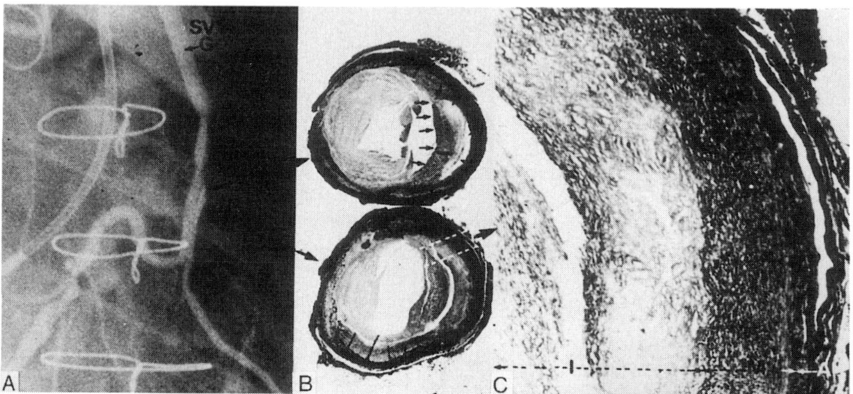

Figure 8 Angiographic-morphologic-histologic correlation at the site of angioplasty dissection 2 months before graft excision. A: Angiographic frame of saphenous vein bypass graft (SVBG) following transluminal balloon angioplasty showing a line of dissection. B: Corresponding morphologic segments of SVBG in area of angiographic dissection showing severe luminal cross-sectional area narrowing with an "intimal flap" (small arrows) and a partially healed intimal "fracture." C: Higher magnification (×80) of boxed area in B showing the intimal (I) fracture site. The intimal thickening is composed of fibrocollagenous tissue, foam cells, and cholesterol clefts (M = media; A = adventitia) (elastic stains). (From Ref. 9, with permission.)

area luminal reduction by intimal thickening occurred in segments 3, 5, and 6. Histologically, the intimal thickening in segments 4 to 6 consisted of foam cells, cholesterol clefts, fibrocollagenous tissue, foci of myofibroblasts, and calcific deposits characteristic of atherosclerotic plaque (Figure 8). Intimal thickening of segments 1 to 3 and 7 was predominantly fibrocollagenous in nature except for occasional foci of foam cells, cholesterol clefts, and calcium. The site of angioplasty dissection (segments 4 to 6) (Figure 8) had partial separation of the intima from the media. This "intimal flap" had begun to reattach to the wall of the graft, representing healing of a localized plaque "tear" or "fracture."

VI. CLINICAL-MORPHOLOGIC CORRELATIONS

Each of the patients just described had one or more clinically successful percutaneous transluminal angioplasty dilations of a stenotic saphenous vein bypass graft *early* (2 months) or *late* (52 and 54 months) after graft insertion.

Angiographic similarities between the early and late saphenous vein grafts included an increase in luminal diameter associated with a decrease in mean transstenotic pressure gradient following angioplasty, and restenosis of the graft at the site of previous dilation 1 or 2 months later. *Angiographic differences* between the grafts included the absence of "cracks," "breaks," or "splits" following dilation in the early graft, but the presence of an intimal "split" following the second angioplasty procedure in the late graft. An additional angiographic difference between the grafts was the location of stenosis. The site of stenosis in the early graft was at the proximal end of the graft (aortic anastomosis), whereas the site of stenosis in the late graft was in the graft body (midportion).

Morphologic similarities between the grafts included diffuse intimal thickening by fibrocollagenous tissue with fibrotic medial and adventitial layers. *Morphologic differences* between the grafts were distinctive: The early graft had thickened intima without atherosclerotic plaque changes or calcific deposits and no morphologic evidence of previous dilations, whereas the late graft had thickened intima typical of atherosclerotic plaque with focal calcific deposits and morphologic evidence of PBA injury.

VII. THERAPEUTIC IMPLICATIONS FOR SAPHENOUS VEIN ANGIOPLASTY DERIVED FROM MORPHOLOGIC OBSERVATIONS

The fate of an aortocoronary saphenous vein bypass graft appears to be dependent on several factors relevant to the time interval from bypass grafting to graft obstruction. Graft occlusion developing *within 1 month* of bypass graft insertion is almost invariably secondary to graft thrombosis related to technical factors, such as stenosis at aortic or coronary anastomotic sites, intraoperative vein trauma, and poor distal runoff secondary to severe atherosclerosis or reduced caliber of the distal native vessel. These technical factors and the nature of the obstruction material (thrombus) appear to limit the role of PBA in successfully relieving saphenous vein graft obstruction occurring within 1 month of bypass operation.

Functionally significant graft stenoses developing *between 1 month and 1 year* following graft insertion nearly always are characterized by intimal thickening histologically composed of cellular or acellular fibrocollagenous tissue. The venous medial and adventitial layers become fibrotic, and the graft resembles a thick, fibrous tube. Focally stenotic lesions produced by this intimal thickening appear amenable to dilation by PBA, as illustrated in the first patient described earlier. However, in view of the histologic composition of the intima, the dilating mechanism is probably not "intimal compression" but,

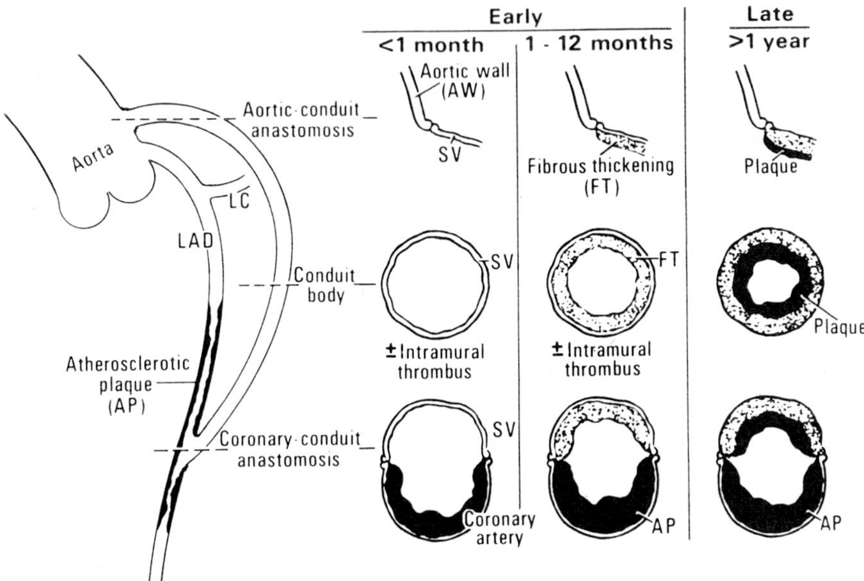

Figure 9 Diagram illustrating possible mechanisms of luminal balloon angiography in stenotic aortocoronary saphenous vein (SV) bypass grafts. Two types of lesions characterize the SV stenoses, depending on the interval from graft insertion to early obstruction. *Early* (≤1 year) grafts (a, left) contain intimal thickening composed primarily of fibrocollagenous tissue without calcium, and dilation is accomplished by conduit "stretching." *Late* (≥1 year) grafts (a, b, c, right) contain intimal thickening composed of atherosclerotic plaque and calcium, and dilation is accomplished by "plaque compression" (unlikely), graft "stretching," or plaque "fracture" or "break" (most likely). (Ao = aorta; LAD = left anterior descending coronary artery; LC = left circumflex coronary artery; LM = left main coronary artery). (From Ref. 9, with permission.)

rather, graft "stretching" (Figure 9). Depending on the degree of graft stretching, the dilating procedure may have limited therapeutic success (weeks to months), with graft "restenosis" representing gradual "restitution of tone" of an overstretched graft segment.

Saphenous vein graft stenoses occurring *beyond 1 year* and generally after 3 years following graft insertion usually consist of atherosclerotic plaque in addition to intimal fibrous thickening. The atherosclerotic plaque in saphenous vein grafts appears morphologically similar to that observed in native coronary arteries: foam cells, cholesterol clefts, blood product debris, fibrocollagenous tissue, and calcific deposits. Focal stenoses produced by this type of lesion also appear amenable to dilation by PBA, as illustrated in the second patient described earlier. The mechanism(s) of conduit dilation in this setting appear similar to those proposed for coronary artery angioplasty: plaque "splitting," "cracking," or "breaking" with or without localized intimal-medial dissection (Figure 9). Therapeutic limitations in dilating saphenous vein grafts narrowed by atherosclerotic plaque should be similar to those observed in atherosclerotic coronary arteries subjected to PBA.

In addition to the age of the bypass graft, at least two other anatomic factors appear to influence the therapeutic success of PBA of saphenous vein grafts: (a) the *length* of stenosis and (b) the *location* of stenosis. Long stenotic segments of saphenous vein (>15–20 mm) are frequently technically more difficult to dilate and are associated with a lower primary therapeutic success compared with short stenotic segments (<5 mm). Graft stenoses may be located at the *anastomotic sites* (aorta-graft or coronary artery-graft) or *within the body* of the graft. Angiographic studies have suggested that saphenous vein graft stenoses at the coronary artery-graft anastomotic site have the best therapeutic results, followed by lesions in the graft body and at the aorta-graft anastomotic site, respectively. An anatomic factor supporting the relatively high success rate at dilating stenotic coronary artery-graft anastomotic sites is the presence of atherosclerotic plaque in the coronary portion of the anastomosis. Stenoses in the graft body or aortic-graft anastomotic site are less likely to have the potential angioplasty advantage of associated atherosclerotic plaque unless the graft is over 3 years old.

VIII. CLINICAL RESULTS OF PERCUTANEOUS TRANSLUMINAL ANGIOPLASTY OF SAPHENOUS VEIN GRAFTS

The angiographic results of at least 72 saphenous vein bypass grafts subjected to PBA have been reported in three studies. Ford and colleagues [2,3] dilated nine saphenous vein grafts 4–84 months (mean, 46 months) after insertion. Primary angiographic success occurred in six of the nine grafts, with only late success (>9 months) in two of the six initial successes. Of the two late successes, one graft was 18 months old at initial angioplasty and the other was 5 months old. Famularo and colleagues [4] reported morphologic observations in an unsuccessful dilation of a saphenous vein conduit with atherosclerotic plaque. Although the age of the graft was not provided, morphology of the angioplasty site showed intimal tears of atherosclerotic plaque. Douglas and associates [13] reported their angioplasty results in 62 bypass grafts. Of 62 grafts, 40 (65%) were dilated early after insertion (≤1 year) and 22 (35%) were dilated late after insertion (>1 year). Primary success occurred in 37/40 (93%)

of the early grafts and in 21/22 (95%) of the late grafts, with the same restenosis rate (24%). Breakdown of the early and late grafts according to stenosis location revealed that the distal graft stenoses (early and late) had a high initial dilation success and lower restenosis rate. Graft stenoses located in the body or proximal end had a slightly lower initial dilation success, but three times the restenosis frequency compared with the distal sites (39% vs. 13%). The morphologic and histologic observations in grafts from the two patients described earlier provide anatomic support for these clinical results.

REFERENCES

1. Griffith LSC, Bulkley BH, Hutchins GM. Occlusive changes at the coronary artery-bypass graft anastomosis. Morphologic study of 95 grafts. J Thorac Cardiovasc Surg 1977; 73:668–679.
2. Ford WB, Wholey MH, Zikria EA, Miller WH, Samadani SR, Koimattur AG, Sullivan ME. Percutaneous transluminal angioplasty in the management of occlusive disease involving the coronary arteries and saphenous vein bypass grafts. J Thorac Cardiovasc Surg 1980; 79:1–11.
3. Ford WB, Wholey MH, Zikria EA, Somadani SR, Sullivan ME. Percutaneous transluminal dilation of aortocoronary saphenous vein bypass grafts. Chest 1981; 79:529–535.
4. Famularo M, Vasilomanolakis EC, Schrager B, Talbert W, Ellestad MH. Percutaneous transluminal angioplasty of aortocoronary saphenous vein graft: morphologic observations. JAMA 1983; 249:3347–3350.
5. Lee G, Ikeda RM, Joye JA, Bogren HG, DeMaria AN, Mason DT. Evaluation of transluminal angioplasty of chronic coronary artery stenosis. Value and limitations assessed in fresh human cadaver hearts. Circulation 1980; 61:77–83.
6. Lie JT, Lawrie GM, Morris GC Jr. Aortocoronary bypass saphenous vein graft atherosclerosis. Anatomic study of 99 vein grafts from normal and hyperlipoproteinemic patients up to 75 months postoperatively. Am J Cardiol 1977; 40:906–913.
7. Smith SH, Greer JC. Morphology of saphenous vein-coronary artery bypass grafts. Seven to 116 months after surgery. Arch Pathol Lab 1983; 107:13–18.
8. Waller BF. Early and late morphologic changes in human coronary arteries after percutaneous transluminal coronary angioplasty. Clin Cardiol 1983; 6:363–372.
9. Waller BF, Rothbaum DA, Gorfinkel JH, Ulbright TM, Linnemeier TJ, Berger SM. Morphologic observations following percutaneous transluminal balloon angioplasty of early and late aortocoronary saphenous vein bypass grafts. J Am Coll Cardiol 1984; 4:784–792.
10. Waller BF, Roberts WC. Amount of luminal narrowing in bypassed and nonbypassed native coronary arteries in necropsy patients early and late after aorto-coronary bypass operations. In: Mason DT, Collins JT Jr, eds. Myocardial Revascularization. Medical and Surgical Advances in Coronary Disease. New York: Yorke Medical Books, 1981:503–513.

11. Waller BF, Dillon JC, Crowley MH. Plaque hematoma and coronary dissection with percutaneous transluminal coronary angioplasty (PTCA) of severely stenotic lesions: morphologic coronary observations in 5 men within 30 days of PTCA. Circulation 1983; 68(suppl III):III-144.
12. Waller BF, McManus BM, Gorfinkel HJ, Kishel JC, Schmidt EC, Kent KM, Roberts WC. Status of the major coronary arteries 80 to 150 days after percutaneous transluminal coronary angioplasty. Analysis of 3 necropsy patients. Am J Cardiol 1983; 51:81–84.
13. Douglas JS Jr, Gruentzig AR, King SB III, Holman J, Ischinger T, Meier B, Craver JM, Jones EL, Waller JL, Bone DK, Guyton R. Percutaneous transluminal coronary angioplasty in patients with prior coronary bypass surgery. J Am Coll Cardiol 1983; 2:745–754.

Editors' Note: For additional information on this subject, see:

Saber RS, Edwards WD, Holmes DR Jr, Vliestra RE, Reeder GS. Balloon angioplasty of aortocoronary saphenous vein bypass grafts: a histopathologic study of six grafts from five patients, with emphasis on restenosis and embolic complications. J Am Coll Cardiol 1988; 12:1501–1509.

14
Reoperation for Patients with Vein Graft Atherosclerosis

Bruce W. Lytle
The Cleveland Clinic Foundation, Cleveland, Ohio

Coronary artery bypass surgery has been an extremely successful treatment for patients with severe coronary artery disease. A myriad of studies have documented the effective symptom relief achieved by coronary bypass surgery, and both observational and randomized prospective studies have identified subsets of patients for whom bypass surgery prolongs the long-term survival rate [1–4]. However, most advances in medical technology create new problems for physicians to confront, and bypass surgery is not an exception to this principle. Cardiologists and cardiac surgeons are currently facing the problems of diagnosis and treatment for patients who have undergone previous bypass surgery [5–12].

For perspective, it is important to remember that the magnitude of these problems are related to the success of bypass surgery. The excellent survival rate after primary operations has generated a large population of patients with an atherogenic diathesis that survive because the adverse effect of their proximal coronary artery obstructions on life expectancy has been decreased by surgery. Because coronary surgery does nothing to lessen atherogenesis, patients post–bypass surgery may develop late complications of atherosclerosis (diffuse distal coronary artery disease and severe noncardiac atherosclerosis) that were uncommon in the pre–bypass surgery era, because such patients often succumbed at an earlier age to myocardial infarction.

For most patients who have had bypass surgery, at least part of their revascularization has been achieved by using segments of reversed greater saphenous vein as bypass grafts from the aorta to the coronary arteries. There is a time-related attrition of those grafts [13–17]. Randomized prospective studies of saphenous vein grafts in patients treated with platelet inhibitors have shown that the 1-year patency rate of saphenous vein to coronary grafts is approximately 90% [18–20]. Prospective patency rate data concerning patients treated with platelet inhibitors does not extend more than 5 years after operation, but observational data indicate that approximately 30% of vein grafts known to be patent 1 year after operation will become occluded by 10 postoperative years, and another 30% will have some evidence of stenoses by that time. Thus, by 10 postoperative years, overall vein graft patency rates are 50–70%, and they continue to decline between 10 and 20 years after surgery, even though at 16–20 postoperative years, 46% of vein grafts are still functioning [4]. The causes of late vein graft failure are multiple, but intrinsic pathologic changes in vein grafts play a major role.

Patients who develop vein graft failure often become candidates for reoperation, and that issue is the subject of this chapter. We will examine the changes that develop in vein grafts, the reasons patients present for reoperation, specific issues that patients with vein graft failure present at the time of reoperation, and the indications for coronary reoperation.

I. VEIN GRAFT PATHOLOGY

To understand coronary reoperations it is necessary to understand the characteristics and the behavior of vein graft pathology. Although this subject is addressed in detail elsewhere in this text, we will review it briefly here.

Within a few weeks of operation virtually all saphenous vein to coronary artery grafts exhibit some degree of intimal fibroplasia, a reaction that is initially cellular but that becomes more fibrous with the passage of time. Intimal fibroplasia is superficial, diffuse (extending the entire length of the graft), concentric, and ubiquitous and produces a relatively smooth, nonfriable graft lining (Figure 1) [3]. Although intimal fibroplasia may produce vein graft stenoses and occlusions, it does not commonly do so [3,14,16].

Within 3–5 years after operation it becomes common for vein graft lesions to exhibit evidence of lipid infiltration, and it appears to be lipid infiltration combined with the basic structure of intimal fibroplasia that produces vein graft atherosclerosis [14,16,21]. Vein graft atherosclerosis is also superficial, diffuse, and concentric, although stenotic lesions may be eccentric. In addition, in the fully developed form it is unencapsulated, friable, and often associated with mural thrombus (Figure 1). Although these characteristics may also be associated with native vessel atherosclerosis, they usually are not. In fact, unencapsulated, thrombus-producing native coronary artery lesions are thought to be the subset of atherosclerotic plaques that are "active" lesions

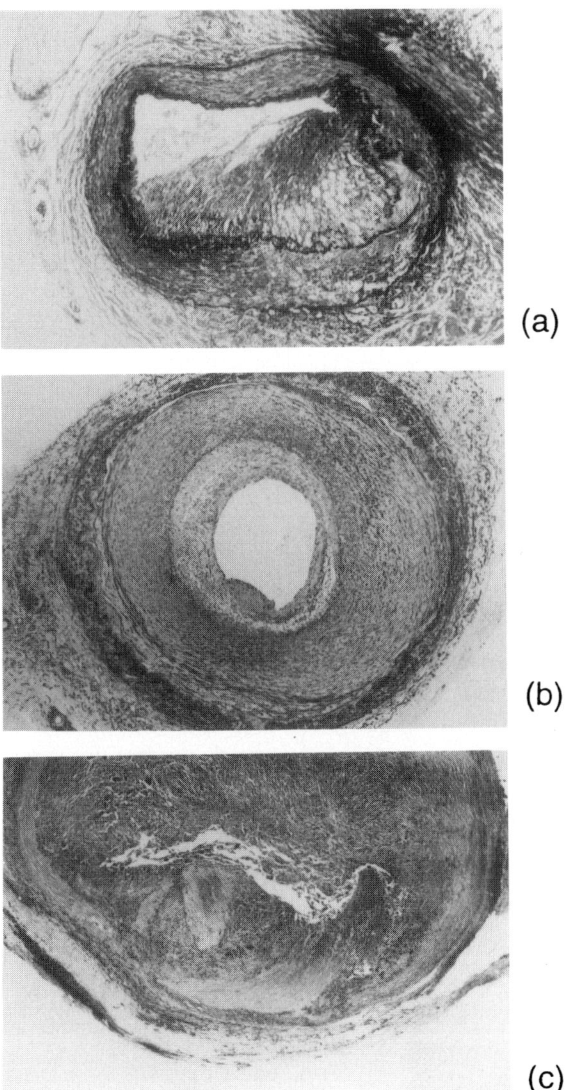

Figure 1 Native coronary artery atherosclerosis (a) tends to be an eccentric and segmental lesion. Early vein graft stenoses are usually caused by intimal fibroplasia (b), a concentric and relatively stable lesion. Vein graft atherosclerosis is friable, disordered, and prone to thrombogenesis. (Reprinted with permission from Ref. 3.)

responsible for producing many episodes of unstable angina and native coronary thrombosis. Thus, the common characteristics of vein graft atherosclerosis are those that are associated with "event-producing" native coronary lesions.

The friability of vein graft atherosclerosis has contributed to the dangers associated with reintervention for those patients. Embolization of atherosclerotic debris into distal coronary vessels causing myocardial infarction has been clearly documented, both at the time of percutaneous procedures and during reoperation [22,23]. In addition, the active nature of vein graft atherosclerosis may predispose to graft thrombosis and embolization, perhaps accounting for some episodes of unstable angina and myocardial infarction in patients with previous bypass surgery.

II. INCIDENCE AND CAUSES OF REOPERATION

Examination of patients undergoing primary bypass surgery during the 1970s has shown that the annual incidence of reoperation was 1.1% at 5 postoperative years, increasing to a rate of 3.9% by 10 postoperative years, and producing a cumulative incidence of reoperation of 2.7%, 11.4%, and 17.3% at 5, 10, and 12 postoperative years, respectively [24]. These patients differed from today's patients who undergo primary bypass surgery in that they were younger and had a higher incidence of limited (single- or double-vessel) coronary artery disease. Also, their primary operation did not routinely involve use of the internal thoracic artery (ITA) as a bypass graft. Multivariate testing of the determinants of the likelihood of reoperation (Table 1) showed that the factors associated with increased risk of reoperation included variables associated with living for a long time (young age, normal left ventricular function, single- or double-vessel disease) and variables associated with the development of recurrent ischemia (incomplete revascularization and not having an ITA).

We have carried out a longitudinal series of studies of patients undergoing a first coronary reoperation and found that over the years the anatomic reasons that patients undergo repeat coronary surgery have changed [5–7]. During the 1967–1978 time frame the mean interval between primary surgery and reoperation was only 45 months, and in 55% of cases the need for reoperation was caused by progression of atherosclerosis in native vessels that had not been jeopardized or grafted at the primary operation. When reoperation was carried out for graft failure, it was often early graft failure (mean interval 26 months between operations) caused by technical errors, including the failure to use the ITA graft. The combination of improved surgical skills and the advent of percutaneous techniques for the treatment of coronary artery disease has made reoperation for early graft failure fairly uncommon.

Table 1 Risk Factors for Reoperations

Risk factors	p Value
Young age	<.0001
No ITA graft	<.0001
Incomplete revascularization	.0004
NYHA Function Class III/IV	.003
Normal LV function	.003
Single-/double-vessel disease	.005

Multivariate testing of patient-related and operation-related variables associated with an increased risk of reoperation after primary coronary bypass surgery.
From Ref. 24.

Examination of our most recent cohort of reoperative patients (1,663 patients undergoing a first reoperation during the years 1988–1991) has shown that the mean interval between operations has increased to 116 months [7]. Graft failure constitutes at least part of the angiographic indications for reoperation in 92% of cases. In addition, only 28% of patients had normal left ventricular function at reoperation, and only 12% had single- or double-vessel coronary artery disease. Left main stenosis was present in 27% of patients, the mean age at reoperation was 62 years, and 21% of patients were 70 or more years old. To sum up then, today's candidates for reoperation usually had triple-vessel disease at the time of the first procedure, underwent an operation that was initially successful, and now are more than 10 years after their primary operation. A combination of progression of native vessel coronary artery disease and late graft failure, usually caused by vein graft atherosclerosis, has produced the need for reoperation. In addition, progression of atherosclerosis has often produced diffuse distal coronary artery disease and significant noncardiac atherosclerosis.

III. RISKS OF CORONARY REOPERATIONS: OPERATIVE STRATEGIES

Data from the nationwide Society for Thoracic Surgeons database documents the heightened in-hospital risks associated with reoperations. For the years 1991–1993, elective primary coronary bypass operations had a 1.74% in-hospital mortality, compared with 5.66% for elective reoperations. Emergency primary operations had a 5.03% risk, compared to 12.95% for emergency reoperations [25]. All authors that have reviewed any significant numbers of reoperations have documented an increased risk of in-hospital mortality compared with that associated with primary bypass operations. And in serial studies of patients undergoing a first reoperation at The Cleveland Clinic Foundation from 1967 through 1991, the in-hospital mortality rate has been between 3% and 4% [5–7]. Those risks and the risks documented by the STS database apply to reoperations in general, not just to repeat surgery for patients with vein graft stenoses. The reasons that reoperations have a higher risk are related to some factors that are unique to reoperations and to other problems that also occur during primary cases but that are more frequent and more difficult to manage in reoperative situations.

The most important unique characteristic of patients undergoing reoperations is that they usually derive their myocardial blood supply from multiple sources, including the native coronary circulation, patent ITA grafts, atherosclerotic vein grafts, and patent vein grafts. This situation complicates myocardial protection. Whereas patients who are undergoing primary surgery derive their entire myocardial blood supply from native coronary circulation (and, therefore, antegrade delivery of cardioplegia into the aortic root duplicates the preoperative situation), antegrade cardioplegia delivery may not protect areas supplied by patent arterial grafts in the reoperative setting and may create atherosclerotic embolization into the distal coronary circulation when delivered down atherosclerotic vein grafts.

Studies of reoperations conducted in the past have noted a specific increase in risk associated with the presence of stenoses in vein grafts. Perrault et al. [10] documented an in-hospital mortality rate of 7%, 17%, and 29% for patients with 1, 2, and 3 or more stenotic vein grafts. In a study we will examine in detail later, when we specifically examined patients with stenotic vein grafts we noted a difference in the risk of reoperation that was dependent upon the age of those stenotic grafts. Patients with early stenoses in vein grafts (<5 years after previous operation) had no mortality at reoperation, whereas those with late stenoses (≥5 years after primary operation) had a mortality rate that was 5.1% overall and 8.5% for patients with late stenosis in a left anterior descending (LAD) vein graft [26].

A major advance in the technique of myocardial protection during reoperations has been the advent of retrograde (coronary sinus) cardioplegia delivery [27–30]. With the use of this technique it is possible to minimize the use of antegrade cardioplegia and, therefore, to minimize the risk of atherosclerotic coronary embolization from atherosclerotic vein grafts. We found that with the use of retrograde cardioplegia in the 1988–1991 time frame, the in-hospital mortality dropped to 4.0% for patients with any late vein graft stenosis and to 3.6% for patients with LAD vein graft stenoses. There was still a trend toward an increased risk for patients with multiple stenotic vein grafts, but their 6.1% mortality rate was not significantly different from 3.7% risk for the entire group of 1663 patients undergoing reoperation [7].

Reoperations for patients with both stenotic vein grafts and patent, angiographically "normal" vein grafts raised the question of the management of "normal"-looking vein grafts. For patients undergoing early reoperations (<5 years after primary surgery), angiographically normal–looking vein grafts are not replaced. For patients undergoing reoperation more than 5 years after primary surgery our general rule is that all vein grafts, stenotic as well as angiographically patent, are replaced at that operation. Most patients with vein graft atherosclerosis that causes stenosis in one graft will have involvement of the other grafts, with the atherosclerotic process producing the risk of atherosclerotic embolization at the time of reoperation and the risk of the development of accelerated postoperative failure of those vein grafts if they are not replaced.

However, having stated that general principal, we must realize that in specific cases there are many exceptions. The use of retrograde cardioplegia has decreased the intraoperative dangers of atherosclerotic embolization. Furthermore, patients do not have unlimited bypass conduits, and the use of those bypass conduits to replace normal-looking vein grafts must take into consideration the age of the patient and the likelihood of further surgery. When replacing vein grafts, we usually deliver antegrade cardioplegia for the induction dose through the aortic root and then disconnect the vein grafts to be replaced and use a combination of retrograde cardioplegia and delivery down newly constructed vein grafts after that time.

The presence of patent left ITA grafts is another technical hurdle that has been cited as a factor increasing the risk of reoperations [12]. Here again, the use of retrograde cardioplegia has been a tremendous advantage for it has allowed protection of those areas of myocardium supplied by patent ITA grafts. In addition, surgical experience helps to avoid damage to patent arterial grafts. In our very early experience there was a trend toward increased mortality and a significant danger of graft damage for patients with patent left ITA grafts [31]. However, that risk has dropped in our more recent series of patients to a mortality rate of 3.7% and a risk of ITA damage of 3.5% for patients with patent left ITA grafts [7]. Although reoperations for patients with patent left ITA grafts are still difficult, they are not riskier.

Reoperations for patients with right ITA grafts are a lot more difficult and a little riskier [7,32]. Strategies for reoperations in this setting must be individualized and have included reoperation through a left thoracotomy to avoid a repeat median sternotomy [33] (thus decreasing the risk of damage to the right ITA graft), use of a small right thoracotomy to dissect the patent right ITA graft away from the sternum prior to repeat median sternotomy, and deep hypothermia with circulatory arrest [32].

Problems that are not unique to reoperation but are more common in the reoperative setting include lack of bypass conduits and diffuse noncardiac atherosclerosis. The use of multiple arterial grafts has been developed not only as a way to provide alternative conduits for patients whose saphenous veins have already been removed, but also as a potential solution to the problem of vein graft atherosclerosis and late vein graft failure. The advantages of arterial grafts are that they are often available and that they may offer long-term protection against atherosclerosis. The disadvantages are that they are smaller bypass conduits than vein grafts and they make a reoperation longer, more extensive, and more technically demanding.

The left and right ITAs are the most proven arterial bypass conduits [13, 34–38]. Angiographic study of patients who might be candidates for reoperation should include ITA angiograms, to ensure their availability and freedom from atherosclerosis, either involving the ITA itself or the subclavian artery. When the left ITA is available at reoperation, it is used routinely, usually as a graft to the LAD coronary artery. Use of the right ITA at reoperation as an in situ graft can be difficult, because scarring of the endothoracic fascia may make it troublesome to obtain length on the pedicle. Thus, it is frequently necessary to use the right ITA as a "free graft." This requires a proximal anastomosis that can be constructed either to the aorta or to a new or old left ITA graft [39].

One of the goals of our most recent review of our reoperative experience was to ask whether or not the use of ITA grafts increased the risks of reoperation. When we divided the patients into subgroups based on the number of ITA grafts done at primary operation and the number done at reoperation, we found that the more ITA grafts that were used the *lower* the in-hospital mortality rate at reoperation. Since that was not a randomized study, there were substantial differences in patient-related variables among those subgroups, but with logistic regression analysis it still appeared that not having an ITA graft at either the first or second operation was the factor most associated with in-hospital mortality. Although a multivariate analysis does not turn a retrospective nonrandomized study into a randomized prospective study, we can reasonably say that the use of ITA grafts did not appear to increase the risk of reoperation [7].

Another concern about the use of ITA grafts has been the risk of wound complication. Large studies have shown that the use of simultaneous bilateral ITA grafts does increase the risk of wound complication in diabetic patients but not in nondiabetics [40]. However, when a single ITA graft was used at a primary operation and a second ITA graft was used at reoperation, we have not noted an increase in wound complications, even in diabetic patients [7].

The right gastroepiploic artery (RGEA) has also been used at reoperation, almost always as an in situ graft to the right coronary artery system. When compared to the ITAs, the RGEA is less consistent in size, more friable, and more prone to spasm. However, midterm patency data regarding RGEA grafts is very encouraging at 2 postoperative years, and anecdotal patency at 5 years after operation has been documented [41]. A major advantage of the RGEA is that a proximal anastomosis is not needed. RGEA grafts are technically more difficult to perform, but we have not noted an increase in morbidity or mortality associated with the use of this graft.

The inferior epigastric artery (IEA) runs posterior to the rectus muscle within the abdominal wall and has been used as a free graft to coronary arteries. Data concerning the long-term patency rate of this graft is scanty but encouraging at 2 years [42]. The radial artery was used as an alternative bypass conduit in the early years of the coronary surgery era but was largely abandoned because of poor patency rates. Its use has been revived in combination with treatment with calcium channel blockers designed to prevent spasm. The early patency data (within a year of operation) are reasonable [43]. However, only time will prove its efficacy.

Assessment of bypass conduit availability is important when evaluating reoperative strategies, particularly when patients have had multiple previous operations. We perform lower extremity venous Doppler mapping studies of reoperative candidates in preference to phlebography, and also use Doppler imaging to evaluate the inferior epigastric and radial arteries. Angiography of the ITAs is very helpful, particularly if ITA use is critical. We rarely perform celiac angiography.

The use of free arterial grafts requires a proximal anastomosis, and at reoperation the scarring and thickening of the reoperative aorta may make an arterial graft to aortic anastomosis difficult. We have often used the hood of a new or old vein graft as the site of a proximal arterial anastomosis during repeat surgery. Another alternative is to construct a proximal anastomosis of a new free arterial graft to a new left ITA graft (T-graft) or to a previously constructed and patent left ITA to LAD graft.

Diffuse noncoronary atherosclerosis, particularly aortic atherosclerosis, is not unique to patients undergoing reoperation, but it is more common in the reoperative setting. The importance of aortic atherosclerosis is that it complicates cannulation for cardiopulmonary bypass and creates the risk of embolization of atherosclerotic debris from the aorta, a cause of stroke, myocardial infarction, and peripheral organ failure [44,45]. The ability to identify the presence of ascending aortic atherosclerosis with echocardiography has been a major help in avoiding these serious complications.

Managing severe aortic atherosclerosis is more difficult than identifying it. Aortic endarterectomy and graft replacement of the ascending aorta can be used to treat severe aortic atherosclerosis. But to accomplish these maneuvers safely requires deep hypothermia and circulatory arrest, and to use those techniques requires cardiopulmonary bypass. Just establishing cardiopulmonary bypass and achieving circulatory arrest has risks when severe ascending aortic atherosclerosis is present. We have used axillary artery cannulation to establish bypass and retrograde (superior vena cava) cerebral perfusion during circulatory arrest to allow the management of aortic atherosclerosis and to treat possible cerebral embolization, with encouraging results in these difficult situations [46,47].

IV. THE EFFECT OF REOPERATION ON THE SURVIVAL OF PATIENTS WITH STENOTIC VEIN GRAFTS

None of the randomized studies of the treatment of coronary artery disease have included patients with previous bypass surgery. Furthermore, few observational studies are available that document the life expectancy for patients with recurrent ischemic syndromes after bypass surgery. The prediction of outcome for patients with prior surgery is complex, because that outcome will depend upon the behavior of many types of pathology rather than just on the behavior of native coronary artery disease alone. Our understanding of the "natural history" and therefore of the indications for therapy for patients post-bypass surgery is in its infancy. In an attempt to start to gain some insight into the management of patients post–bypass surgery, we undertook two studies of patients who had had bypass surgery and who then underwent a postoperative angiogram.

Our first study involved the retrospective comparison of 723 patients who had a documented stenosis (20–99%) in at least one vein-to-coronary bypass graft with 573 patients who had an angiogram after bypass surgery that showed no stenotic vein grafts [48]. Patients who underwent reoperation or angioplasty within a year of this postoperative angiogram were excluded from the study. The analysis of late outcome via univariate and multivariate analyses showed that late vein graft stenoses ($\geq$5 years after operation) were more dangerous than early vein graft stenoses (<5 years after operation), and that a late stenosis in a vein graft to the LAD coronary artery was a predictor of a decreased long-term survival and event-free survival.

Our second study, also a retrospective, nonrandomized study, was designed to answer the question of whether or not reoperation prolonged the survival of patients with stenotic vein grafts [26]. In this study, the 723 patients from our first study with stenotic vein grafts were considered the medically treated group (MED group). They did not undergo reoperation or PTCA within a year after their angiogram (intention to treat medically) but could undergo repeat surgery at a later date. They were compared to 394 patients who were found to have a stenotic vein graft and who underwent reoperation within 1 month of their catheterization (intention to treat surgically, REOP group). There were some obvious biases present in the selection of therapy for these patients. Patients in the REOP group had a higher prevalence of high-risk characteristics such as late vein graft stenoses, severe symptoms, abnormal left ventricular function, left main stenoses, and they had fewer patent saphenous vein grafts and ITA grafts. Thus, there was a tendency to suggest reoperation for higher-risk patients and medical therapy for patients who seemed to be in a situation where they might be alright without reoperation.

The reoperations for the REOP group were carried out during the late 1970s and early 1980s, and the in-hospital risks reflected the risks for patients with stenotic vein grafts at that time. There was no mortality for patients with early vein graft stenoses and a 5.1% risk (17 of 335) for patients with late stenoses in vein grafts, including an 8.5% risk for patients with a late stenosis in an SVG–LAD graft. With our current methods of myocardial protection, the in-hospital mortality for patients with a late stenosis in an LAD vein graft is less than 4% [7].

Multiple variables were tested for their influence on long-term outcome (including in-hospital mortality) via univariate and multivariate testing. Not surprisingly, the results were complex. Patients with early stenoses in vein grafts did not appear to have an improved survival with reoperation. Table 2 shows the results of that multivariate model. Comparison of the univariate survival

Table 2 Multivariate Models of Variables Influencing Survival for Patients with Early and with Late Vein Graft Stenoses

Early (<5 years) vein graft stenoses		
	p Value	Relative risks
Variables *decreasing* survival:		
LVG (moderate/severe)	.0001	2.55
Age (at catheterization)	.0001	1.04
Angina at catheterization	.0408	1.54
Occluded SVG–LAD	.0286	2.03
3 VD/LM[a]	.0287	1.57
Late (≥5 years) vein graft stenoses		
	p Value	Relative risks
Variables *decreasing* survival:		
LVG (moderate/severe)	.0001	2.58
Age (at catheterization)	.0001	1.04
3 VD/LM	.0011	2.87
LAD vein graft stenosis (20–99%)	.0019	1.90
Variables *increasing* survival:		
Reoperation	.0007	0.51

3 VD/LM = triple-vessel disease and/or left main coronary artery stenosis; LVG = left ventriculogram.
From Ref. 26.

curves of the MED and REOP groups of patients with early stenoses shows that survival was good for the REOP group but that the medically treated patients also did well (Figure 2). Patients in the reoperation subgroup started out being much more symptomatic than patients in the medically treated group, and reoperation was a very effective way of improving their symptoms. It should also be noted that of the medically treated patients with early vein graft stenoses, 33% eventually underwent reoperation. However, it did appear that patients with early vein graft stenoses could be safely treated on the basis of their symptoms and that mildly symptomatic patients with early stenoses were not at a high risk of death if treated without surgery.

It was a different story for patients with late vein graft stenoses. Multivariate testing (Table 2) showed that a late stenosis in an LAD vein graft was a specific factor decreasing survival and that reoperation was a specific factor increasing survival. Univariate comparisons of the REOP and MED groups with late vein graft stenoses are shown in Figure 3. The positive effect of reoperation is more evident in the multivariate model because the patients in the REOP group had a higher incidence of unfavorable characteristics.

Univariate comparisons for patients with late stenoses in SVG–LAD grafts are shown in Figure 4. It was this subgroup where the long-term benefit of reoperation was most obvious, despite a slightly increased in-hospital risk of reoperation, mainly because this subgroup did very poorly with medical treatment. When patients were divided into subgroups based on the severity

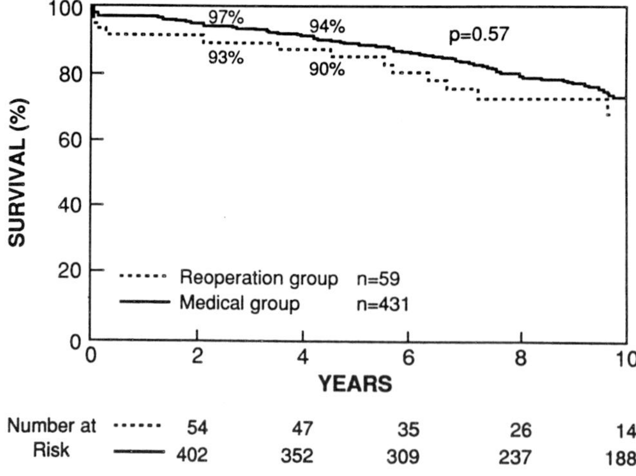

Figure 2 There was no difference in the survival of patients with early (<5 postoperative years) stenoses in vein grafts treated medically or surgically (p = not significant). (From Ref. 26.)

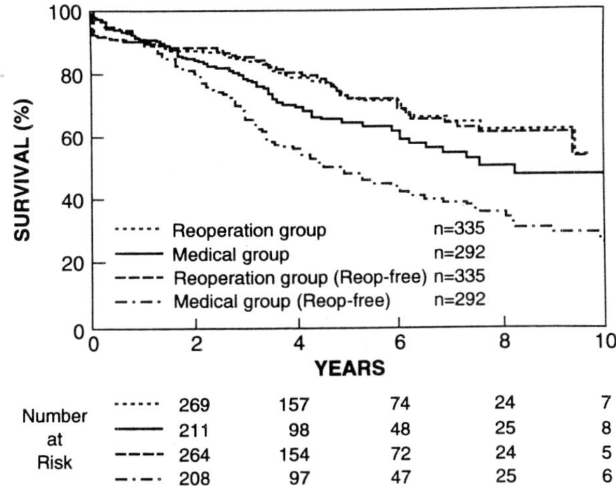

Figure 3 Survival and reoperation-free survival of patients with late (≥5 years) stenoses in saphenous vein grafts. Patients undergoing reoperation had improved survival. Patients in the group initially treated medically had reoperation-free survival of only 48% at 5 years. (From Ref. 26.)

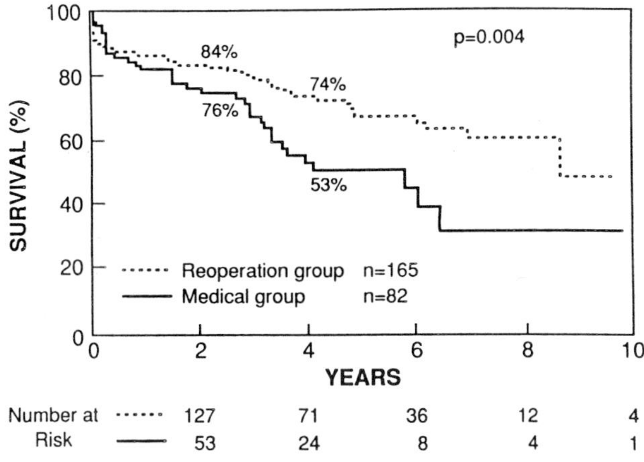

Figure 4 Patients with late stenoses in saphenous vein grafts to the LAD coronary artery had improved survival when compared to patients treated without initial reoperation. (From Ref. 26.)

of an LAD vein graft stenosis, the benefit of surgery was obvious throughout the follow-up period for patients with severe (50–99%) stenoses. Patients with mild to moderate stenoses (20–49%) in LAD vein grafts initially did well with medical management, but deaths began to occur within a year after operation. And for the entire period of this study there was a trend toward improved survival for the REOP group, even for patients with mild to moderate stenoses (Figure 5).

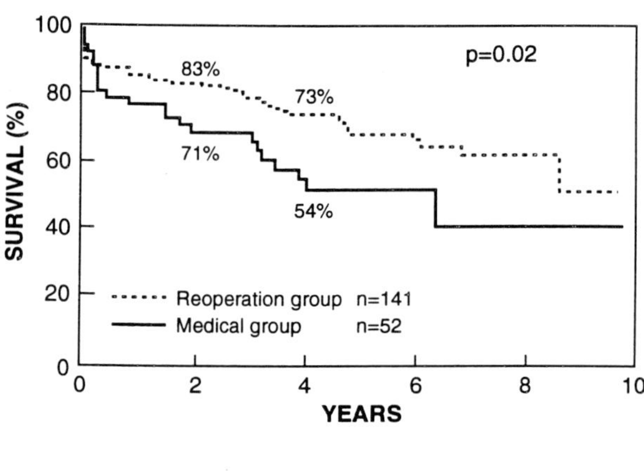

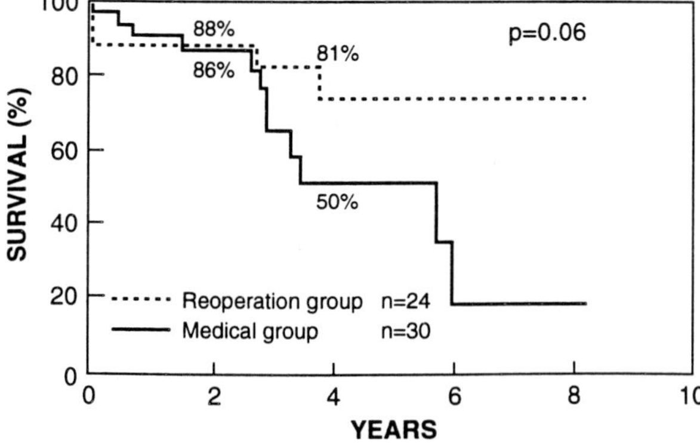

Figure 5 Survival of patients with stenotic saphenous vein to LAD grafts. Patients with severe stenoses (50–99%) (top graph) had superior survival for patients in the reoperation group. For patients with moderate stenoses (bottom), survival of medically treated patients was initially favorable but deteriorated abruptly after 2 years. (From Ref. 26.)

The improvement in survival with reoperation did not appear to be dependent upon severe symptoms. When the subgroup of patients with late vein graft stenoses and mild (NYHA I or II) angina was examined as a subgroup, multivariate testing still indicated that reoperation improved survival. Again, a stenosis in the LAD vein graft was a specific factor decreasing survival.

The one subgroup of patients with late vein graft stenoses for whom reoperation did not appear to improve survival was patients who had a patent ITA graft to the LAD coronary artery in addition to a stenotic vein graft (Figure 6). Both the MED and REOP groups of patients with patent ITA grafts had very favorable late survival. Again, it is important to realize that patients with severe symptoms and large amounts of myocardium in jeopardy were concentrated in the group that underwent reoperation. However, it appears that patients who have a patent ITA–LAD graft, are not severely symptomatic, and do not have large areas of myocardium in jeopardy may be safely treated without surgery, at least initially.

We do not consider these studies to be the last word in how to treat patients with previous bypass surgery. However, they are a start. The study of patients after bypass surgery is complex, since outcome appears to be related not only to ventricular function and the amount of myocardium in jeopardy, but to the vessel and pathology that jeopardizes that myocardium. A stenosis

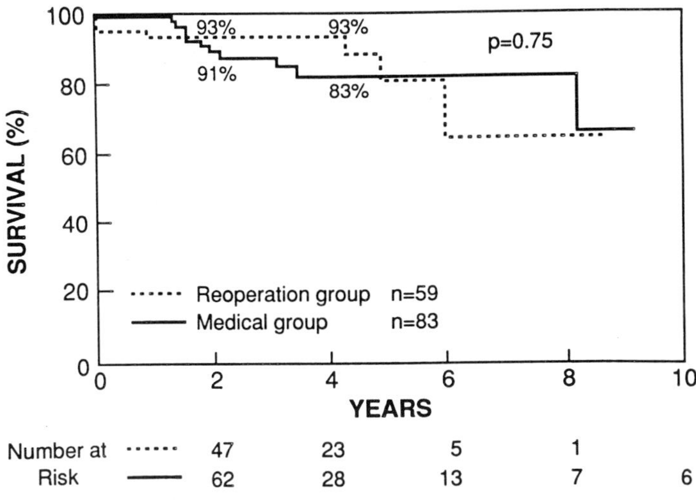

Figure 6   The survival of patients with patent ITA grafts to the LAD in addition to at least one stenotic vein graft was equivalent for the MED and REOP groups. (From Ref. 26.)

in a native coronary artery has a different natural history than a stenosis in an IMA graft, and both are different from a stenosis in a vein graft. Therefore, patients with stenoses in vein grafts are a very heterogeneous group. Some subgroups will have a good outcome without any treatment, and some must undergo repeat surgery or they are faced with a high likelihood of death. Patients with early stenoses in vein grafts usually can be treated according to their symptomatic status: If they are not highly symptomatic, they do not appear to be faced with a high risk of short-term mortality if they don't undergo repeat surgery. When they are symptomatic, reoperation is relatively safe and provides consistent symptom relief. On the other hand, patients with late stenoses in vein grafts are in significant danger without repeat surgery, and reoperation does appear to improve their long-term survival even if they are not severely symptomatic. This principle is particularly true for patients with late stenoses in LAD vein grafts. The exception to that principle is that patients with patent ITA grafts to the anterior descending coronary artery appear to have reasonably favorable survival without reoperation.

The availability of percutaneous means of treating vein graft stenoses makes decision making today even more difficult. Articles elsewhere in this text address the details of the results of interventional treatment for vein grafts. The role of percutaneous treatment is hard to assess because of the lack of risk-stratified patient-based studies and few long-term data regarding the angiographic outcome of vein grafts after interventional treatments. However, some observations are worth noting.

Percutaneous treatments of vein grafts are safer when early lesions are involved, and the recurrence rate of early lesions is much less than the recurrence rate of late atherosclerotic lesions. Atherosclerotic vein grafts have a high risk of recurrence after percutaneous treatments, and, if the occurrence of a stenosis anywhere in the graft is used as the index of recurrence, the risk of recurrence continues to rise even beyond the 6 months to 1 year period after angioplasty. Thus, the long-term angiographic outcome after percutaneous treatments of late stenoses of vein grafts remains very uncertain.

For these reasons it is most logical to use percutaneous treatments for symptomatic patients who are not in a severely life-threatening situation. Such patients include those with early vein graft stenoses and patients with late vein graft stenoses and discrete vein graft lesions, good ventricular function, single stenotic vein grafts not involving the LAD coronary artery, and those with patent ITA grafts. In other words, patients who are likely to tolerate treatment failure. Surgery is probably most effectively applied to patients with life-threatening anatomy. Those include patients with late stenoses in multiple vein grafts, vein grafts to the anterior descending coronary artery or jeopardizing large amounts of myocardium, and those with poor left ventricular function.

REFERENCES

1. Varnauskas E, The European Coronary Study Group. Twelve-year follow-up of survival in the randomized European Coronary Surgery Study. N Engl J Med 1988; 319:332–337.
2. CASS Principle Investigators. Myocardial infarction and mortality in the Coronary Artery Surgery Study (CASS) randomized trial. N Engl J Med 1984; 310:750–758.
3. Lytle BW, Cosgrove DM. Coronary artery bypass surgery. In: Wells SA, ed. Current Problems in Surgery. Philadelphia: W. B. Saunders, 1992 (Oct):733–807.
4. Lawrie GM, Morris GC Jr, Earle N. Long-term results of coronary artery bypass surgery. Analysis of 1698 patients followed 15 to 20 years. Ann Surg 1991; 213:377–385.
5. Lytle BW, Loop FD, Cosgrove DM, Taylor PC, Goormastic M, Peper W, Gill CC, Golding LAR, Stewart RW. Fifteen hundred coronary reoperations: results and determinants of early and late survival. J Thorac Cardiovasc Surg 1987; 93:847–859.
6. Loop FD, Lytle BW, Cosgrove DM, Woods EL, Stewart RW, Golding LAR, Goormastic M, Taylor PC. Reoperation for coronary atherosclerosis: Changing practice in 2509 consecutive patients. Ann Surg 1990; 212:378–386.
7. Lytle BW, McElroy D, McCarthy PM, Loop FD, Taylor PC, Goormastic M, Stewart RW, Cosgrove DM. The influence of arterial coronary bypass grafts on the mortality of coronary reoperations. J Thorac Cardiovasc Surg 1994; 107:675–683.
8. Salomon NW, Page US, Bigelow JC, Krause AH, Okies JE, Metzdorff MT. Reoperative coronary surgery. Comparative analysis of 6591 patients undergoing primary bypass and 508 patients undergoing reoperative coronary artery bypass. J Thorac Cardiovasc Surg 1990; 100:250–260.
9. Verheul HA, Moulijn AC, Hondema S, Schouwink M, Dunning AJ. Late results of 200 repeat coronary artery bypass operations. Am J Cardiol 1991; 67:24–30.
10. Perrault L, Carrier M, Cartier R, Leclerc Y, Hebert Y, Diaz OS, Pelletier C. Morbidity and mortality of reoperation for coronary artery bypass grafting: significance of atherosclerotic vein grafts. Can J Cardiol 1991; 7:427–430.
11. Galbut DL, Traad EA, Dorman MJ, DeWitt PL, Larsen PB, Kurlansky PA, Carrillo RG, Gentsch TO, Galbut B, Ebra G. Bilateral internal mammary artery grafts in reoperative and primary coronary bypass surgery. Ann Thorac Surg 1991; 52:20–28.
12. Akins CW, Buckley MJ, Daggett WM, Hilgenberg AD, Vlahakes GJ, Torchiana DF, Austen WG. Reoperative coronary grafting: changing patient profiles, operative indications, techniques, and results. Ann Thorac Surg 1994; 58:359–365.
13. Lytle BW, Loop FD, Cosgrove DM, Ratliff NB, Easley K, Taylor PC. Long-term (5 to 12 years) serial studies of internal mammary artery and saphenous vein coronary bypass grafts. J Thorac Cardiovasc Surg 1985; 89:248–258.
14. Bourassa MG, Campeau L, Lesperance J. Changes in grafts and coronary arteries after coronary bypass surgery. Cardiovasc Clin 1991; 21:83–100.
15. Neitzel GF, Barboriak JJ, Pintar K, Qureshi I. Atherosclerosis in aortocoronary bypass grafts. Morphologic study and risk factor analysis 6 to 12 years after surgery. Arteriosclerosis 1986; 6:594–600.

16. Solymoss BC, Leung TK, Pelletier LC, Campeau L. Pathologic changes in coronary artery saphenous vein grafts and related etiologic factors. Cardiovasc Clin 1991; 21:45–65.
17. Fitzgibbon GM, Leach AJ, Kafka HP, Keon WJ. Coronary bypass graft fate: long-term angiographic study. J Am Coll Cardiol 1991; 17:1075–1080.
18. Chesebro JH, Fuster V, Elveback LR, Clements IP, Smith HC, Holmes DR Jr, Bardsley WT, Pluth JR, Wallace RB, Puga FJ. Effect of dipyridamole and aspirin on late vein graft patency after coronary bypass operations. N Engl J Med 1984; 310:209–214.
19. Goldman S, Copeland J, Moritz T, Henderson W, Zadina K, Ovitt T, Doherty J, Read R, Chesler E, Sako Y. Saphenous vein graft patency 1 year after coronary artery bypass surgery and effects of antiplatelet therapy. Circulation 1989; 80: 1190–1197.
20. Gavaghan TP, Gebski V, Baron DW. Immediate postoperative aspirin improves vein graft patency early and late after coronary artery bypass graft surgery. A placebo-controlled, randomized study. Circulation 1991; 83:1526–1533.
21. Ratliff NB, Myles JL. Rapidly progressive atherosclerosis in aortocoronary saphenous vein grafts. Possible immuno-mediated disease. Arch Pathol Lab Med 1989; 113:772–776.
22. Jain U, Sullivan HJ, Pifarre R, Winters G, Grieco J, Calandra D, Hinkamp T. Graft atheroembolism as the probable cause of failure to wean from cardiopulmonary bypass. J Cardiolthorac Anesthesia 1990; 4:476–480.
23. Keon WJ, Heggtveit HA, Lecluc J. Perioperative myocardial infarction caused by atheroembolization. J Thorac Cardiovasc Surg 1982; 84:849–855.
24. Cosgrove DM, Loop FD, Lytle BW, Gill CC, Golding LAR, Gibson C, Stewart RW, Taylor PC, Goormastic M. Predictors of reoperation after myocardial revascularization. J Thorac Cardiovasc Surg 1986; 92:811–821.
25. Clark RE, The Ad Hoc Committee. Data Analyses of The Society of Thoracic Surgeons National Cardiac Surgery Database, January 1994.
26. Lytle BW, Loop FD, Taylor PC, Goormastic M, Stewart RW, Novoa R, McCarthy PM, Cosgrove DM. The effect of coronary reoperation on the survival of patients with stenoses in saphenous vein to coronary bypass grafts. J Thorac Cardiovasc Surg 1993; 105:605–614.
27. Buckberg GD. Strategies and logic of cardioplegic delivery to prevent, avoid and reverse ischemic and reperfusion damage. J Thorac Cardiovasc Surg 1987; 93:127–139.
28. Menasche P, Kural S, Fauchet M. Retrograde coronary sinus perfusion: a safe alternative for ensuring cardioplegic delivery in aortic valve surgery. Ann Thorac Surg 1982; 34:647–658.
29. Gundry SR, Razzouk AJ, Vigesaa RE, Wang N, Bailey LL. Optimal delivery of cardioplegic solution for "redo" operations. J Thorac Cardiovasc Surg 1992; 103:896–901.
30. Partington MT, Acar C, Buckberg GD, Julia PL. Studies of retrograde cardioplegia. II. Advantages of antegrade/retrograde cardioplegia to optimize distribution in jeopardized myocardium. J Thorac Cardiovasc Surg 1989; 97:613–622.
31. Baillot RG, Loop FD, Cosgrove DM, Lytle BW. Reoperation after previous grafting with the internal mammary artery: technique and early results. Ann Thorac Surg 1985; 40:271–273.

32. Joyce FS, McCarthy PM, Taylor PC, Cosgrove DM, Lytle BW. Cardiac reoperation in patients with bilateral thoracic artery grafts. Ann Thorac Surg 1994; 58:80–85.

33. Ungerleider RM, Mills NL, Wechsler AS. Left thoracotomy for reoperative coronary artery bypass procedures. Ann Thorac Surg 1985; 40:11–15.

34. Loop FD, Lytle BW, Cosgrove DM, Stewart RW, Goormastic M, Williams GW, Golding LAR, Gill CC, Taylor PC, Sheldon WC, Proudfit WL. Influence of the internal-mammary-artery graft on 10-year survival and other cardiac events. N Engl J Med 1986; 314:1–6.

35. Dion R, Verheist R, Rousseau M, Goenen M, Ponlot R, Kestens-Servaye Y, Chalant CH. Sequential mammary grafting. Clinical, functional and angiographic assessment 6 months postoperatively in 231 consecutive patients. J Thorac Cardiovasc Surg 1989; 98:80–88.

36. Sargeant P, Lasaffre E, Flameny W. Internal mammary artery: methods of use and their effect on survival. Eur J Cardiothorac Surg 1990; 4:72–78.

37. Galbut DL, Traad EA, Dorman WJ, DeWitt PL, Larsen PB, Kirlansky PA, Button JH, Ally JM, Gentsch TO. Seventeen-year experience with bilateral internal mammary artery grafts. Ann Thorac Surg 1990; 4:195–201.

38. Fiore AC, Naunheim KS, Dean P, Kaiser GC, Pennington G, Willman VL, McBride LR, Barner HB. Results of internal thoracic artery grafting over 15 years: single vs. double grafts. Ann Thorac Surg 1990; 49:202–208.

39. Tector AJ, Amundsen S, Schmahl TM, Kress DC, Peter M. Total revascularization with T grafts. Ann Thorac Surg 1994; 57:33–39.

40. Loop FD, Lytle BW, Cosgrove DM, Mahfood S, McHenry MC, Goormastic M, Stewart RW, Golding LAR, Taylor PC. Sternal wound complications after isolated coronary artery bypass grafting: early and late mortality, morbidity and cost of care. Ann Thorac Surg 1990; 49:179–187.

41. Suma H, Wanibuchi Y, Terada Y, Fukuda S, Takayama T, Furuta S. The right gastroepiploic artery graft: clinical and angiographic midterm results in 200 patients. J Thorac Cardiovasc Surg 1993; 105:615–623.

42. Buche M, Schroeder E, Gurné O, Chenu P, Paquay JL, Marchandise B, Eucher P, Louagie Y, Dion R, Schoevaerdts JC. Coronary artery bypass grafting with the inferior epigastric artery. Midterm clinical and angiographic results. J Thorac Cardiovasc Surg 1995; 109:553–560.

43. Acar C, Jebara VA, Portoghese M, Beyssen B, Pagny JY, Grare P, Chachques JC, Fabiani JN, Deloche A, Guermonprez JL, Carpentier AF. Revival of the radial artery for coronary artery bypass grafting. Ann Thorac Surg 1992; 54:652–660.

44. Barzilai B, Marshall WG Jr, Saffitz JE, Kouchoukos N. Avoidance of embolic complications by ultrasonic characterization of the ascending aorta. Circulation 1989; 80(suppl I):I275–I279.

45. Blauth CI, Cosgrove DM, Webb BW, Ratliff NB, Boylan M, Piedmonte MR, Lytle BW, Loop FD. Atheroembolism from the ascending aorta: an emerging problem in cardiac surgery. J Thorac Cardiovasc Surg 1992; 103:1104–1112.

46. Sabik JF, Lytle BW, McCarthy PM, Cosgrove DM. Axillary artery: an alternative site of arterial cannulation for patients with extensive aortic and peripheral vascular disease. J Thorac Cardiovasc Surg 1995; 109:885–891.

47. Lytle BW, McCarthy PM, Meaney KM, Stewart RW, Cosgrove DM. Systemic hypothermia and circulatory arrest combined with arterial perfusion of the superior vena cava: effective intraoperative cerebral protection. J Thorac Cardiovasc Surg 1995; 109:738–743.
48. Lytle BW, Loop FD, Taylor PC, Simpfendorfer C, Kramer JR, Ratliff NB, Goormastic M, Cosgrove DM. Vein graft disease: the clinical impact of stenoses in saphenous vein bypass grafts to coronary arteries. J Thorac Cardiovasc Surg 1992; 103:831–840.

15

Acute Myocardial Infarction in Patients with Prior Revascularization Surgery

Charles Maynard and W. Douglas Weaver*
University of Washington School of Medicine, Seattle, Washington

I. INTRODUCTION

During the 1970s and '80s, there were dramatic increases in the use of coronary artery bypass surgery (CABS) [1]. More recently, with the widespread availability and use of coronary angioplasty, there have been significant changes in the characteristics of patients undergoing CABS. These include an increase in the average age of patients, including an increase in octogenarians, a greater proportion of patients with severe, multivessel, complex coronary artery disease, and more patients with severe left ventricular dysfunction. In addition, there is evidence that the number of reoperations increased during the early 1980s [1].

As a result of the relatively frequent use of CABS performed in this country over the past 20 years, an increasing proportion of patients hospitalized with acute myocardial infarction (AMI) have histories of prior CABS. Although there is considerable information about the epidemiology, treatment, and outcome of patients with AMI, comparatively little is known about the subgroup of patients with prior CABS, including the efficacy and outcome of acute reperfusion therapies in these patients.

Current affiliation: Henry Ford Healthcare System, Detroit, Michigan.

II. PURPOSE AND ORGANIZATION

The purpose of this chapter is first to review existing information about the epidemiology, treatment, and short- and long-term outcome of patients with AMI who have undergone prior CABS. A second objective is to report new findings concerning patients from the Myocardial Infarction Triage and Intervention (MITI) registry; this database includes all individuals who were admitted to coronary care units in all hospitals in the Seattle metropolitan area (King County, Wash.) during the years 1988–1993. In examining the subset of patients who had the diagnosis of AMI at discharge or death, patients with and without prior CABS will be compared with respect to baseline characteristics, treatment, and outcome, including hospital mortality, prolonged angina, reinfarction, new congestive heart failure, and long-term survival.

III. EXISTING KNOWLEDGE

A. Epidemiology

Investigations from institutions in three major metropolitan areas in the United States and Canada have provided considerable information about the prevalence of CABS in patients with AMI and have characterized these patients with respect to age, gender, prior medical histories, and presenting features. In the earliest series (1977–1982) from the Montreal Heart Institute, 77 (4%) of 2,000 consecutive patients with AMI had undergone previous CABS and developed AMI 2 or more months after revascularization [2]. The average time from previous CABS to the index AMI was 4.5 years in the 77 patients who were younger than 70 years of age. In comparison to 77 control patients with AMI, patients with previous CABS were more often men and more often had a history of previous myocardial infarction. The two groups were similar with respect to other cardiac histories, including hypertension and congestive heart failure.

In a follow-up report (1978–1986), 205 (5%) of 4,051 patients with AMI had previous revascularization and were younger than 70 years [3]. In comparison to their counterparts who were not revascularized prior to developing AMI, patients with previous CABS were predominantly male and more often had histories of previous myocardial infarction. In Montreal the prevalence of previous CABS in patients with AMI increased from 2.3% in the late 1970s to 6.7% in 1980–81, and to 11.2% in 1982–84 [4].

In a more recent report of patients with AMI from San Diego, Calif., Vancouver, British Columbia, and Geneva, Switzerland, 219 (9%) of 2,494 hospitalized between 1984 and 1989 had previous bypass surgery [5]. Patients with previous CABS were more often male and more frequently had evidence

these therapies in patients with previous revascularization. Reperfusion therapies were used at about half the rate that they were in patients without previous bypass surgery; in the population from San Diego and other cities, 11% received thrombolysis, coronary angioplasty, or bypass surgery within 2 days of infarction, whereas 20% of patients without previous revascularization received these interventions. In the MITI registry, thrombolytic therapy, angioplasty, and bypass surgery were employed prior to hospital discharge in 20%, 14%, and 12%, respectively, of patients with previous revascularization. Only coronary angioplasty was used more frequently (20%) in the group without revascularization; the use of other reperfusion therapies was similar. In MITI, 38% of patients with previous bypass surgery had at least one intervention; in addition, cardiac catheterization prior to hospital discharge was used in 54% of these patients, whereas in San Diego 49% of similar patients underwent coronary angiography within 60 days of infarction.

Despite the frequent use of thrombolytic therapy and primary angioplasty in patients with previous surgical revascularization, little is known about the efficacy of these therapies. This statement is particularly true with respect to thrombolytic therapy, since patients with bypass grafts were excluded from most randomized trials of thrombolytic agents. Our current understanding of the efficacy of thrombolytic therapy in patients with bypass grafts is from several studies in which fewer than 12 patients with bypass grafts received intracoronary or intravenous thrombolytic therapy [7,9–11].

In the review by Grines et al., 11 of the 50 patients received intravenous thrombolytic therapy (streptokinase or urokinase); infarct vessel patency was achieved in three of three native coronary arteries but in only two of eight patients with vein grafts [7]. A more direct approach of emergency cardiac catheterization with intragraft thrombolytic therapy was successful in restoring patency in 8 of 10 occluded saphenous veins; in some instances, thrombolytic drugs were followed with balloon angioplasty. The authors concluded that the large mass of thrombus and minimal or absent flow in the graft may have necessitated larger doses of intravenous agents, or the use of intragraft thrombolysis, or mechanical means of reperfusion, including angioplasty or bypass surgery.

Conversely, Kleiman et al. reported successful reperfusion with intravenous thrombolytic therapy [recombinant tissue plasminogen activator (rt-PA)] in four of five patients with bypass grafts [9]. In a series of 40 patients with previous CABS who were treated with angioplasty and/or thrombolytic therapy, Kavanaugh and Topol reported that in four patients treated with intravenous thrombolytic therapy only, three patients had successful reperfusion with rt-PA; the one patient who was not reperfused had an occluded native coronary artery [10]. Unfortunately, given the small numbers of patients in these series, it is difficult to make definitive statements about the efficacy of thrombolytic therapy in patients with bypass grafts. Rt-PA *may* be a better agent for these patients. As in the study by Grines et al. [7], only urokinase and streptokinase were used, and they did not perform as well as in the studies where rt-PA was used. But the numbers of patients studied were small and therefore not conclusive. In the MITI registry, many more patients with bypass grafts received thrombolytic therapy; however, information about the reperfusion status of these patients was not available, because few patients received 90-minute angiography. In addition, the relevant angiograms have not been collected and centrally released.

There is somewhat more evidence about the efficacy of coronary angioplasty during AMI for patients with previous bypass grafts. One group of investigators suggested that angioplasty of totally occluded venous bypass grafts should not be attempted because of the high rate of reocclusion [12], although this conclusion was based on results in only 15 patients. Alternatively, others have not encountered such difficulty and instead report favorable results with direct angioplasty or a combination of lytic therapy and angioplasty [7,8,10]. In a relatively large series of patients with bypass grafts, 72 patients (26 anterior, 46 inferior) underwent direct coronary angioplasty during AMI [8]. These patients were 12% of all patients with AMI at the Mid-American Heart Institute from 1981 through 1989. Direct angioplasty without antecedent thrombolytic therapy was successful in 85% of vein grafts and in 100% of native arteries. The authors concluded that prior bypass surgery should not preclude reperfusion therapy by direct coronary angioplasty, for it can be performed safely and result in excellent short- and long-term survival. Since direct coronary angioplasty was the predominant mode of reperfusion therapy for all patients with AMI at this institution, it was not possible to compare the results of direct angioplasty with those achieved by thrombolytic therapy.

Finally, there are few published reports about the use of other intracoronary devices (e.g., stents, atherectomy catheters) for AMI in patients with previous bypass grafts [13]. There is a role for coronary artery bypass surgery as reperfusion therapy for patients with previous bypass grafts, and there is a body of literature concerning emergency CABS for patients with AMI [14]. However, patients with previous bypass grafts who undergo CABS within 30 days of AMI are at extremely high risk; in one study their risk of death was three times that of patients with AMI who were undergoing their first bypass operations [15].

D. Outcomes

In both San Diego and Seattle, patients with previous CABS who were hospitalized with suspected AMI had mortality similar to their counterparts who did not have bypass grafts. In Seattle, hospital mortality was 10.5% for the group with previous CABS and was 9.9% for those without, whereas in San

Diego it was 7% and 9%, respectively. Also at the Montreal Heart Institute, hospital mortality was similar for patients with previous bypass grafts and for selected controls with AMI. In the MITI registry, the occurrence of complications such as recurrent chest pain, new congestive heart failure, and cardiac arrest was similar in the two groups.

Of interest in the MITI registry was the result that patients with previous CABS who received reperfusion therapies experienced higher hospital mortality than did their counterparts who did not have previous bypass grafts yet received these therapies. For patients receiving thrombolytic therapy, hospital mortality was higher for patients with previous bypass surgery (11.3%) than it was for those who did not have bypass grafts prior to infarction (5.4%). Similar findings were noted for patients undergoing coronary angioplasty (11.9% vs. 5.0%) and coronary artery bypass surgery (16.7% vs. 7.7%) at any time prior to hospital discharge. Among those patients who had one or more interventions during hospitalization, prior bypass surgery was a statistically significant predictor of hospital mortality, even after adjusting for the fact that patients with bypass grafts had considerably higher levels of risk than their counterparts. This finding is indicative of the relatively high risk of patients with prior surgery and the extremely low risk of patients without grafts who received reperfusion therapies [16].

Finally, the long-term prognosis after AMI in patients with prior CABS has been assessed by investigators from Montreal and San Diego [3,5]. For patients treated at the Montreal Heart Institute, cumulative mortality 5 years after discharge was similar in the postbypass and control groups (30% vs. 25%); however, patients with previous surgery more often had reinfarction, more hospital admissions for unstable angina, and more revascularization procedures. In San Diego, 1-year cardiac mortality was higher for patients with prior CABS (16% vs. 8%); yet after adjustment for risk factors associated with mortality, prior bypass surgery was only of borderline statistical significance in predicting 1-year mortality. The adjusted odds ratio of death at 1 year for patients with prior CABS as opposed to those without a history of surgery was 1.3 (95% confidence interval = 1.0, 1.7).

E. Summary

The prevalence of previous coronary artery surgery in patients with AMI increased from 4% in the late 1970s to over 10% in the late 1980s. This is not surprising, given the rapid increase in the number of patients undergoing CABS in the late '70s and early '80s and given the fact that the mean time from surgery to AMI was about 7 years. Despite having higher levels of risk, as evidenced by increased congestive heart failure, history of previous infarction, and angina, patients with bypass grafts had hospital mortality similar to that of patients who had AMI but did not have previous CABS. This discrepancy could be explained by the fact that patients with previous CABS generally have smaller infarcts [4]. In addition, the long-term prognosis for patients with previous grafts is not as good, mainly because of increased severity of disease and reduced left ventricular function [5].

Even in the mid-1990s, our understanding of the mechanism of AMI in patients with previous bypass grafts is deficient. The exclusion of these patients from randomized trials of thrombolytic therapy and angioplasty is in part responsible for this deficiency. Unfortunately, little is known concerning optimal methods for treating patients with bypass grafts who develop AMI; current knowledge is based on studies with small numbers of patients or insufficient numbers to allow for meaningful comparisons of strategies. As seen in the MITI registry, patients with previous CABS who received reperfusion therapy were generally at higher risk than typical patients who were at relatively low risk. Unfortunately, current findings say little about which reperfusion strategies might be more effective for patients with previous surgery; for example, there are no published, controlled comparisons, let alone randomized ones, of angioplasty vs. thrombolytic therapy in these patients. Given that 10% of patients with AMI have previous bypass grafts—a considerable number of patients nationwide—the need for knowledge of optimal treatment strategies for these patients is imperative.

IV. NEW FINDINGS FROM THE MITI REGISTRY

A. The MITI Registry

The MITI registry of all patients admitted to coronary care units in metropolitan Seattle was implemented in part to provide perspective to the MITI randomized trial of prehospital vs. hospital-initiated thrombolytic therapy [17]. In addition, the registry has produced important information about the treatment and outcomes of all patients with AMI. Since the trial considered for enrollment only those patients eligible for thrombolytic therapy (25–40% of all patients with acute infarction), project investigators believed it was essential that more be known about those not eligible for therapy as well as about those eligible but not enrolled in the trial.

Enrollment in the registry began in January 1988. Patients were identified from coronary care unit admission logs, and information from hospital charts was abstracted to MITI data collection forms by project personnel. Since the inception of the registry, demographic and outcome data have been collected for all patients admitted to coronary care units for suspected AMI. As of December 1993, over 45,000 patients with suspected AMI had been admitted to coronary care units in 19 hospitals in King County, Wash., which includes the city of Seattle and suburban areas. The diagnosis of AMI was established from information contained in patients' medical records and coronary care unit logs.

Variable collection for patients with AMI has changed over the years of the registry. Initially, a six-page form containing detailed information concerning prior medical histories, symptoms on admission to the hospital, laboratory data, hospital course, and therapies, including thrombolytic therapy and angioplasty, was employed for all patients with AMI. However, in 1991 a more detailed data collection form was used for select subsets of patients, including those receiving thrombolytic therapy or coronary angioplasty within 6 hours of hospital admission. In 1993, a simplified form, replacing all previous instruments, was used for all admissions. As of December 1993, the registry included 11,000 patients who developed AMI prior to hospital discharge or death. June 1994 was the last month patients were entered in the registry, because funding for this project has been discontinued.

To date, investigators have produced a variety of published reports using information from the registry. The effects of age [18,19], prior bypass surgery [6], gender [20], race [21,22], cardiac catheterization [23], and coronary angioplasty [24] on outcomes associated with AMI have been examined. In addition, results concerning hospital mortality [16], electrocardiographic readings [25], and most recently changes in the use of thrombolytic therapy over the past 5 years [26] have been published.

B. Patient Population

From January 1988 to December 1993, 11,055 patients with AMI were admitted to coronary care units in 19 hospitals in the metropolitan Seattle area; of these patients, 1,094—or almost 10%—had previous bypass grafts. As can be seen in Figure 1, the proportion of patients with previous CABS was constant over the 6-year period. The mean time from surgery to hospital admission was 7.8 ± 4.1 years in those 497 patients for whom the year of previous surgery was collected.

The distinctive baseline characteristics of AMI patients with prior bypass surgery are shown in Table 1. There was a higher proportion of men in the group with previous CABS, although the two groups did not differ with respect to age. As in previous studies, patients with previous bypass grafts had more complicated cardiac histories; over half of these patients had myocardial infarction prior to the index hospitalization, and over 70% had a history of angina pectoris. In addition, the prevalence of previous congestive heart failure was twice that in the group without previous surgery. Also, of note was the fact that almost 30% of patients with previous CABS had diabetes mellitus, whereas only 19% of patients without previous surgery had this condition. Finally, 15% of patients with previous CABS had coronary angioplasty prior to hospital admission; this was almost five times more than their counterparts without surgery had.

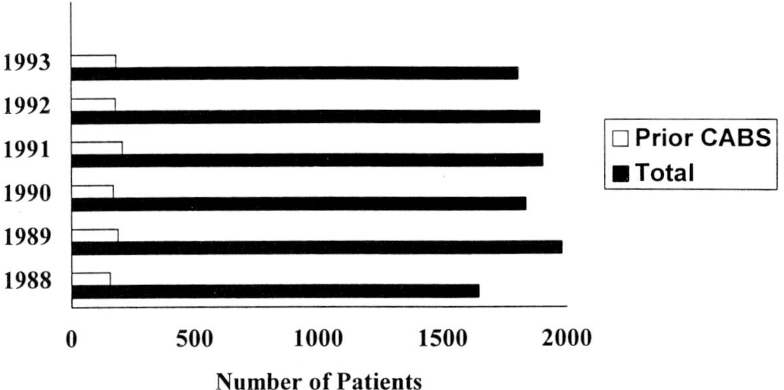

Figure 1 Myocardial infarction in the Myocardial Infarction Triage and Intervention registry, 1988–1993. The open bars display the total number of patients, and the solid bars show the number of patients with previous bypass surgery. CABS = coronary artery bypass surgery.

With respect to symptoms on admission, a slightly higher proportion of patients with previous bypass surgery had chest pain at the time of hospital admission. The incidence of cardiogenic shock was similar in the two groups, and the median time from symptom onset to hospital arrival was 2 hours in both groups (25th and 75th percentiles = 1, 5 hours). Despite more extant coronary artery disease, the use of 911 and emergency medical services was similar for patients with prior CABS and for those without surgery—about half in both groups. Finally, the two groups differed with respect to initial electro-cardiographic characteristics, in that patients with prior surgery less often had acute changes (ST elevation).

C. Treatments

In the two groups, there were statistically significant differences in the use of various treatments, including acute reperfusion therapies (thrombolysis or an-gioplasty) within 6 hours of hospital arrival. As seen in Table 2, thrombolysis at any time prior to hospital discharge was used in 14% of patients with pre-vious CABS and in 24% of other patients. Coronary angioplasty prior to hos-pital discharge was also employed less frequently in patients with previous CABS (17% vs. 24%), although the use of CABS prior to hospital discharge was similar in the two groups (12% vs. 11%). The use of cardiac catheterization prior to hospital discharge was also similar in the two groups of patients.

Table 1 Prior Bypass Surgery and AMI: Patient Characteristics

Variable	Prior surgery ($n = 1,094$)	No prior surgery ($n = 9,960$)	p
Demographics:			
Age	66.1 ± 10.1	66.2 ± 13.6	.78
Women	20.2%	36.0%	<.0001
Race:			
White	94.8%	91.6%	
Black	2.3%	3.9%	
Asian	2.3%	3.7%	
Other	0.6%	0.8%	
History of:			
AMI	57.3%	17.3%	<.0001
CHF	19.0%	10.5%	<.0001
Angina	71.9%	29.5%	<.0001
Hyperlipidemia	29.6%	21.3%	<.0001
Hypertension	45.0%	46.7%	.67
Thrombolysis	3.0%	1.1%	<.0001
Angioplasty	15.2%	3.4%	<.0001
Diabetes	29.5%	18.6%	<.0001
Smoking	21.5%	28.7%	.002
Signs and symptoms on admission:			
Chest pain	94.7%	91.4%	.003
Cardiogenic shock	1.6%	1.6%	.99
Heart rate (beats per minute)	81 ± 20	81 ± 22	.76
Systolic blood pressure (mm Hg)	142 ± 30	143 ± 30	.82
Diastolic blood pressure (mm Hg)	83 ± 18	85 ± 19	.07
Initial ECG findings:			
ST elevation	34%	53%	<0.0001
ST depression	32%	16%	
Bundle branch block	27%	25%	
Normal	1%	2%	
Indeterminate	6%	3%	

AMI = acute myocardial infarction; CHF = congestive heart failure; ECG = electrocardiogram.

Thrombolytic therapy within 6 hours of hospital admission was administered to 11% of patients with previous CABS and to 19% of remaining patients. However, the use of coronary angioplasty within 6 hours of admission was similar in the two groups (6% vs. 8%). Coronary artery surgery within 48 hours of admission was performed in 3% of both groups of patients. Finally, cardiac catheterization within 6 hours of hospital admission was performed in 18% of all patients, and was similar in the two groups.

Table 2 Prior Bypass Surgery and AMI Interventions and Outcomes

Variable	Prior surgery ($n = 1{,}094$)	No prior surgery ($n = 9{,}960$)	p
Treatments:			
Thrombolysis	14.4%	23.7%	<.0001
Thrombolysis <6 hr from hospital arrival	11.4%	19.2%	<.0001
Cardiac catheterization	56.6%	57.2%	.64
Cardiac catheterization <6 hr from hospital arrival	17.9%	18.2%	.85
Angioplasty	17.1%	23.6%	.0001
Angioplasty <6 hr from hospital arrival	6.0%	8.1%	.05
Bypass surgery	12.4%	11.3%	.53
Bypass surgery <48 hr from admission	3.2%	2.6%	.28
Outcomes:			
Recurrent chest pain	26.6%	21.6%	.12
New CHF	21.7%	21.8%	.97
Reinfarction	4.6%	4.0%	.50
Cardiac arrest	10.4%	8.7%	.27
Any stroke	1.8%	2.0%	.77
Hemorrhagic stroke	0.6%	0.0%	.16
Hospital death	10.8%	9.3%	.26

AMI = acute myocardial infarction; CHF = congestive heart failure.

Multivariate logistic regression was used to identify factors associated with receiving thrombolytic therapy, coronary angioplasty, or CABS in the 1,094 patients with previous bypass grafts. Younger age, having undergone coronary angioplasty prior to the index event, and the absence of a history of congestive heart failure were associated with receiving one or more of these treatments. In addition, separate analyses were conducted to identify predictors of (a) intravenous thrombolytic therapy within 6 hours of hospital admission, (b) coronary angioplasty within 6 hours of hospital admission, (c) CABS within 48 hours of hospital admission, (d) coronary angioplasty at any time prior to hospital discharge, and (e) CABS at any time prior to hospital discharge. Similar sets of predictors were identified for each type of therapy. In general, patients who did not receive these therapies were older, more often had previous congestive heart failure, and less often had previous angioplasty.

Patients with previous CABS who received reperfusion therapies differed from their counterparts who did not receive these treatments in two other important ways. In general, patients undergoing these therapies more often had ST-segment elevation on their admission electrocardiograms and had larger infarcts as indicated by peak (CK) and peak CK MB values. For example, 79% of patients receiving thrombolytic therapy had ST-segment elevation on their baseline electrocardiograms, whereas only 29% of patients who did not receive thrombolytic therapy, angioplasty, or bypass surgery did. Similarly, 83% of those receiving thrombolytic therapy had peak CK elevations exceeding twice the upper limit of normal, and 85% had abnormal peak CK MB values. In contrast, only 61% of patients not receiving these therapies had elevated CK values, and 70% had abnormal CK MB readings. These differences were also noted for patients undergoing angioplasty or bypass surgery prior to hospital discharge. Unfortunately, electrocardiographic information was known for only one-third of patients, and enzyme information was known for only two-thirds of those with previous CABS. However, based on this limited information, it is likely that patients with bypass grafts who received thrombolytic therapy, angioplasty, or bypass surgery more often had ST-segment elevation and developed larger infarcts than their counterparts who did not receive these therapies.

D. Hospital Mortality and Other Short-Term Outcomes

Despite having higher levels of risk, patients with previous bypass surgery had outcomes that were similar to those patients who did not have previous bypass surgery. As seen in Table 2, hospital mortality was similar in the two groups of patients; it was 10.8% for patients with previous surgery and 9.3% for those without prior surgery. Again, this result is consistent with findings from previous studies, including the earlier report from the MITI registry. In addition, the occurrence of in-hospital complications, including recurrent chest pain, new congestive heart failure, reinfarction, and cardiac arrest, did not differ according to previous surgical status. Length of hospital stay was 8.0 ± 6.0 days for patients with previous CABS and 8.2 ± 8.0 days for remaining patients.

However, for patients with previous CABS who received thrombolytic therapy, coronary angioplasty, or repeat bypass surgery prior to discharge, hospital mortality was higher than that experienced by their counterparts without previous surgery who received similar therapies. As seen in Figure 2, for patients receiving thrombolytic therapy within 6 hours of hospital admission, hospital mortality was considerably higher for patients with previous CABS (16.9% vs. 5.6%); the same result was true for those patients undergoing coronary angioplasty within 6 hours of hospital admission (15.0% vs. 6.3%) and for those undergoing coronary artery bypass surgery within 48 hours of admission (15.2% vs. 6.1%). Although mortality was lower in patients undergoing late angioplasty (>6 hours from hospital admission), it was still higher in patients

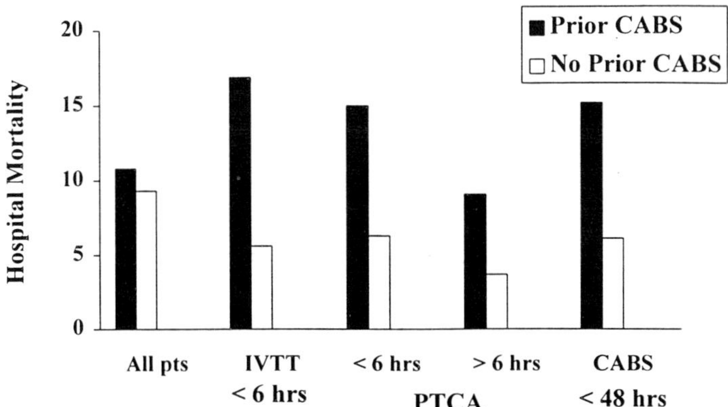

Figure 2 Hospital mortality in patients with and without prior coronary artery bypass surgery according to treatment. Thrombolytic therapy refers to treatment within 6 hours of admission, and bypass surgery refers to surgery within 48 hours of admission. CABS = coronary artery bypass surgery; hrs = hours; IVTT = intravenous thrombolytic therapy; PTCA = percutaneous transluminal coronary angioplasty.

with bypass grafts (9.1% vs. 3.7%), as shown in Figure 2. Similar mortality differences were also noted for those patients who received intravenous thrombolytic therapy at any time (15.6% vs. 5.7%), coronary angioplasty at any time (10.7% vs. 4.6%), or those who underwent CABS at any time (15.0% vs. 6.2%). For the group that did not receive these therapies at any time during hospitalization, patients with previous CABS actually had lower hospital mortality (9.6% vs. 12.7%).

In the 5,150 patients who received thrombolytic therapy, angioplasty, or bypass surgery, hospital mortality was 12.9% for patients with previous CABS and 5.6% for the remainder of patients. Since patients with previous CABS had higher levels of risk, it would be important to know if this mortality differential persisted after adjustment for these factors. After adjusting for advanced age, female gender, history of congestive heart failure, and absence of elevated lipids, patients with prior surgery were almost three times as likely to die as their counterparts who received reperfusion therapies but did not have previous surgery (odds ratio = 2.6, 95% confidence interval = 1.8, 3.7). Clearly, those with previous CABS who received early or late therapies prior to discharge had a much higher risk of death than their counterparts who received these therapies but did not have previous bypass grafts.

In the 1,094 patients with previous bypass surgery, it was somewhat puzzling that hospital mortality was worse for patients who received thrombolytic therapy, angioplasty, or bypass surgery. These individuals were younger and less often had congestive heart failure than did patients who did not receive these therapies, yet they also had more ST-segment elevation and larger infarct size, as indicated by peak CK and CKMB values. It is the latter factor that probably accounts for the higher hospital mortality in the group of patients receiving both early and late reperfusion therapies.

The use of high-risk treatments may be necessary to reduce morbidity and mortality in patients with previous grafts who develop AMI. This may be true particularly with respect to acute reperfusion therapies. In Seattle area hospitals, 169 patients (15%) with previous bypass grafts received either intra-

Table 3 Prior Bypass Surgery and AMI Intravenous Thrombolytic Therapy vs. Direct Coronary Angioplasty

Variable	IVTT ($n = 114$)	Direct PTCA ($n = 55$)	p
Demographics:			
Age	63.2 ± 8.7	61.1 ± 10.1	.18
Women	15.8%	20.0%	.49
History of:			
AMI	58.8%	49.1%	.49
CHF	12.3%	7.3%	.61
Angina	71.1%	65.5%	.07
Hyperlipidemia	31.6%	36.4%	.33
Hypertension	36.8%	36.4%	.47
Thrombolysis	5.3%	5.5%	.96
Angioplasty	9.6%	32.7%	.002
Diabetes	14.1%	5.9%	.35
Smoking	32.4%	32.4%	.99
Symptoms on admission:			
Chest pain	99.1%	96.4%	.20
Cardiogenic shock	2.6%	1.8%	.74
Initial ECG findings:			.04
ST elevation	78%	52%	
ST depression	6%	15%	
Bundle branch block	15%	32%	
Indeterminate	4%	3%	
Outcomes:			
Recurrent angina	37.7%	34.5%	.69
Reinfarction	3.5%	1.8%	.54
New CHF	17.9%	20.0%	.70
Death	15.0%	9.1%	.28

CHF = congestive heart failure; ECG = electrocardiogram; IVTT = intravenous thrombolytic therapy; PTCA = percutaneous transluminal coronary angioplasty.

venous thrombolytic therapy (n = 114) or direct coronary angioplasty only (n = 55) within 6 hours of hospital admission. Patients receiving direct coronary angioplasty were not treated with thrombolytic therapy prior to or during the intervention. As can be seen in Table 3, the two groups were similar with respect to baseline characteristics, except that a much higher proportion of patients in the direct angioplasty group had undergone a previous angioplasty. Although hospital mortality was worse in the group treated with thrombolytic therapy, the difference was not statistically significant, and could in part be explained by the higher prevalence of diabetes in the group with thrombolytic therapy. It appears that the two therapies were equally effective, although critical angiographic evidence was not available to fully evaluate these two therapies.

E. Long-Term Survival

With vital status information from the National Death Index, it was possible to determine long-term survival status for patients in the MITI registry. Long-term survival was significantly better for patients without previous CABS, as can be seen in Figure 3. Two-year survival was 72% for patients with previous CABS and 77% for those without prior surgery. Even after adjusting for higher

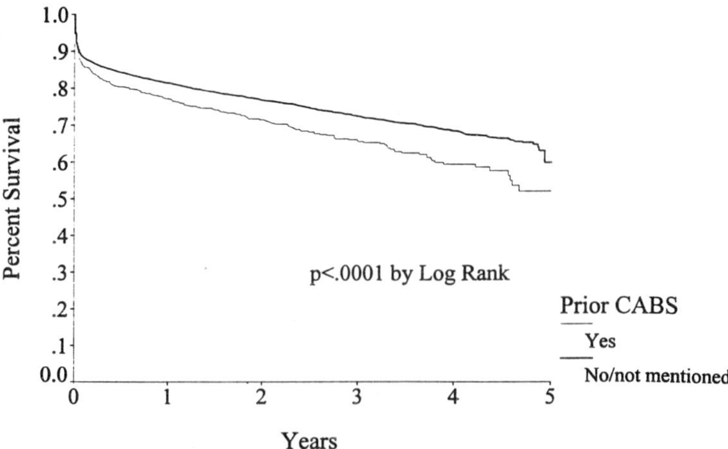

Figure 3 Cumulative survival in patients with previous coronary bypass surgery (n = 1,094) and without it (n = 9,960). The difference in survival was highly statistically significant (p < .0001 by the log rank statistic) and remained so after adjustment for baseline differences in the two groups by Cox proportional hazards regression. CABS = coronary artery bypass surgery.

risk in patients with previous CABS, previous bypass surgery was a predictor of adverse long-term survival ($p < .0001$). The results of Cox proportional hazards regression indicated that after adjusting for advanced age, history of previous infarction, history of congestive heart failure, hypertension, and absence of elevated lipids, the adjusted risk of death was 30% higher in patients with previous CABS (hazard ratio = 1.30, 95% confidence interval = 1.15, 1.48).

Whereas hospital mortality was worse for patients with prior surgery who underwent reperfusion therapies prior to hospital discharge, this was not the case for long-term survival. In fact, long-term survival was improved for patients who received reperfusion therapy (Figure 4). Two-year survival was 78% for patients receiving thrombolytic therapy, angioplasty, or coronary artery bypass surgery at any time prior to hospital discharge, while it was 68% for patients not receiving these therapies ($p = .002$). As seen in Figure 4, survival was similar for patients who received emergent or late therapy, where emergent therapy was defined as the administration of thrombolytic therapy or coronary angioplasty within 6 hours of hospital admission or bypass surgery within 48 hours of admission. However, when the higher level of risk in patients

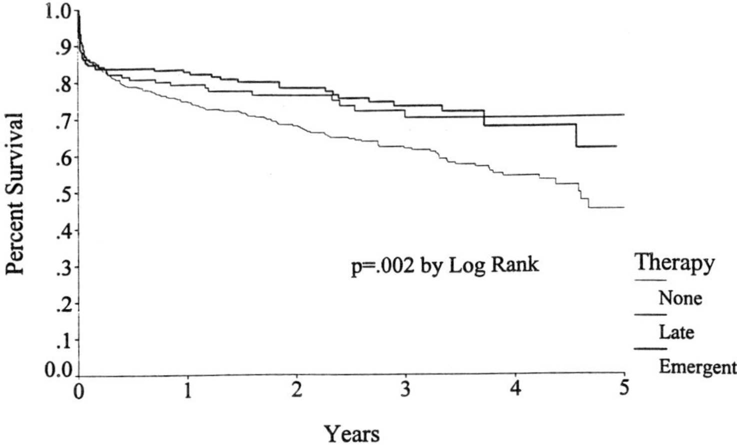

Figure 4 Cumulative survival in patients with previous coronary artery bypass surgery. Patients are categorized according to emergent, late, and no reperfusion therapy. Survival was improved for those receiving either early or late therapies, although patients who had no therapy had worse survival ($p = .002$). Two-year survival was 78% for patients receiving either early or late therapy ($n = 412$), but was only 68% for patients not receiving therapy ($n = 684$). After adjustment for differences in baseline characteristics by Cox regression, the survival difference was no longer statistically significant ($p = .28$).

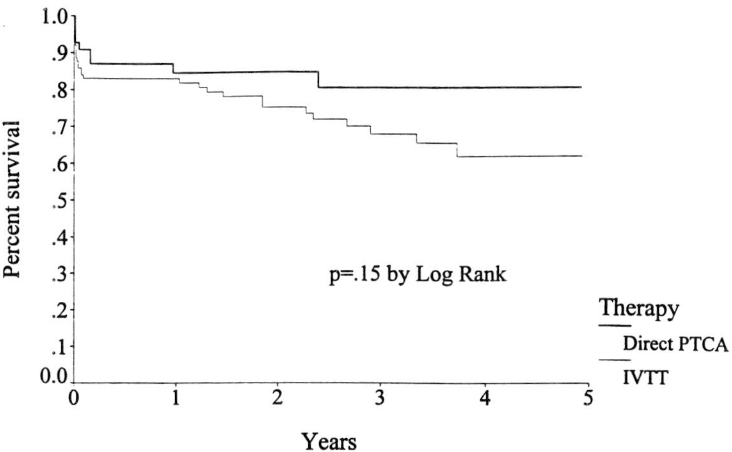

Figure 5 Cumulative survival in patients with previous coronary artery bypass surgery who received direct angioplasty ($n = 55$) or intravenous thrombolytic therapy within 6 hours of hospital admission ($n = 114$). There was no difference in survival ($p = .15$ by log rank statistic). IVTT = intravenous thrombolytic therapy; PTCA = percutaneous transluminal coronary angioplasty.

not receiving these therapies was considered, the survival difference was no longer statistically significant ($p = .28$).

In the select group of patients undergoing immediate direct coronary angioplasty or thrombolytic therapy, long-term survival tended to be better in those receiving direct coronary angioplasty (Figure 5). Two-year survival was 75% for patients receiving thrombolytic therapy and was 85% for those undergoing direct angioplasty ($p = .15$). After adjustments for covariates by Cox regression, the association between survival and type of treatment remained statistically not significant ($p = .26$). Small numbers of patients in the two groups decreased the chance of detecting a statistically significant difference.

V. CONCLUSION

Over the past 20 years, the prevalence of previous coronary artery surgery in patients with AMI has increased more than twofold. Despite having higher levels of risk, patients with previous CABS had hospital mortality that was similar to that of patients who developed AMI but did not have previous CABS. These similar outcomes may be the result of smaller infarcts experienced by patients with previous surgery. However, the finding of similar short-term outcomes may be illusory, for long-term survival for patients with previous surgery was considerably worse than it was for patients without previous surgery. In fact, after adjusting for the higher level of risk in patients with previous bypass surgery, the risk of death was 30% higher in these patients.

In the group of patients with previous bypass surgery, those patients who received thrombolytic therapy, angioplasty, and/or coronary artery bypass surgery prior to hospital discharge had worse hospital mortality than their counterparts who did not receive these therapies. The reason for this finding was that patients who received these therapies had evolved larger infarctions than their counterparts with previous CABS who did not receive these therapies. Despite the higher in-hospital mortality rate, subsequent survival was better for patients who received these therapies than for those who did not. This finding suggests that more needs to be known about the mechanism of AMI in patients with previous bypass grafts, so that these therapies can be offered to those patients who can benefit the most from them. In particular, how these therapies work in native as opposed to bypass grafts needs to be better understood. In addition, more needs to be known about the efficacy of thrombolytic therapy versus direct coronary angioplasty, because, to date, current studies have been hampered by small numbers of patients or the lack of well-designed comparative studies. Nevertheless, increased understanding of how these therapies work and for whom they are most effective is sorely needed, for there does appear to be long-term benefit associated with the use of reperfusion therapies in patients with previous bypass grafts.

REFERENCES

1. Loop FD, Lytle BW, Gill CC, Golding LA, Cosgrove DM, Taylor PC. Trends in selection and results of coronary re-operations. Ann Thorac Surg 1983; 133:380–388.
2. Waters DD, Pelletier GB, Hache M, Theroux P, Campeau L. Myocardial infarction in patients with previous coronary artery bypass surgery. J Am Coll Cardiol 1984; 3:909–915.
3. Wiseman A, Waters DD, Walling A, Pelletier GB, Roy D, Theroux P. Long-term prognosis after myocardial infarction in patients with previous coronary artery bypass surgery. J Am Coll Cardiol 1988; 12:873–880.
4. Crean PA, Waters DD, Bosch X, Pelletier GB, Roy D, Theroux P. Angiographic findings after myocardial infarction in patients with previous bypass surgery: explanations for smaller infarcts in this group compared with control patients. Circulation 1985; 71:693–698.
5. Dittrich HC, Gilpin E, Nicod P, Henning H, Cali G, Ricou F, Ross J. Outcome after acute myocardial infarction in patients with prior coronary artery bypass surgery. Am J Cardiol 1993; 72:507–513.

6. Maynard C, Weaver WD, Litwin PE, Martin JS, Cerqueira MD, Kudenchuk PJ. Acute myocardial infarction and prior coronary artery surgery in the Myocardial Triage and Intervention Registry. Coronary Artery Disease 1991; 2:443–448.

7. Grines CL, Booth NC, Nissen SE, Gurley JC, Bennett KA, O'Connor WN, DeMaria AN. Mechanism of acute myocardial infarction in patients with prior coronary artery bypass grafting and therapeutic implications. Am J Cardiol 1990; 65:1292–1296.

8. Kahn JK, Rutherford BD, McConahay DR, Johnson W, Giorgi LV, Ligon R, Hartzler GO. Usefulness of angioplasty during acute myocardial infarction in patients with prior coronary artery bypass grafting. Am J Cardiol 1990; 65:698–702.

9. Kleiman NS, Berman DA, Gaston WR, Cashion WR, Roberts R. Early intravenous thrombolytic therapy for acute myocardial infarction in patients with prior coronary artery bypass grafts. Am J Cardiol 1989; 63:102–104.

10. Kavanaugh KM, Topol EJ. Acute intervention during myocardial infarction in patients with prior coronary bypass surgery. Am J Cardiol 1990; 65:924–926.

11. Salinger MH, Lopez A, Frohlich TG, McDonough TJ, Heuter DC, Stagl RD. Systemic and local saphenous vein graft thrombolysis using a tissue plasminogen activator. Cath Cardiovasc Diag 1990; 19:198–201.

12. de Feyter PJ, Serruys P, van den Brand M, Meester H, Beatt K, Suryapranata H. Percutaneous transluminal angioplasty of a totally occluded venous bypass graft: a challenge that should be resisted. Am J Cardiol 1989; 64:88–90.

13. Lasorda DM, Incorvati DL, Randall RR. Extraction atherectomy during myocardial infarction in a patient with prior coronary artery bypass surgery. Cath Cardiovasc Diag 1992; 26:117–121.

14. Pirwitz MJ, Hillis LD. Emergency coronary artery bypass surgery for acute myocardial infarction. Coronary Artery Disease 1994; 5:385–391.

15. Kennedy JW, Ivey TD, Misbach G, Allen MD, Maynard C, Dalquist JE, Kruse S, Stewart DK. Coronary artery bypass graft surgery early after acute myocardial infarction. Circulation 1989; 79:I-73–I-78.

16. Maynard C, Weaver WD, Litwin PE, Martin JS, Kudenchuk PJ, Dewhurst TA, Eisenberg MS, Hallstrom AP, Chambers J. Hospital mortality in acute myocardial infarction in the era of reperfusion therapy. Am J Cardiol 1993; 72:877–882.

17. Weaver WD, Cerqueira M, Hallstrom AP, Litwin PE, Kudenchuk PJ, Eisenberg MS. for the MITI Project Investigators. Prehospital-initiated vs. hospital-initiated thrombolytic therapy. JAMA 1993; 270:1211–1216.

18. Weaver WD, Litwin PE, Martin JS, Kudenchuk PJ, Maynard C, Eisenberg MS, Ho MT, Cobb LA, Kennedy JW, Wirkus MS. Effect of age on the use of thrombolytic therapy and mortality in acute myocardial infarction. J Am Coll Cardiol 1991; 18:657–662.

19. Maynard C, Litwin PE, Martin JS, Weaver WD. Treatment and outcome of acute myocardial infarction in women 75 years and older. Cardiology in the Elderly 1993; 1:121–125.

20. Maynard C, Litwin PE, Martin JS, Weaver WD. Gender differences in the treatment of acute myocardial infarction. Arch Intern Med 1992; 152:972–976.

21. Maynard C, Litwin PE, Martin JS, Cerqueira M, Kudnechuk PJ, Ho MT, Kennedy JW, Cobb JA, Schaeffer SM, Hallstrom AP, Weaver WD. Characteristics of black

patients admitted to coronary care units in metropolitan Seattle. Am J Cardiol 1991; 67:18–23.

22. Maynard C, Every NR, Litwin PE, Martin JS, Weaver WD. Outcomes in African American women with suspected acute myocardial infarction. J Natl Med Assoc 1995; 87:339–344.

23. Every NR, Larson EB, Litwin PE, Maynard C, Fihn S, Eisenberg MS, Hallstrom AP, Martin JS, Weaver WD. The effect of on-site catheterization facilites on utilization of cardiac procedures and mortality after acute myocardial infarction. N Engl J Med 1993; 329:546–551.

24. Weaver WD, Litwin PE, Martin JS. The use of direct angioplasty for treatment of patients with acute myocardial infarction in hospitals with and without on-site cardiac surgery. Circulation 1993; 88:2067–2075.

25. Kudenchuk P, Ho MT, Weaver WD, Litwin PE, Martin JS, Eisenberg MS, Hallstrom AP, Cobb LA, Kennedy JW. Accuracy of computer interpreted electrocardiography in selecting patients for thrombolytic therapy. J Am Coll Cardiol 1991; 17:1486–1491.

26. Maynard C, Litwin PE, Martin JS, Hallstrom AP, Weaver WD. Changes in the use of thrombolytic therapy in Seattle area hospitals from 1988 to 1992. J Thrombosis Thrombolysis 1995; 1:195–199.

16
Evaluating the Cost of Coronary Surgery and Coronary Angioplasty

William S. Weintraub, Patrick D. Mauldin,*
and Edmund R. Becker
Emory University, Atlanta, Georgia

I. INTRODUCTION

In considering the choice of coronary revascularization, either with catheter-based intervention or surgery, it is reasonable to question both the cost and the relationship of cost to outcome. In the recent past it was sufficient to show that a form of therapy was effective. Thereafter providers could charge the usual and customary charge and expect insurance companies and Medicare to pay. The escalating costs of medical care as well as other pressures within our society have made this untenable. Thus, we have seen and will see in the future that new forms of therapy, and perhaps existing ones, have to be justified on economic grounds as well as on efficacy grounds. This has given birth to a new discpline called *clinical microeconomics*. As with many new fields, the goals of this field are not entirely well defined and the methods are still being developed. The problems of assessment of costs and comparison with efficacy are especially relevant when considering expensive forms for therapy that are commonly used and have multiple complex and interrelating indices of outcome. In perhaps no single form of therapy are these issues as relevant as with coronary revascularization.

**Current affiliation*: Medical University of South Carolina, Charleston, South Carolina.

II. PURPOSES AND GOALS OF ECONOMIC ANALYSES

Economic analyses in medicine can involve macroeconomic policy issues or microeconomic assessment of any aspect of health care. This review will concentrate on microeconomic assessment of therapy as applied to coronary artery bypass surgery and coronary angioplasty. Assessment of therapy can involve assessment of cost, assessment of efficacy or the relationship between cost and efficacy. The goal may be to assess the cost of therapy or to compare two forms of therapy. For instance, the goal of a study may be to assess the cost of coronary angioplasty, as compared with the goal of comparing the costs of angioplasty and coronary surgery. The comparison of two forms of therapy may occur within the structure of a prospective randomized controlled trial or may make use of existing databases. A randomized trial will allow quite different questions to be addressed compared with database studies. A randomized trial will permit comparison in a matched population that is free of selection bias. Database studies will permit comparison in populations of greater breadth and variety, but will always suffer from selection bias.

When two competing forms of therapy are considered, then the relative efficacies and relative costs may be considered. There are three related forms of analysis that may be used. The first is cost-effectiveness analysis, in which the costs of the two forms of therapy are measured as well as the relative effectiveness of the two forms of therapy [1]. This form of analysis assumes that one measure of effectiveness can be achieved, often survival. This method breaks down when there are multiple measures of effectiveness. The second is cost–utility analysis in which the cost is measured as above, while all measures of effectiveness are incorporated into one measure called *utility* [2]. There are clear-cut and well-known limitations to determining utility. Approaches to measuring utility will be addressed in the following section. A third, and somewhat less popular form of analysis, is cost–benefit analysis, in which measures of cost and effectiveness are reduced to a single measure, generally dollars (or other currency) [3]. Clinicians often find this form of analysis to be confusing (or perhaps just more confusing than cost-effectiveness and cost–utility analyses). In principle these types of analyses can provide measures of cost per unit increase in effectiveness (or utility).

How should these analyses be used? In principle, all that is needed is to choose the therapy that costs less per unit increase in effectiveness than any other therapy. However, even if the biases in selection of populations as well as limitations in measurement and analytic techniques could be overcome, considerable problems in interpretation would remain. This is because there are different shareholders with different stakes in the outcome. Physicians and patients have traditionally been more concerned about effectiveness. Hospitals and especially insurance companies have been concerned about costs. The interpretation of cost-effectiveness requires a societal perspective. Thus, if one form of therapy can be convincingly shown to be both more effective and less expensive than a competing form of therapy, there can be little argument. On the contrary, if one form of therapy is more effective, but at a higher cost, then it is a societal decision as to whether the therapy in question is worth spending money on. When efficacy and costs are uncertain, as is often the case, the decision is even harder. Needless to say, society has done a poor job in selecting which forms of therapy to invest in. Why has this process been so difficult in medicine? The separation of concerns over effectiveness and costs to different shareholders has removed the normal market mechanism governed by willingness to pay [4–7]. In the traditional fee-for-service system, demand for services continues to increase, consuming ever more resources. *Health care reform* is essentially a euphemism for controlling costs, and involves increasing the role of those who pay the bills to help control costs, hopefully with some limitations to prevent abuse by the payers who might attempt to limit ligitimate services in order to save money. This process may make medicine more market oriented.

The forgoing discussion reveals the limitations of economic analysis. Cost-effectiveness analyses cannot in and of themselves set policy. If only effectiveness is important, then the most effective therapy will be chosen, regardless of cost. If only saving money is important, then the least expensive therapy will be chosen. Cost-effectiveness analyses are naturally of greatest interest to policymakers who must weigh selection of therapy given limited resources.

III. METHODS FOR DETERMINING COSTS

A. Hospital Costs

Medical costs for a procedure such as coronary surgery can be naturally broken down into three components: in-hospital direct costs, follow-up direct costs, and indirect costs. In-hospital costs comprise hospital costs and professional billings. Follow-up direct costs include those for physician office visits, outpatient testing, medications, home health providers, and additional hospitalizations. Indirect costs reflect opportunity costs from loss of work or other economic losses to the patient, family, and business. If only coronary surgery is considered, without an alternative form of therapy, it is probably not meaningful to try to figure out just which costs in follow-up are related to the procedure. Thus for bypass surgery alone, or any procedure alone, it is reasonable to consider in-hospital direct costs only. However, if surgery is considered in contrast to another form of therapy, such as coronary angioplasty, then it is certainly meaningful to consider costs after the hospitalization. This is actually necessary, because there may well be very different levels of consumption of services after discharge.

The most common source of data for hospital costs is hospital charges. Hospital charges may be gathered either from line-item charges of every single item consumed or from grouped charges generally prepared by hospital finance departments. The most commonly used source in nonfederal hospitals is the UB-82 (now updated to UB-92), in which the charges are grouped into categories. This is a uniform billing statement used by all third-party carriers. Charges are available for, but not limited to, such services as the surgical suite, cardiac catheterization laboratory, intensive care unit, postoperative or postprocedural floor care, respiratory therapy, physical therapy, pulmonary function, anesthesia, recovery room, medical and surgical supplies, laboratory, pharmacy, ECG, telemetry and social services. The data elements were determined by the National Uniform Billing Committee, which included representatives from HCFA, Blue Cross, and multiple other national organizations.

However, there is a very real difference between hospital charges and costs [8]. While hospitals will generally follow guidelines of the American Hospital Association in setting charges, charges are known to vary widely. Hospitals will set their charges to maximize profits. This does not always mean setting the highest price for a service, but it does mean that the relationship of cost to charges is tenuous. What is the cost of a service? When considering hospital services, it generally means resources utilized. There is another point of view, that reimbursements are really the cost, because this is cost to the payer. There is no uniformly agreed-to principle of whether resources consumed or cost to the payer most accurately reflect cost. Most work has centered on resources consumed. Resource consumption may, in principle, be determined if the relationship between what a resource costs and what is charged for the resource is known. All attempts at this are approximations, since the costs of services are shared in ways that may be very difficult to separate. For instance, how much of a pharmacist's time goes into dispensing an aspirin? Worse yet, how much of the operating room expense can be meaningfully applied to one patient undergoing cholecystectomy? Accountants try to determine the separation of costs from charges using either "top-down" or "bottom-up" methods. In top-down methods, all of the costs of a particular department, such as the operating room, are determined and then all of the charges. By dividing the total costs by the total charges, a fraction is produced. For any one patient, the cost in the operating room would be the charge multiplied by this ratio. This method may be criticized as too broad to describe differing services. For instance, a chest x-ray would not be expected to have the same cost-to-charge ratio as an intravenous pyelogram. More sophisticated bottom-up accounting approaches are being developed and slowly implemented in hospitals in which the resource utilization for each procedure is accounted for [9–12]. This issue of determining cost accurately is of differing importance to differing audiences. The health services research community may be well satisfied with approximations using department cost-to-charge ratios, understanding that there is considerable error. However, to hospital administrators who must set prices, the issue of defining cost more accurately becomes crucial as profit margins narrow. Inherent in the problem is the inevitable cross-subsidization that occurs in a business that offers multiple products. When a business offers many products, it is not possible to determine cost definitively.

Another issue in considering hospital costs is *marginal cost*. Average costs include all resources used, including fixed resources whose costs would not be decreased if not utilized. Marginal costing accepts fixed costs as a given and focuses only on those additional resources consumed by each additional patient. However, there is no certain method of separating marginal from fixed costs. For instance, the cost of the building may be sunk, or fixed. However, how does one determine the marginal cost of operating room staff? If coronary surgery decreases as angioplasty becomes more common, do the operating room nurses remain on staff in the operating room, or will they be assigned to other duties? Hlatky et al. [13] have developed four methods of reducing charges to costs: (1) cost of supplies, (2) cost of personnel and supplies, (3) average direct costs, and (4) average direct costs plus hospital overhead. While these researchers never established any one of these scales as the best measure of marginal costs, they maintained that any one of these is superior to the use of hospital charges. The importance of marginal costs may also vary with the audience. For instance, policy planners may be more interested in average costs because that is what they pay. Hospital administrators may be more interested in marginal costs, because it is the cost relative to reimbursement for the next patient that determines whether a patient can be operated on profitably. However, the difficulties in measuring marginal costs are formidable, and almost all hospital cost studies use average costs.

B. Professional Costs

Assessing professional costs for procedures presents additional challenges. It is not adequate to consider the surgeon's or the angiplasty operator's fee alone, for there are other professionals who provide services in each of these cases. The goal must be to capture *all* of the professional services for a procedure. For coronary surgery this may include fees for the surgeon, the assistants, the cardiologist, anaesthesia, radiology, clinical pathology, professional components of any other testing, and any other consultants. Thus, the goal is first to create a profile of the professional services consumed and then to assess the cost. As a quick simulation method, the Medicare reimbursement schedule for a DRG and the fee for the primary physician, such as an angioplasty operator, has been used to estimate cost. This is probably not valid, because the DRG may not adequately describe a hospitalization, and a DRG will not adequately describe the profile of the multiple physician charges associated with a hospitalization besides that of the primary physician. Simulated hospital charges may, at times, be needed where data are not available. However, the simulated estimate should be based on real data from as similar a hospitalization as possible. In any case, real data will always be more compelling than simulations based on uncertain sources, and simulations seem unlikely to be able to assess the profile of professional services.

Professional charges have not historically been subject to the same type of accounting scrutiny as hospital charges. In fact, a substantial amount of health economics literature documents the distortions in the market for physician services and the fact that this market does not satisfy the economic conditions for being reasonably competitive on physician prices [14]. If a surgeon charges $5,000 for coronary surgery, is this a reasonable estimate of the charge or the cost? In 1991, the Health Insurance Association of America collected mean surgical charges for a three-vessel CABG and found the physician charges were: New York City—$8,189; Philadelphia—$6,118; Atlanta—$4,656; Chicago—$5,902; Denver—$4,499; Dallas—$2,461; and Los Angeles—$6,375 [15]. The range in physician charges for the three-vessel CABG among these seven major U.S. cities is $5,728. Few health care researchers would be confident that the wide variation is due to significant cost differences. Consequently, there is no theoretical basis for efforts to determine physician costs from charges. Furthermore, using physician payments as a gauge of costs does little to improve the estimates. Given the widespread variation in insurance arrangements, physician payments are still significantly distorted and biased.

There has been an effort to rationalize physician payments by developing a set of scales for services. This system, called the *resource-based relative value scale (RBRVS)* was developed over a period of years and included many physician consultants to try to assess the relative time, physical, and cognitive efforts associated with physician services [16–17]. Each service is assigned a number called its *relative value units (RVUs)*. If the profile of physician services for a procedure or hospitalization is known, then RVUs for each service may be used to develop a proxy for the physician costs. The total RVUs may be converted to a dollar figure by a conversion factor. The Health Care Financing Agency has a standard conversion factor. The appeal of the RBRVS is that it is a relative weighting system that assigns unique weights for physician work and practice costs for each physician service by CPT-4 code. As a result, after assigning a conversion factor, standardized estimates of the costs can be calculated and used as a gauge of physician costs. While there are still some problems with this approach and experience is limited, especially for the practice cost values in the RBRVS, it holds considerable promise and overcomes some of the major drawbacks in physician charge data [18]. A significant challenge in using RBRVS is to get a complete and accurate profile of physician services for any hospitalization or procedure.

C. Follow-Up Costs

Charges during follow-up present a different set of challenges. To determine costs during follow-up, it is essential to determine patient utilization of services, including follow-up direct costs and indirect costs. Direct costs include those for medical services such as additional hospitalizations, physician office visits, medications, procedures and testing, rehabilitation, nursing home stays, and home health services. While the particular services used may be assessed by mailout questionnaire or telephone interview, patients will not have a realistic view of how much they spend for services. This is complicated by insurance, because patients cannot be expected to respond reliably about how much they paid out of pocket for services and how much the insurance company paid for services. Because there is no central database to which to appeal to find their expenses, the only reasonable approach is to try to identify the services. A profile of the costs of each type of service and medication can then be built. Follow-up hospitalizations may be assessed by obtaining the charges as discussed earlier, or these costs may be estimated from similar hospitalizations where data are available. Office visits and other services may be similarly estimated. Medications may be estimated by compiling a list of medication prices from several pharmacies. Using these cost estimates, a partial simulation of postdischarge direct cost may be determined. In determining services utilized, random repeat sampling of some fraction of the population should be performed to determine validity of the data set.

Indirect costs include missed time from work by the patient or family members. Follow-up indirect costs are probably the most difficult to determine, and are often excluded as unmeasurable. In any case, it is not possible to measure directly all of the indirect costs and to define perfectly the boundaries of these costs. For instance, if an executive in a company has coronary surgery and is out of work for 6 weeks, there may or may not be loss of pay. In any case, there was an effect on the business that cannot readily be determined. Indirect costs, if measured at all, are often confined to family loss of income. There are two possible methods, direct survey and a simulation. The direct survey will have errors, in that there will be uncertainty as to income loss and patients may be uncomfortable revealing this information. If this method is used, income loss should be validated against another source, and this may be difficult or impossible. At the very least, a number chosen at random should be resurveyed to determine reproducibility. Alternatively, a simulation could be constructed in which lost time is estimated and a dollar cost attached based on type of job. Sources of data to construct such a simulation will require validation. Indirect costs of either of these types create a bias, in that higher-paying jobs become more valued. The loss of work of a laborer may create a much bigger problem for that individual and family than would loss of work for the higher-paid business executive. In any case, if indirect costs are estimated, the numbers must be examined with both interest and skepticism as to their accuracy.

IV. ASSESSING VALIDITY

In all studies there is a concern about the validity of underlying data. In clinical studies, the investigator is responsible for assessing and attesting to the validity of the data. This is much more difficult in economic studies. Even in a single institution the investigators must use data provided from hospital or professional financial services. Much of the data are not subject to checking because there may be no secondary source to audit against and no way of repeating data collection. Furthermore, the methods used to assess cost from the underlying data are necessarily based on a set of assumptions. Furthermore, inflation undermines the strict dollar values determined. Cost may be inflated or deflated by multiplying by a constant to convert from any one year to another, based on the medical inflation rate, but this is just one more assumption that adds artificiality to the calculations. Thus, in considering cost it is not reasonable or possible to determine one final bottom-line dollar figure. Rather, all cost estimates must be considered an attempt to estimate a value that cannot truly be measured.

V. PUBLISHED ESTIMATES OF COST

What are the costs of these procedures? National trends of CABG can be determined from discharge data for nonfederal hospitals in the United States, compiled by the National Center for Health Statistics with procedures determined from ICD-9-CM codes. There were 170,000 CABG procedures in 1982, 202,000 in 1984, 284,000 in 1986, and 368,000 in 1989. Current length of stay has a median value of 7 days. While adequate estimates of the cost of CABG are not available, if we accept an estimate of $30,000 per CABG, then the national total is about $11 billion. For PTCA the direct costs are less, in part because length of stay is considerably shorter than it is for CABG and because the use of resources during the initial hospitalization is lower. However, restenosis may limit the cost advantage of PTCA. National PTCA data are first available for 1983, when 32,300 procedures were performed. This increased to 46,000 in 1984, to 133,000 in 1986, and to 156,000 in 1987. As for coronary surgery, an adequate estimate of costs is not available. If we accept an estimate of $15,000 for a PTCA and the number of PTCA procedures is around 400,000, then an estimate would be approximately $6 billion. Thus, $17 billion is probably a reasonable estimate for the total direct initial annual "cost" for coronary revascularization.

The determinants of the costs of PTCA have been analyzed in several studies. Mark [19] has proposed analyzing the cost determinants of PTCA in four major categories: patient-specific, hospital-specific, treatment-specific, and geographic-economic. For patient-specific factors, Topol et al. [20] found that the charges for PTCA were higher in older patients, in female patients, and in patients with a history of prior myocardial infarction. Regarding hospital-specific factors, they found that teaching hospitals had significantly lower charges for PTCA than nonteaching hospitals except in the Midwest region of the United States. Considering geographic factors, the West had the highest charges and the Midwest the lowest. As might be expected, complications increase costs. Reeder et al. [21] found that unsuccessful PTCA more than doubled hospital charges compared with an initially successful procedure. Barbash et al. [22] found higher charges for nonelective procedures, for procedures in patients with more severe symptoms, and in older patients. Guzman et al. [23] compared the hospital cost of atherectomy ($n = 126$) to angioplasty ($n = 126$). Atherectomy, at $9,345 ± 8,856, cost 28% more than angioplasty, at $7,301 ± 4,637. Cohen et al. [24] reduced charges to costs, using departmental cost-to-charge ratios. Costs of angioplasty ($n = 113$), atherectomy ($n = 34$), stenting ($n = 64$), and coronary surgery ($n = 89$) were compared using 1991 costs (Table 1). Costs of stenting were higher than those for angioplasty or atherectomy, but none of the procedures were as expensive as coronary surgery. Dick et al. [25] also found atherectomy and stenting to be more expensive than balloon angioplasty. None of these studies included professional costs.

Hospital costs of coronary surgery have been under investigation since the 1970s. Return to work has been extensively studied. At Emory University, 66% of a cohort of 1,593 patients returned to work after CABG [26]. Return to work was higher in patients with complete revascularization, without chest pain at follow-up, in younger patients, in patients with higher educational levels, in patients who were not disabled before surgery, and in patients with preserved left ventricular function. Weintraub et al. [27] examined length of stay after coronary surgery at Emory. Length of stay could be related to preoperative factors, but postoperative complications predominated, despite

Table 1 Hospital Costs and Charges for Revascularization

	PTCA	Atherectomy	Stenting	CABG
Hospital length of stay (days)	2.6 ± 1.7	2.3 ± 1.5	5.5 ± 2.6	9.3 ± 3.6
ICU length of stay (days)	0.2 ± 0.6	0.1 ± 0.7	0.3 ± 1.1	2.5 ± 2.0
Mean charge	$8,639	$8,391	$12,670	$27,739
Mean cost	$5,369	$5,726	$7,878	$20,937

From Ref. 24.

their relatively infrequent occurrence. This suggests that complications may have a major effect on determining outliers with high in-hospital costs. Length of stay after CABG was found to have a modal value at 7 days, with a long tail out to 180 days. Hemenway et al. [28], in a study from the early 1980s, estimated the cost of coronary surgery, including preoperative catheterization, at $28,000. In the more recent literature, Mauldin et al. [29] predicted hospital costs for first-time CABG patients in 1990 from preoperative and postoperative variables. The mean cost to the hospital for the 382 patients who underwent a first-time CABG with no complications was $16,776. For patients with one complication the mean costs increased to $17,794. After one complication, costs continued to increase as the number of complications increased, with the most expensive complications being adult respiratory distress syndrome and septicemia. Smith et al. [30] specifically studied preoperative predictors of costs, and found higher costs with several factors, especially older age, lower ejection fractions, and prior surgery.

Several studies have compared data using the charges for PTCA with CABG. Given the methodological problems in these investigations (use of charges to estimate costs, problems in measuring charges/costs, length of follow-up periods, potential bias in samples, dates of analysis, differences among institutions, etc.), any summary comparisons across these studies must be viewed with skepticism. Length of stay is considerably shorter with PTCA than it is for CABG, and the use of resources during the initial hospitalization is two to three times less for uncomplicated PTCA [21,31–33]. While the charges at 1 year are also lower, restenosis may limit the cost advantage of PTCA [21]. The major factors in the cost of PTCA that contributed to overall costs were the early failure rate (30%) (with early crossover to CABG) and the 33% restenosis rate. Over 80% of these patients required repeat revascularization. Of these nonrandomized comparative charge studies, only the study of Black et al. [33] specifically considered patients with multivessel disease. Black et al. studied direct hospital and professional charges for 100 PTCA patients and 100 CABG patients (Table 2). While the charges for angioplasty were lower than those for coronary surgery, charges were used as a proxy for costs and indirect costs were not calculated. Weintraub et al. [27] estimated costs for 787 two-vessel CAD patients treated with either PTCA or CABG. The authors found a cumulative increase in costs for the PTCA group over time but, at 5 years the overall costs of PTCA were still significantly lower than CABG costs. In a study from the Netherlands, van den Brand et al. [34] noted the initial cost of coronary surgery to be more than twice that of angioplasty, but the numbers had pulled closer together by 1 year due to additional procedures in the angioplasty patients. Hlatky et al. [35] examined in-hospital resource utilization in patients underoing CABG and PTCA. These investigators developed four scales to compare economic costs of the two procedures: (1) cost of supplies,

Table 2 Hospital Stay and Initial Cost

	PTCA		CABG	
	Mean	Range	Mean	Range
Hospital stay (days)	5	3–25	13	7–16
Hospital charges:				
Procedure charge ($)	2,761	1,423–5,379	4,368	2,821–6,671
Room charge ($)	1,301	470–9,005	4,236	1,112–16,967
Miscellaneous ($)	2,123	467–13,889	6,769	3,628–29,792
Total hospital charges ($)	6,185	2,825–24,370	15,372	9,153–51,396
Physician charges ($)	2,953	1,607–12,311	7,398	3,146–15,771
Total charges ($)	9,138	4,820–33,820	22,771	15,601–66,322

From Ref. 33.

(2) cost of personnel and supplies, (3) average direct costs, and (4) average direct costs plus hospital overhead. They note that the difference in cost between CABG and PTCA is overstated when charges are used as a proxy for economic costs when compared with any of these accounting methods. Second, the estimated differences between CABG and PTCA are smaller the more stringent the definition of marginal costs; i.e., the differences are smallest using scale 1 and greatest using scale 4. Mark et al. [36] noted that in comparable patients, return to work was earlier with angioplasty than with surgery, but by 1 year there was no difference.

At present, there are two randomized, controlled trials in the United States currently studying the short- and long-term cost differences of PTCA and CABG in multivessel CAD: the Emory Angioplasty vs. Surgery Trial (EAST) [37] and the Bypass Angioplasty Revascularization Investigation Substudy of Economics and Quality of Life (BARI SEQOL) [38]. EAST is a 392 patient trial conducted at Emory in which eligible patients with multiple-vessel coronary disease were randomized to angioplasty or coronary surgery. There was no difference between treatment arms at 3 years in either the primary composite endpoint of death, Q-wave myocardial infarction, or large ischemic thallium defect or in any component of the primary endpoint. There was a large difference between the treatment arms, however, in the additional revascularization procedures, with much higher rates of additional coronary surgery and coronary angioplasty in the group randomized to angioplasty. The costs were measured as hospital costs plus professional charges. Hospital costs were derived from charges by applying departmental cost-to-charge ratios, reducing the charge from each department to costs, and then adding up the derived costs. The sum of hospital costs and professional charges was $16,223 ± 11,552 for the angioplasty group and $24,005 ± 6,222 for the surgery group, in 1987 dollars ($p <$ .0001). If these numbers were inflated to 1993 dollars, the figure for angioplasty would be \$24,821 ± 17,675 and for surgery would be \$36,728 ± 9,520. Follow-up charge data for procedures were collected in similar detail to the initial charges. At 3 years the sum of professional charges and hospital costs was \$23,734 ± 15,798 (median \$19,059) for coronary angioplasty and \$25,310 ± 7,480 (median \$23,572) for coronary surgery, in 1987 dollars, numbers that were close although statistically different ($p <$ .0001). Inflated to 1993 dollars the sum for angioplasty would be \$36,313 ± 24,171 (median \$29,160) and for surgery would be \$38,724 ± 11,444 (median \$36,065). Thus most, although perhaps not all, of the initial cost advantage of angioplasty over surgery was lost by 3 years due to additional procedures in the angioplasty group. The EAST study is continuing. Results to 8 years will be investigated as well as the use of RBRVS [18] to assess professional fees. Quality of life and nonprocedural costs are also being studied.

BARI is a multicenter trial with 1,800 patients and includes prospective information on economic costs and quality of life, which is expected in late 1995. Two European randomized trials of PTCA and CABG are also including economic endpoints. The Randomized Intervention Treatment of Angina (RITA) is a British trial with 1,011 patients [39,40]. In RITA, a partial simulation revealed that the initial cost of angioplasty was 50% that of surgery, while at 2 years the cost of angioplasty was 80% that of surgery, with a difference of £1,011. The German Angioplasty Bypass Intervention study (GABI) has 358 patients [41]. In the GABI trial, the initial procedural costs were \$16,562 for CABG and \$5,000 for PTCA. After 1 year, the authors found that there was little increase in cumulative costs in the CABG group, while the cumulative costs for PTCA were \$11,250. Similarly, in the Argentine randomized trial of percutaneous transluminal coronary angioplasty versus coronary artery bypass surgery, the in-hospital and 1-year costs of surgery were higher than those for angioplasty [42]. None of these trials provided information on how cultural differences in the practice of medicine may influence costs.

Generalization of the results from any of these studies to other populations is difficult and of uncertain validity. In particular, in patients with prior coronary surgery in whom either redo coronary surgery or coronary angioplasty is contemplated, there are essentially no data. In one small study from the United Kingdom the cost of 15 first-time coronary procedures was compared with that of five reoperative procedures [43]. In this study there was a trend to high cost for reoperative procedures. Nonetheless, it seems likely that angioplasty will be less expensive initially, but that additional procedures in the angioplasty group will narrow the cost difference. As patients returning for procedures after prior surgery are in general a higher-risk population with severe disease, complications will be higher and costs will be correspondingly greater.

health improvement, can be related to clinical variables, including choice of therapy, as well as to cost. The use of the MIMIC model in assessing coronary surgery remains, at present, experimental, with essentially no published literature. The MIMIC model is currently being developed for the EAST study.

VII. CURRENT AND FUTURE TRENDS AND POLICY IMPLICATIONS

Microeconomic analyses in clinical medicine offer a powerful set of methods that may be used for clinical decision making as well as for policy. To date, most cost-effectiveness analyses have been simulations. The formidable difficulties in determining cost and utility have delayed the introduction of these tools into the clinical arena, where cost-effectiveness analyses could be part of many clinical trials or routinely applied to observational databases. Econometric methods offer potential, although unproven ability, to overcome the difficulties in measurement of traditional approaches. With the current changes in health care, accountability and cost are becoming more important. Thus, we can expect to see an increasing number of studies using these methods. Although we must maintain a level of skepticism, given sources of error and theoretical limitations, clinical microeconomic analyses should help guide medical decision making in many areas in the future. In an era of great changes in medicine, the economics of revascularization must be seen as a "moving target." Coronary surgery is changing the least, while angioplasty continues to undergo methodologic change. Although intervention in the coronaries today includes new devices, the impact on overall results has been variable [57–59]. The effect of changes in interventional procedures on cost has been of some interest. Recent data have shown that the impact of new devices is relatively small, except for coronary stents, and that stents increase cost primarily through prolonged length of stay [24,60]. While in the EAST trial 38% of the angioplasties were performed as staged procedures, at present this figure would be much lower [37]. In fact, recent data from Emory suggest that whereas resource use after intervention in the coronaries is falling, as measured by length of stay and emergency surgery, the hospital cost, measured in 1994 dollars, has not changed over an 8-year period [61]. Nonetheless, professional fees are falling. Hospitals are currently making great efforts to become more efficient, and length of stay is decreasing. Furthermore, the impact of managed care and capitation on costs is, at present, unknown. Presumably, capitation will result in increased efficiency. Thus, interpretation of economic data requires the perspective of changes in hospital and professional economic trends as well as secular inflationary trends. The real cost savings are unlikely to come about through increased efficiency but, rather, through avoiding expensive procedures in patients in whom they are not needed.

REFERENCES

1. Drummond MF, Stoddart GL, Torrance GW. Methods for the Economic Evaluation of Health Care Programmes. Oxford: Oxford University Press, 1990, pp. 74–111.
2. Drummond MF, Stoddart GL, Torrance GW. Methods for the Economic Evaluation of Health Care Programmes. Oxford: Oxford University Press, 1990, pp. 112–148.
3. Drummond MF, Stoddart GL, Torrance GW. Methods for the Economic Evaluation of Health Care Programmes. Oxford: Oxford University Press, 1990, pp. 149–167.
4. Machina MJ. Choice under uncertainty: problems solved and unsolved. J Econ Perspectives 1987; 1:121–154.
5. Cook PJ, Graham DA. The demand for insurance and protection: the case of irreplaceable commodities. Quarterly J Econ 1977; 91:143–156.
6. Fuchs VR, Zeckhauser R. Valuing health—a "priceless" commodity. Am Econ Review 1987; 77:263–268.
7. Graham DA. Cost-benefit analysis under uncertainty. Am Econ Review 1981; 71:715–725.
8. Finkler SA. The distinction between cost and charges. Ann Intern Med 1982; 96:102–109.
9. Finkler SA. Cost finding for high-technology, high-cost services. Health Care Manage Rev 1980; 5:17–29.
10. Shuman J, Wolfe H, Perlman M. Model for hospital microcosting. Industrial Engineering 1973; 39–43.
11. Cooper R, Kaplan RS. Measure costs right: make the right decisions. Harvard Business Review 1988; 5:96–103.
12. Dearden J. Cost accounting comes to service industries. Harvard Business Review 1978 (September-October):132–140.
13. Hlatky MA, Lipscomb J, Nelson C, Califf RM, Pryor D, Wallace AG, Mark DB. Resource use and cost of initial coronary revascularization: coronary angioplasty versus coronary bypass surgery. Circulation 1990; 82(suppl IV):IV-208–IV-213.
14. Feldstein PJ. Health Care Economics. 2d ed. New York: Wiley, 1983, pp. 169–197.
15. Health Insurance Association of America. Source Book of Health Insurance Data, 1991. Washington, DC: HIAA, 1991, p. 55.
16. Hsiao WC, Braun P, Yntema D, Becker ER. Estimating Physicians' Work for a Resource-Based Relative Value Scale. N Engl J Med 1988; 319:835–841.
17. Becker ER, Dunn D, Hsiao WC. Relative cost differences among physicians' specialty practices. JAMA 1988; 260:2397–2402.
18. Becker ER, Mauldin PD, Weintraub WS, King SB III. Physician profiles of coronary revascularization in the Emory Angioplasty vs Surgery Trial: understanding physician differences using Resource-Based Relative Values. J Am Coll Cardiol 1995; 25:344A.
19. Mark D. Medical economics and health policy issues for interventional cardiology. In: Topol E, ed. Textbook of Interventional Cardiology. 2d ed. Philadelphia: W.B. Saunders, 1993.

20. Topol EJ, Ellis SE, Cosgrove DM, Bates ER, Muller DWN, Shork NJ, Shork MA, Loop FD. Analysis of coronary angioplasty practice in the United States with an insurance-claims database. Circulation 1993; 87:1489–1497.

21. Reeder GS, Krishan I, Nobrega FT, Naessens J, Kelley M, Cristianson JB, McAfee MK. Is percutaneous coronary angioplasty less expensive than bypass surgery? N Engl J Med 1984; 311:1157–1162.

22. Barbash GI, Rabkin MT, Kane NM, Baim DS. Coronary angioplasty under the prospective payment system: the need for a severity-adjusted payment scheme. J Am Coll Cardiol 1986; 8:784–790.

23. Guzman LA, Simpfendorfer C, Fix J, Franco I, Whitlow PL. Comparison of costs of new atherectomy devices and balloon angioplasty for coronary artery disease. Am J Cardiol 1994; 74:22–25.

24. Cohen DJ, Breall JA, Kalon KL, Weintraub RM, Kuntz RE, Weinstein MC, Baim DS. Economics of elective coronary revascularization: comparison of costs and charges for conventional angioplasty, directional atherectomy, stenting and bypass surgery. J Am Coll Cardiol 1993; 22:1052–1059.

25. Dick RJ, Popma JJ, Muller DW, Burek KA, Topol EJ. In-hospital costs associated with new percutaneous coronary devices. Am J Cardiol 1991; 68:879–885.

26. Almeida D, Bradford JM, Wenger NK, King SB, Hurst JW. Return to work after coronary bypass surgery. Circulation 1983; 68(suppl II):205–213.

27. Weintraub WS, Jones EL, Craver J, Guyton R, Cohen CL. Determinants of prolonged length of hospital stay after coronary bypass surgery. Circulation 1989; 80: 276–284.

28. Hemenway D, Sherman H, Mudge GH Jr, Flatley M, Lindsey NM, Goldman L. Comparative costs versus symptomatic and employment benefits of medical and surgical treatment of stable angina pectoris. Medical Care 1985; 23:133–141.

29. Mauldin PD, Weintraub WS, Becker E. Predicting hospital charges and costs for coronary surgery from pre-operative and post-operative variables. Am J Cardiol 1994; 74:772–775.

30. Smith LR, Milano CA, Molter BS, Elbeery JR, Sabiston DC Jr, Smith PK. Preoperative determinants of postoperative costs associated with coronary artery bypass graft surgery. Circulation 1994; 90(5 Pt 2):II124–II128.

31. Kelly ME, Taylor GJ, Moses HW, Mikell FL, Dove JT, Batchelder JE, Wellons HA Jr, Schneider JA. Comparative cost of myocardial revascularization: percutaneous transluminal angioplasty and coronary artery bypass surgery. J Am Coll Cardiol 1985; 5:16–20.

32. Jang GC, Black PC, Cowley MJ, Gruentzig AR, Dorros G, Holmes DR Jr, Kent KM, Leatherman LL, Myler RK, Sjolander SME, Stertzer SH, Vetrovec GW, Willis WH, Williams DO. Relative cost of coronary angioplasty and bypass surgery in a one-vessel disease model. Am J Cardiol 1984; 53:52C–55C.

33. Black AJR, Roubin GS, Sutor C, Moe N, Jarboe JM, Douglas JS Jr, King SB III. Comparative costs of percutaneous transluminal coronary angioplasty and coronary artery bypass grafting in multivessel coronary artery disease. Am J Cardiol 1988; 62:809–811.

34. van den Brand M, van Halem C, van den Brink F, de Feyter P, Serruys P, Suryapranata H, Meeter K, Bos E, van Dalen FJ. Comparison of costs of percutane-

ous transluminal coronary angioplasty and coronary bypass surgery for patients with angina pectoris. Eur Heart J 1990; 11:765–771.

35. Hlatky MA, Lipscomb J, Nelson C, Califf RM, Pryor D, Wallace AG, Mark DB. Resource use and cost of initial coronary revascularization: coronary angioplasty versus coronary bypass surgery. Circulation 1990; 82(suppl IV):IV-208–IV-213.

36. Mark DB, Lam LC, Lee KL, Jones RH, Pryor DB, Stack RS, Williams RB, Clapp-Channing NE, Califf RM, Hlatky MA. Effects of coronary angioplasty, coronary bypass surgery, and medical therapy on employment in patients with coronary artery disease. A prospective comparison study. Ann Intern Med 1994; 120: 111–117.

37. King SB III, Lembo NJ, Weintraub WS, Kosinski AS, Barnhart HX, Kutner MH, Alazraki NP, Guyton RA, Zhao XQ. A randomized trial comparing coronary angioplasty with coronary bypass surgery: the Emory Angioplasty versus Surgery Trial. N Engl J Med 1994; 331:1044–1050.

38. Protocol for the Bypass Angioplasty Revascularization Investigation. Circulation 1991; 84(suppl V):V-1–V-27.

39. Hampton JR, Henderson RA, Julian DG, and the RITA trial participants. Coronary angioplasty versus coronary artery bypass surgery: the Randomized Intervention Treatment of Angina (RITA) trial. Lancet 1993; 341:573–580.

40. Sculpher MJ, Seed P, Henderson RA, Buxton MJ, Pocock SJ, Parker J, Joy MD, Sowton E, Hampton JR. Health service costs of coronary angioplasty and coronary artery bypass surgery: the Randomized Intervention Treatment of Angina (RITA) trial. Lancet 1994; 344(8927):927–930.

41. Hamm CW, Reimers J, Ischinger T, Rupprecht HJ, Berger J, Bleifeld W for the German Angioplasty Bypass Surgery Investigation. N Engl J Med 1994; 331: 1037–1043.

42. Rodriguez A, Boullon F, Perez-Balino N, Paviotti C, Liprandi MI, Palacios IF. Argentine randomized trial of percutaneous transluminal coronary angioplasty versus coronary artery bypass surgery in multivessel disease (ERACI): in-hospital results and 1-year follow-up. J Am Coll Cardiol 1993; 22:1060–1067.

43. Dougenis D, Naik S, Brown AH. Is repeated coronary surgery for recurrent angina cost effective? Eur Heart J 1992; 13:9–14.

44. Ferguson CE. Microeconomic Theory. 6th ed. Homewood, Ill: Richard D. Irwin, 1968.

45. Alchian A. The meaning of utility measurement. Am Econ Review 1953; 43:26–50.

46. Harsanyi JC. Cardinal welfare, individualistic ethics, and interpersonal comparisons of utility. J Pol Econ 1955; 63:309–321.

47. Pliskin JS, Shepard DS, Weinstein MC. Utility functions for life years and health status. Operations Research 1980; 28:206–224.

48. Sackett DL, Torrance GW. The utility of different health states as perceived by the general public. J Chronic Dis 1978; 31:697–704.

49. Churchill DN, Morgan J, Torrance GW. Quality of life in end-stage renal disease. Peritoneal Dialysis Bull 1984; 4:20–23.

50. Kaplan RM, Bush JW, Berry CC. Health status: types of validity of the index of well-being. Health Services Research 1976; 11:478–507.

51. Loomes G, McKenzie L. The use of QALYs in health care decision making. Soc Sci Med 1989; 28:299–308.

52. McNeil BJ, Weichselbaum R, Pauker SG. Speech and survival: tradeoffs between quality and quantity of life in laryngeal cancer. N Engl J Med 1981; 305:982–987.
53. Weinstein MC, Stason WB. Cost effectiveness of coronary artery bypass surgery. Circulation 1982; 66(suppl III):56–65.
54. Joreskog KG, Goldberger AS. Estimation of a model with multiple indicators and multiple cause of a single latent variable. J Amer Stat Assoc 1975; 70:631–639.
55. Van de Ven, Wynard PMM, Van Der Gaag J. Health as an unobservable: a MIMIC-model of demand for health care. J Health Econ 1982; 1:157–183.
56. Van De Ven, Wynard PMM, Hooijmans EM. The MIMIC health status index (what it is and what it does). In: Economics of Health Care. Kluwer Academic Publishers, 1992:19–29.
57. Baim DS, Kent KM, King SB III, Safian RD, Cowley MJ, Holmes DR, Roubin GS, Gallup D, Steenkiste AR, Detre K. Evaluating new devices. Acute (in-hospital) results from the New Approaches to Coronary Intervention Registry. Circulation 1994; 89:471–481.
58. Topol EJ, Leya F, Pinkerton CA, Whitlow PL, Hofling B, Simonton CA, Masden RR, Serruys RW, Leon MB, Williams DO, King SB III, Mark KB, Isner JM, Holmes DR Jr, Ellis SG, Lee KL, Keeler GP, Berdan LG, Hinohara T, Califf RM for the CAVEAT study group. A comparison of directional atherectomy with coronary angioplasty in patients with coronary artery disease. N Engl J Med 1993; 329:221–227.
59. Fischman DL, Leon MB, Baim DS, Schatz RA, Savage MP, Penn I, Detre K, Veltri L, Ricci D, Nobuyoshi M, Cleman M, Heuser R, Almond D, Teirstein PS, Fish RD, Colombo A, Brinker J, Moses J, Shaknovich A, Hirshfeld J, Bailey S, Ellis S, Rake R, Goldberg S for the Stent Restenosis Study Investigators. A randomized comparison of coronary-stent placement and balloon angioplasty in the treatment of coronary artery disease. N Engl J Med 1994; 331:496–501.
60. Weintraub WS, Waksman R, Benard J, Hicks F, Canup D, Becker E, Mauldin P, King SB III. The influence of new devices on the costs of interventional procedures (abstr). Circulation 1994; 90:I-44.
61. Weintraub WS, Ghazzal ZMB, Scott N, Douglas JS Jr, Benard J, Mauldin P, Becker N, King SB III. Declining resource utilization in interventional cardiology (abstr). J Am Coll Cardiol 1995; 25:81A.

Index

About the Editors

ERIC R. BATES is Professor of Medicine and Director of the Cardiac Catheterization Laboratory at the University of Michigan Medical Center, Ann Arbor, Michigan. He is the author of *Thrombolysis and Adjunctive Therapy in Acute Myocardial Infarction* (Marcel Dekker, 1993). Dr. Bates is a Fellow of the American College of Physicians, the American College of Cardiology, the American College of Chest Physicians, the American College of Angiology, and the American Heart Association. He received the B. A. degree (1972) from Princeton University, New Jersey, and the M.D. degree (1976) from the University of Michigan, Ann Arbor.

DAVID R. HOLMES, Jr. is Professor of Medicine at the Mayo Medical School, Mayo Clinic, Rochester, Minnesota. Additionally, he is Consultant to the Department of Internal Medicine, Division of Cardiovascular Diseases, Mayo Clinic and Mayo Foundation; and Director of the Cardiac Catheterization Laboratory, Mayo Clinic. Dr. Holmes is Editor of the *International Journal of Cardiology*. A Fellow of the American College of Cardiology, the Council on Circulation of the American Heart Association, and the Society for Cardiac Angiography and Interventions, he is a member of the American Heart Association and the Interventional Andreas Gruentzig Society. Dr. Holmes received the M.D. degree (1971) from the Medical College of Wisconsin, Milwaukee.